CESAREAN DELIVERY

Edited by **Raed Salim**

Cesarean Delivery
Edited by Raed Salim

Published by InTech
Janeza Trdine 9, 51000 Rijeka, Croatia

Publishing Process Manager Marina Jozipovic

Technical Editor Teodora Smiljanic

Cover Designer InTech Design Team

Additional hard copies can be obtained from orders@intechopen.com

Cesarean Delivery, Edited by Raed Salim
p. cm.
ISBN 978-953-51-0638-8

For EU product safety concerns:
IN TECH d.o.o., Prolaz Marije Krucifikse Kozulić 3, 51000 Rijeka, Croatia,
info@intechopen.com or visit our website at intechopen.com.

Meet the editor

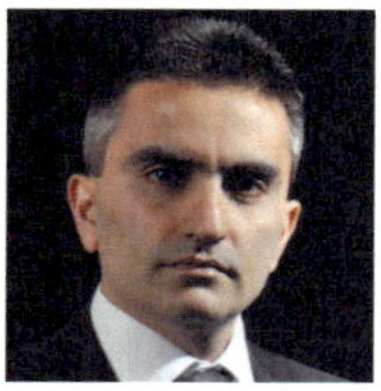

Dr Raed Salim, MD at the Hebrew University, Hadassah Medical School, Jerusalem, Israel. Director, delivery ward, Emek Medical Center, Afula and Senior lecturer, Ruth and Bruce Rappaport Faculty of Medicine, Technion, Haifa Israel. Dr Raed Salim serves as a reviewer for several international professional journals in obstetrics and gynecology. His research includes several publications on cesarean delivery with special interest in timing of elective cesarean delivery and related health implications, placenta accreta developing following cesarean delivery, interventions for reducing the rate of infection following cesarean delivery and labor progress among women attempting a trial of labor after cesarean.

Contents

Preface

Child birth is a natural process, but in certain circumstances, cesarean delivery is necessary to save the life of a child or mother. This issue is more acute in low income countries, where cesarean delivery rates are well below the acceptable minimum standard of 5% outlined by the World Heath Organization. In this book, the authors describe how poor healthcare access, underdeveloped healthcare infrastructure, geographical inaccessibility, cultural mistrust, poverty, and paucity of human health resources can become barriers for providing cesarean deliveries to all women who need them. Several studies in West Africa emphasized this gap by demonstrating increased maternal mortality due to a smaller proportion of deliveries performed by caesarean delivery.

On the other hand, rates of cesarean delivery, especially in high income countries, have risen dramatically over the last 30 years and the worldwide increase in the cesarean delivery rate has become a major public health concern. Reasons for the dramatic increase in the cesarean delivery rate are complex. This increase was driven in part by the increased incidence of multiple gestations and the decreased incidences of vaginal births after cesarean and vaginal breech deliveries. However, lifesaving indications for cesarean delivery represent only a small proportion of this increase in the cesarean delivery rate. Much of the increase comes from unproven conjectures concerning the advantages of caesarean delivery. It seems that the cesarean delivery has become a modern standard of care, though, much controversy still exists. Recently, demands for elective cesarean delivery have increased due to concern regarding pelvic floor disorders following vaginal delivery, a reduction in cesarean complication rates and women having fewer children.

As more women are delivering by cesarean, new concerns have emerged regarding long term maternal risks particularly placenta accreta and uterine rupture following a trial of labor. Regarding the short term complications, the rate of maternal mortality and severe morbidity that include thromboembolic events, major puerperal infection, severe hemorrhage, intestinal obstruction, injuries to the urinary tract and operative interventions after delivery is significantly more frequent among women undergoing cesarean delivery than vaginal delivery. Due to the worldwide dramatic increase in obesity during the past 20 years, these complications are expected to rise.

Additionally, more women are postponing pregnancy into the fourth and fifth decades of life for a variety of reasons. Older women are more likely to have cesarean delivery without labor. Severe complications for women older than 35 years are more frequent than for younger women. Since the rate of cesarean delivery is constantly increasing for mothers of all ages, races, and ethnic groups a growing number of women are expected to experience at least some of these complications.

In view of that, this book provides on the one hand evidence based reports and practical steps that may be adopted in an effort to reduce the cesarean delivery rate, and on the other hand, the book provides the best and up to date perioperative guidelines (where available) and tips to help improve health care quality among women undergoing cesarean delivery with special attention to obese women.

Pregnant women require special consideration when anesthesia is provided. Airway problems and difficult tracheal intubation are 10 times more frequent in the parturient than in the general population and are a major cause of maternal morbidity and mortality. Additionally, the increased use of regional anesthesia in the last decades has resulted in a lack of experienced anesthesiologists for providing general anesthesia in the emergent obstetric setting. Due to the considerable importance of this issue, broad coverage of the issue of obstetric anesthesia is provided. The book includes guidelines and a systematic review that anesthesia providers should know in obstetrics and a friendly-user review of anesthesia care for obstetric patients.

Cesarean surgery is strongly associated with delayed early breastfeeding, poorer infant suckling, more formula supplementation, and a shorter duration of breastfeeding. The book provides tips and guidelines of how to help establish and maintain exclusive breastfeeding shortly after the procedure including in cases of multiple gestation.

In conclusion, this book provides a convenient source that will aid to answer several questions related to the procedure; for example what is an "appropriate" cesarean delivery rate? Can the cesarean delivery rate be safely reduced? What are the obstacles for an acceptable cesarean delivery rate in the sub-Saharan African countries? When to perform an elective cesarean at term? Which anesthetic technique to use? What are the difficulties and complications that are related to obstetric anesthesia? How to perform the procedure in 15 minutes? Why morbidly obese women need special attention? And is it feasible to breastfeed directly after a cesarean? The authors answer all these questions through practical evidence based, comprehensive review of the clinical, social, ethical, and economic considerations.

To succeed in these selected objectives, distinguished experts from different disciplines were selected to ensure accurate coverage of the recent scientific and clinical advances to bring to care providers and purchasers up to date and essential information to help improve health care quality. I am very grateful to all my colleagues who have contributed to this valuable book.

Last, I am very grateful to all the "InTech team" for their help and support with this project. It has been a privilege and a pleasure to work with these dedicated personals.

Dr. Raed Salim
Department of Obstetrics and Gynecology, Emek Medical Center, Afula,
Rappaport Faculty of Medicine, Technion, Haifa,
Israel

1

How to Manage Labor Induction or Augmentation to Decrease the Cesarean Deliveries Rate

Shi-Yann Cheng
China Medical University Beigang Hospital
Taiwan

1. Introduction

There are many indications for term labor inductions and more than 15% of all gravid women require aid in cervical ripening and labor induction. That their labor courses are longer than that of spontaneous labor is the most common met problem. The prolonged course of spontaneous labor among nulliparous women is another common problem. They can result in a negative birth experience (Waldenstrom et al. 2004; Nystedt et al. 2006) and can be associated with non-reassuring fetal hear rate (FHR) resulting in emergency cesarean delivery (Bugg et al. 2006; Florica et al. 2006). When we think over the root cause of these problems, the immature cervix is the greatest barrier, which results in more concerned and unnecessary cesarean deliveries. Therefore, how to break through the immature cervix is the critical point. Misoprostol, a synthetic prostaglandin E1 analogue, was initially used to treat peptic ulcers caused by prostaglandin synthetase inhibitors, and was approved by the U.S. Food and Drug Administration for obstetric use in April 2002 (ACOG Committee Opinion. Number 283, May 2003. New U.S. Food and Drug Administration labeling on Cytotec (misoprostol) use and pregnancy 2003). Because the misoprostol has powerful uterotropic and uterotonic effect, there have been many researches to conduct clinical trials to learn how to administrate this agent under consideration of safety for labor induction since 1992 (Keirse 1993; Sanchez-Ramos et al. 1993; Hofmeyr et al. 1999; Wing 1999). The fetal hypoxia resulted from uterine hyperstimulation under administration of misoprostol is always a concern (Bennett et al. 1998; Kolderup et al. 1999; Hofmeyr &Gulmezoglu 2001; Shetty et al. 2001, 2002a; Shetty et al. 2002b; Alfirevic &Weeks 2006). The recommended dosage of misoprostol so far is 50 mcg per 4 hours via oral route (Alfirevic &Weeks 2006) or 25 mcg per 4 hours via vaginal route (Weeks &Alfirevic 2006), but the induction interval is too long. In consideration of individuals with different metabolism and response, the fixed-dosage of misoprostol will give risk of fetal hypoxia. Therefore, the individualized administrating method of titrated oral misoprostol against uterine response was developed (Cheng et al. 2008; Ho et al. 2010).

2. Principle of titrated oral misoprostol administration according to uterine response and pharmacokinetics

After misoprostol is absorbed, it undergoes rapid de-esterification to its free acid, which is responsible for its clinical activity and is detectable in plasma (Zieman et al. 1997). Because the minimal effect and toxicity of serum concentration of misoprostol acid for uterus at term are unknown, the rationale for titrated administration stems from the proven efficacy and pharmacokinetics of misoprostol, and the extreme interindividual and intraindividual variation in terms of uterine sensitivity (Cheng et al. 2008). To avoid uterine hyperstimulation and shorten the interval of labor course, the principle is that misoprostol should be administered in small, frequent doses (one dose per hour generally), titrated against uterine response and analogous to the conventional titrated use of oxytocin. The misoprostol is manufactured as an oral tablet 100 or 200 mcg so far and is water-soluble. The oral administration is easier and has greater acceptability among women. Because the absorption is more rapid and possibly more predictable, with a peak serum concentration after oral administration of 34 minutes and a half-life of 20–40 minutes (Zieman et al. 1997), the 1-hour interval between oral administrations and the increasing dosage of 20 mcg every 4 hours from initial 20 mcg are determined based on this mathematical model of the time to peak serum concentration and half-life of oral misoprostol after absorption. This method virtually maintains a steady serum level of misoprostol acid without large fluctuations and increases by one and one third the peak serum concentration of 20 mcg absorptive misoprostol every four hours. This mathematic model is described as figure 1.

times t=34+60n n=0,1,2,3, --- (minutes)

dosage (mcg)	34	94	154	214	274	...
20	P					
20		$P(1/4^0+1/4^1)$				
20			$P(1/4^0+1/4^1+1/4^2)$			
20				$P(1/4^0+1/4^1+1/4^2+1/4^3)$		
40					$P+P(1/4^0+1/4^1+1/4^2+1/4^3+1/4^4)$	
...						

Set the function C=f(t), where

C: concentration of misoprostol acid (pg/ml) in plasma

t: times during the whole process, t= 34+60n (minutes), when intake misoprostol at n=0, 1, 2, 3, ---(hours)

T_{max} (the time to peak plasma concentration of misoprostol acid after absorption): 34 minutes

$T_{1/2}$ (the half-life of misoprostol acid): 30 minutes were already determined according to pharmacokinetics study

When at n=0, intake 20 mcg, t=34 minutes, set the peak plasma concentration of misoprostol acid, C=P

When at n=1, intake 20 mcg, t=34+(60×1)=94 minutes, then $C=P(1/4^0+1/4^1)$

When at n=2, intake 20 mcg, t=34+(60×2)=154 minutes, then $C=P(1/4^0+1/4^1+1/4^2)$

When at n=3, intake 20 mcg, t=34+(60×3)=214 minutes, then $C=P(1/4^0+1/4^1+1/4^2+1/4^3)$

When at n=4, intake 40 mcg, t=34+(60×3)=214 minutes, then $C=P+P(1/4^0+1/4^1+1/4^2+1/4^3+1/4^4)$

...

Therefore, the C=f(t) is convergent series, the upper limit=P/(1-1/4)+P/(1-1/4)+---

=(4/3)P+(4/3)P+---

Fig. 1. Mathematic Model of Titrated Oral Misoprostol

3. Clinical pharmacology of misoprostol

Misoprostol does not affect the hepatic mixed function oxidase enzyme systems. In patients with varying degrees of renal impairment, an approximate doubling of $T_{1/2}$, peak serum concentration (C_{max}), and area under the serum concentration curve were found when compared with normal patients, but no clear correlation between the degree of impairment and area under the serum concentration curve was shown. No routine dosage adjustment is recommended in older patients or patients with renal impairment. Misoprostol does not produce clinically significant effects on serum levels of prolactin, gonadotropin, thyroid-stimulating hormone, growth hormone, thyroxine, cortisol, gastrointestinal hormones, creatinine, or uric acid. Neither gastric emptying, immunologic competence, platelet aggregation, pulmonary function, nor the cardiovascular system is modified by the recommended doses of misoprostol. Therefore, the use of misoprostol is not contraindicated with renal disease, severe anemia, systemic lupus erythematosus, hypertension, or heart disease.

4. Risk of misoprostol administration

The uterine rupture is the unwanted risk no matter what it happen to women with or without previous caesarean surgery. Most study suggest that the use of misoprostol in women with previous caesarean delivery increases the frequency of uterine scar disruption, either described as uterine dehiscence or over uterine rupture (Wing et al. 1998; Blanchette et al. 1999; Choy-Hee &Raynor 2001). There are sporadic reports of spontaneous uterine rupture in women without prior surgery (Bennett 1997; Khabbaz et al. 2001). Grand multiparity seems to be a risk factor, although a report of uterine rupture in a primigravida also exists (Thomas et al. 2003). Therefore, the conditions to give labor induction or augmentation need to be evaluated in advance.

5. Indication and contraindications to administer misoprostol

5.1 Indications and contraindications of labor induction with titrated oral misoprostol

The indications of labor induction with titrated oral misoprostol include postterm pregnancy, preeclampsia, diabetes mellitus, oligohydramnios, intrauterine fetal growth restriction, and abnormal antepartum fetal surveillance results. The contraindications include nonreassuring FHR pattern, uterine scar, grand multiparity($\geqq$5), any contraindication to labor or vaginal delivery or both, suspected placental abruption with abnormal FHR pattern and hypersensitivity to misoprostol or prostaglandin analogues.

5.2 Indicaitons and contraindications of labor augmentation with titrated oral misoprostol

Women with reassuring FHR pattern and developing inadequate uterine contractions (two or fewer contractions per 10 minutes) for at least 30-minute windows during the labor course are indicated for labor augmentation with titrated oral misoprostol. The contraindications include nonreassuring FHR pattern, uterine scar, grand multiparity($\geqq$5), any contraindication to labor or vaginal delivery or both, suspected placental abruption with abnormal FHR pattern and hypersensitivity to misoprostol or prostaglandin analogues.

6. Procedure of preparing oral misoprostol solution and guidelines of administration

Misoprostol is manufactured as an oral tablet and is water-soluble. The uterine activity produced by an oral solution is faster and stronger than that of an oral tablet, or when given via the rectal or vaginal route (Chong et al. 2004). One tablet of misoprostol is 200 mcg and may be dissolved in 200 ml of tap water in a medicine bottle. The misoprostol solution needs to be used completely within 24 hours after preparation or discarded. Women are induced with one basal unit of 20 ml of misoprostol solution (1 mcg/ml) prepared as described above. The determined volume of misoprostol solution will be poured according to obstetrician's discretion at each dosing following the guidelines of labor induction (Cheng et al. 2008) or augmentation (Ho et al. 2010). Initially, the determined volume may be given at obstetrician's order according to the guidelines when the regular uterine contractions are not achieved. Once the regular uterine contractions are achieved, the obstetrician will be called to visit and make decision of next step. Therefore, the individualized administration of misoprostol will avoid the accident issue of fetal hypoxia resulted from uterine hyperstimulation. The flowchart of administration is showed as Figure 2 and the guidelines are also described as the followings.

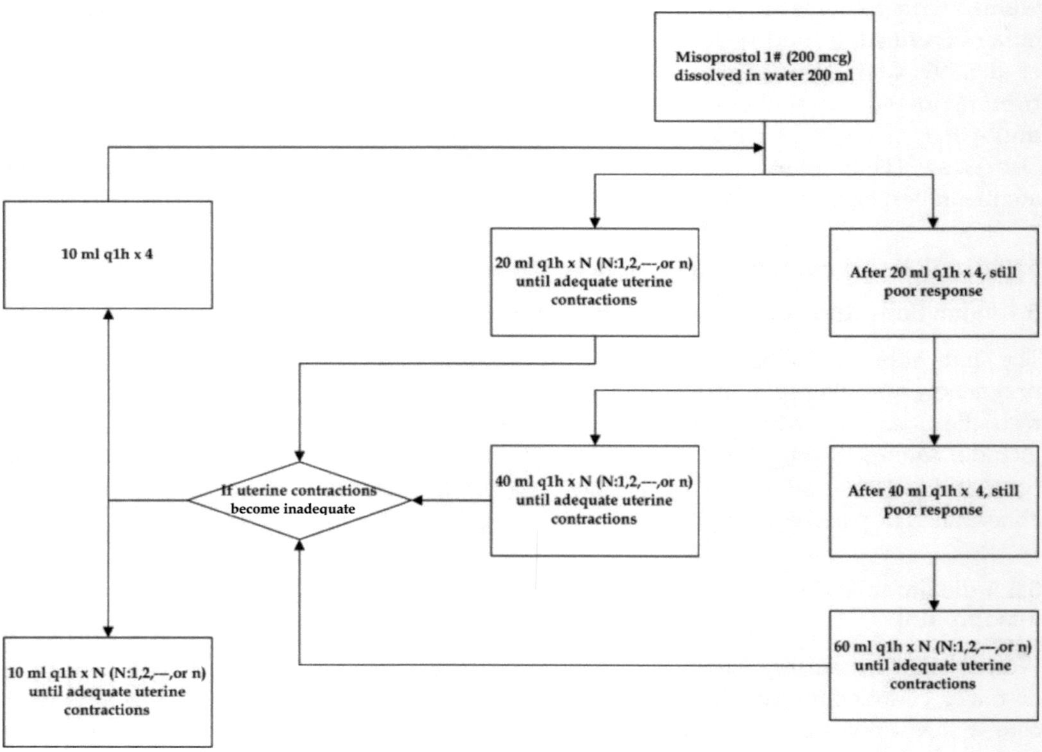

Fig. 2. Flowchart of administration

6.1 The guidelines of titrated oral misoprostol administration in labor induction

1. The initial dose of 20 mcg/h is administered until adequate uterine contractions are achieved. If contractions do not occur after four doses, the dosage is increased to 40 mcg/h and repeated every hour until uterine contractions are achieved, for a maximum of four more doses. If response still remains poor after 8 h, the dosage could be increased to 60 mcg/h until adequate contractions occur. The usual 'nil by mouth' rule is not enforced during the latent phase of the labor course.
2. Adequate uterine contractions are defined as three or more in 10 minutes over 30-minute windows. Once uterine activity is adequate over 1 hour, no further misoprostol is given.
3. If contractions subsequently become inadequate, hourly doses of misoprostol solution are started at 10 mcg/h and could be increased to 20 mcg/h and perhaps 40 mcg/h based on uterine responsiveness. This process is repeated until adequate uterine contractions occur.
4. Fetal heart rate and uterine activity are continuously monitored throughout labor induction.
5. Induction failure is defined as not entering the active phase after 36 h of misoprostol treatment, with a maximum cumulative dosage of 1600 mcg. Failure to progress is defined as the cervical dilation or fetal descent without any progress for 3 hours after entering the active labor phase as augmented by the agent.
6. Intravenous magnesium sulfate (4 g over 30 min) could be given at the physician's discretion if uterine hyperstimulation occur.
7. When the cervix achieved a Bishop score of 9, artificial rupture of the membrane could be performed at the physician's discretion.
8. The active phase is defined as achieving adequate uterine contractions with cervical dilatation greater than 3 cm.
9. Supplemental oxytocin could be used at the physician's discretion when uterine contractions are inadequate or when entering into the active phase with a favorable cervix (Bishop score > 8) because of poor response to misoprostol.
10. Failure to progress is defined as the cervical dilation or fetal descent without any progress for 3 hours after entering the active labor phase as augmented by the agent.
11. Cesarean section will be offered to all patients after induction failure, failure of labor to progress or when nonreassuring FHR occur.

6.2 The guidelines of titrated oral misoprostol administration in labor augmentation

1. Misoprostol is initially administered at a dose of 20 mcg/h until adequate uterine contractions are achieved. If contractions do not occur after 4 hours (four doses), the dosage could be increased to 40 mcg and repeated every hour until uterine contractions occurred. Nothing by mouth, except medication, was allowed during the active phase of labor.
2. Adequate uterine contractions are defined as three or more in 10 minutes over 30-minute windows. Once uterine activity is adequate over 1 hour, no further misoprostol is given.
3. If contractions subsequently become inadequate, hourly doses of misoprostol solution are started at 10 mcg/h and could be increased to 20 mcg/h and to as much as 40 mcg/h based on uterine responsiveness. This process is repeated until adequate uterine contractions occur.

4. Both fetal heart rate and uterine activity are continuously monitored throughout labor augmentation.
5. The maximum cumulative dosage of misoprostol is 1,600 mcg.
6. Intravenous magnesium sulfate (4 g over 30 minutes) could be given at the discretion of the physician if uterine hyperstimulation occur.
7. When the cervix achieved a Bishop score of 9, artificial rupture of the membrane could be performed at the physician's discretion.
8. The active phase is defined as achieving adequate uterine contractions with cervical dilatation greater than 3 cm.
9. Failure to progress is defined as the cervical dilation or fetal descent without any progress for 3 hours after entering the active labor phase as augmented by the agent.
10. Cesarean delivery is offered to all patients after failure of labor to progress or when nonreassuring FHR occur.

7. Efficacy of titrated oral misoprostol

The hourly misoprostol administration which is based on pharmacokinetics proves to be effective from the following studies.

7.1 The efficacy of titrated oral misoprostol for labor induction

There is one randomized controlled trial was to compare titrated oral with vaginal misoprostol for labor induction (Cheng et al. 2008). Women between 34 and 42 weeks of gestation with an unfavorable cervix (Bishop score less than or equal to 6) and an indication for labor induction were randomly assigned to receive titrated oral or vaginal misoprostol. The titrated oral misoprostol group received a basal unit of 20 mL misoprostol solution (1 mcg/mL) every 1 hour for four doses and then were titrated against individual uterine response. The vaginal group received 25 mcg every 4 hours until attaining a more favourable cervix. Vaginal delivery within 12 hours was the primary outcome. The data were analyzed by intention-to-treat. Titrated oral misoprostol was given to 101 (48.8%) women and vaginal misoprostol to 106 (51.2%) women. Completed vaginal delivery occurred within 12 hours in 75 (74.3%) women in the titrated oral group and 27 (25.5%) women in the vaginal group ($P < 0.01$; relative risk [RR] 8.44, 95% confidence interval [CI] 4.52–15.76). Four women (4.0%) in the titrated oral group and 18 (17.0%) women in the vaginal group underwent cesarean deliveries ($P < 0.01$; RR 0.20, 95% CI 0.07–0.62). The incidence of hyperstimulation was 0.0% in the titrated oral group compared with 11.3% in the vaginal group ($P < 0.01$; RR 0.08, 95% CI 0.01- 0.61). Although more women experienced nausea (10.9%) in the titrated oral group ($P < 0.01$; RR 27.07, 95% CI 1.57- 465.70), fewer infants had Apgar scores of less than 7 at 1 minute in the titrated oral group than in the vaginal group ($P < 0.01$; RR 0.10, 95% CI 0.01- 0.76). The conclusion is that titrated oral misoprostol was associated with a lower incidence of uterine hyperstimulation and a lower cesarean delivery rate than vaginal misoprostol for labor induction in patients with unfavorable cervix.

7.2 The efficacy of titrated oral misoprostol for labor augmentation

There is another randomized controlled trial to compare titrated oral misoprostol with intravenous oxytocin for labor augmentation at 36 to 42 weeks of gestation with spontaneous onset of active labor (Ho et al. 2010). Women meeting the general selection criteria with regular contractions and an effaced cervix dilated between 3 and 9 cm, and who had inadequate uterine contractions (two or fewer contractions every 10 minutes) during the first stage of labor, were randomly assigned to titrated oral misoprostol or intravenous oxytocin. Augmentation–to–vaginal delivery interval and vaginal delivery within 12 or 24 hours were the primary outcomes. The data were analyzed by intention-to-treat. Of the 231 women, 118 (51.1%) were randomized to titrated oral misoprostol and 113 (48.9%) to titrated intravenous oxytocin. The median interval from the start of augmentation to vaginal delivery was 5.22 hours (3.77– 8.58 hours, 25th–75th percentile) in the misoprostol group, and 5.20 hours (3.23– 6.50 hours, 25th– 75th percentile) in the intravenous oxytocin group (P=.019). Complete vaginal delivery occurred within 12 hours for 92 (78.0%) women in the misoprostol group and for 97 (85.8%) women in the oxytocin group (P=.121; RR 0.91, 95% CI 0.80 –1.03). There were no significant differences between the two groups who delivered vaginally within 24 hours. Twelve (10.2%) women in the misoprostol group and 13 (11.5%) women in the oxytocin group underwent cesarean deliveries (P=.744; RR 0.88, 95% CI 0.42–1.85). Side effects and neonatal outcomes also did not differ between the two groups. The conclusion is that labor augmentation with titrated oral misoprostol or intravenous oxytocin resulted in similar rates of vaginal delivery within 12 and 24 hours.

7.3 The efficacy of hourly oral misoprostol for terminating midtrimester pregnancies

In addition, there was one pilot study of hourly oral misoprostol for terminating midtrimester pregnancies (Cheng et al. 2010b). Sixteen women with living fetuses, who had undergone pregnancy termination at 12–25 weeks of gestational age, were reviewed. The method of induction was hourly oral administration of misoprostol, given at doses of 200 mcg/hr for the first 12 hours and 400 mcg/hr after 12 hours until delivery. Data including the induction-to-delivery interval and total dosage of misoprostol were recorded and analyzed. All 16 women successfully underwent vaginal termination within 36 hours. The median induction-todelivery interval was 12.0 hours (range, 6.3–30.9 hours), with 13 women (81.3%) undergoing vaginal delivery within 24 hours. The median total dosage of misoprostol was 2,600 mcg. The most common side effect was diarrhea, which was easily relieved by medication. These preliminary results show that oral administration of misoprostol at hourly intervals is a promising method for terminating midtrimester pregnancies.

7.4 The outcomes of labor induction with titrated oral misoprostol between nulliparous and multiparous women

There was one retrospective study to review the medical records of all patients between 37 and 42 weeks of gestation with a Bishop score ≦6 who underwent labor induction with titrated oral misoprostol solution (Cheng et al. 2010a). The women were allocated into two groups: nulliparous and multiparous. The women received one basal unit of misoprostol solution (20 ml, 1 mcg/ml) every hour for four doses; additional doses were titrated against individual uterine response. The interval of latent and active phase and vaginal delivery within 12 hours were the primary outcomes. Of the 112 women included in the study, 49 (43.8%) mulliparae and 63 (56.2%) multiparae underwent labor induction with titrated oral misoprostol solution. Although fewer women delivered vaginally within 12 hours in the nulliparous group than in the multiparous group (42.9% vs 85.7%; P<0.01; RR, 0.54; 95% CI, 0.39–0.76), there was no significant difference between two groups regarding vaginal delivery within 24 hours (87.8% vs 100.0%; P=0.09; RR 0.96; 95% CI 0.90–1.02). Four (8.2%) women in the nulliparous group and none (0.0%) women in the muliparous group underwent caesarean deliveries (P=0.02; RR 1.09; 95% CI 1.00–1.18). All induction intervals, including the latent and active phases, were significantly shorter in the multiparous group (P < 0.01). Induction failure did not occur in any patient in either of the groups. There were no instances of hyperstimulation, which was defined as tachysystole or hypertonus with nonreassuring fetal heart rate pattern, although tachysystole defined as the presence of at least six contractions in 10 min over at least two 10-min windows, occurred in four (8.2%) nulliparous women and in four (6.3%) multiparous women. Hypertonus, defined as a single contraction lasting more than 2 min, did not occur in either group. None of the neonates in either group had an Apgar score of < 7 at 1 min. The conclusion is that titrated oral misoprostol solution is a promising method of labor induction for both nulliparous and multiparous women.

8. Adverse effects of misoprostol

In published case reports (Graber &Meier 1991; Bond &Van Zee 1994; Austin et al. 1997), accidental overdosing with misoprostol resulting in pyrexia, hypoxia, and rhabdomyolysis all occurred with a single intake at a dosage exceeding 3,000 µg. Therefore, these adverse effects are the sign of misoprostol toxicity, which is good indicator when administrating hourly oral misoprostol for terminating midtrimester pregnancies. The other common side effect is the nausea, vomiting or diarrhea. Although it commonly occurs in the course of hourly oral misoprostol for terminating midtrimester pregnancies, it rarely occurs in the course of labor induction or augmentation with titrated oral misoprostol. Furthermore, these side effects are easily relieved by medication.

9. Teratogenicity of misoprostol

A form of congenital facial paralysis known as Mobius syndrome and limb defects have occurred in the infants of women who have taken misoprostol during the first trimester for abortions which failed (Gonzalez et al. 1998; Pastuszak et al. 1998). First trimester exposure to misoprostol is also associated with high incidences of vascular disruption defects in newborns (Vargas et al. 2000). In the Latina American Collaborative Study of Congenital Malformations of 4673 malformed infants and 4980 control infants, an increased frequency of transverse limb defects, ring-shaped constrictions of the extremities, arthrogryposis, hydrocephalus, holoprosencephaly, and bladder exstrophy, but not Mobius syndrome, was found in those infants exposed to misoprostol in utero (Orioli &Castilla 2000). There are no known reports of teratogenicity of misoprostol ingestion when taken after the first trimester.

10. Conclusion

Cesarean birth rates are greater than 20% in many developed countries (Betran et al. 2007). The main diagnosis contributing to the high rate in nulliparous women is dystocia or prolonged labor. Traditionally, a policy of vaginal dinoprostone under immature cervix or early amniotomy with oxytocin administration under mature cervix for the prevention of delay in labor progress is associated with a modest reduction in the rate of cesarean births (O'Driscoll et al. 1984). However, the course of vaginal dinoprostone or misoprostol is tedious, and excessive uterine contractility resulting in fetal distress is always concerned during the oral or vaginal use of the fixed-dosage misoprostol. The oxytocin administration through the intravenous route needs to be under the control of an intravenous pump machine and may be inconvenient in certain settings. Because titrated oral misoprostol solution is easier to administer than titrated intravenous oxytocin, it is worth conducting these treatment regimens for labor induction or augmentation. Additionally, misoprostol offers several advantages over dinoprostone or oxytocin such as longer shelf life, stability at room temperature, and easy administration. It is an ideal alternative to traditional dinoprostone or oxytocin in labor induction or augmentation. In consideration of interindividual or intraindividual variation of drug response during the dosing course, it is reasonable that the titrated oral misoprostol solution replaces the fixed dosage misoprostol via vaginal or oral route in labor induction or augmentation. In aspect of completing vaginal delivery to reduce the cesarean rate, the use of titrated oral misoprostol is also superior to the traditional use of vaginal misoprostol from the above randomized controlled trial.

11. Acknowledgment

The author acknowledges the participation of obstetricians and nursing staff of labor ward of China Medical University Beigang Hospital for their participation in monitoring of subjects of all related studies. The author also thanks China Medical University Biostastistics Center for the data analysis. The studies were supported by grants from the China Medical University Beigang Hospital.

12. References

ACOG Committee Opinion. Number 283, May 2003. New U.S. Food and Drug Administration labeling on Cytotec (misoprostol) use and pregnancy. (2003). *Obstet Gynecol*, Vol.101, No.5 Pt 1, (2003/05/10), pp. 1049-1050, ISSN 0029-7844 (Print)

Alfirevic, Z. & A. Weeks (2006). Oral misoprostol for induction of labour. *Cochrane Database Syst Rev*, No.2, (2006/04/21), pp. CD001338, ISSN 1469-493X (Electronic)

Austin, J., M. D. Ford, A. Rouse & E. Hanna (1997). Acute intravaginal misoprostol toxicity with fetal demise. *J Emerg Med*, Vol.15, No.1, (1997/01/01), pp. 61-64, ISSN 0736-4679 (Print) 0736-4679 (Linking)

Bennett, B. B. (1997). Uterine rupture during induction of labor at term with intravaginal misoprostol. *Obstet Gynecol*, Vol.89, No.5 Pt 2, (1997/05/01), pp. 832-833, ISSN 0029-7844 (Print) 0029-7844 (Linking)

Bennett, K. A., K. Butt, J. M. Crane, D. Hutchens & D. C. Young (1998). A masked randomized comparison of oral and vaginal administration of misoprostol for labor induction. *Obstet Gynecol*, Vol.92, No.4 Pt 1, (1998/10/09), pp. 481-486, ISSN 0029-7844 (Print)

Betran, A. P., M. Merialdi, J. A. Lauer, W. Bing-Shun, J. Thomas, P. Van Look & M. Wagner (2007). Rates of caesarean section: analysis of global, regional and national estimates. *Paediatr Perinat Epidemiol*, Vol.21, No.2, (2007/02/17), pp. 98-113, ISSN 0269-5022 (Print)

Blanchette, H. A., S. Nayak & S. Erasmus (1999). Comparison of the safety and efficacy of intravaginal misoprostol (prostaglandin E1) with those of dinoprostone (prostaglandin E2) for cervical ripening and induction of labor in a community hospital. *Am J Obstet Gynecol*, Vol.180, No.6 Pt 1, (1999/06/16), pp. 1551-1559, ISSN 0002-9378 (Print) 0002-9378 (Linking)

Bond, G. R. & A. Van Zee (1994). Overdosage of misoprostol in pregnancy. *Am J Obstet Gynecol*, Vol.171, No.2, (1994/08/01), pp. 561-562, ISSN 0002-9378 (Print)

Bugg, G. J., E. Stanley, P. N. Baker, M. J. Taggart & T. A. Johnston (2006). Outcomes of labours augmented with oxytocin. *Eur J Obstet Gynecol Reprod Biol*, Vol.124, No.1, (2005/06/16), pp. 37-41, ISSN 0301-2115 (Print)

Cheng, S. Y., C. S. Hsue, G. H. Hwang, W. Chen & T. C. Li (2010a). Comparison of labor induction with titrated oral misoprostol solution between nulliparous and multiparous women. *J Obstet Gynaecol Res*, Vol.36, No.1, (2010/02/25), pp. 72-78, ISSN 1341-8076 (Print) 1341-8076 (Linking)

Cheng, S. Y., C. S. Hsue, G. H. Hwang, L. C. Tsai & S. C. Pei (2010b). Hourly oral misoprostol administration for terminating midtrimester pregnancies: a pilot study. *Taiwan J Obstet Gynecol*, Vol.49, No.4, (2011/01/05), pp. 438-441, ISSN 1875-6263 (Electronic) 1028-4559 (Linking)

Cheng, S. Y., H. Ming & J. C. Lee (2008). Titrated oral compared with vaginal misoprostol for labor induction: a randomized controlled trial. *Obstet Gynecol*, Vol.111, No.1, (2008/01/01), pp. 119-125, ISSN 0029-7844 (Print)

Chong, Y. S., S. Chua, L. Shen & S. Arulkumaran (2004). Does the route of administration of misoprostol make a difference? The uterotonic effect and side effects of misoprostol given by different routes after vaginal delivery. *Eur J Obstet Gynecol Reprod Biol*, Vol.113, No.2, (2004/04/06), pp. 191-198, ISSN 0301-2115 (Print)

Choy-Hee, L. & B. D. Raynor (2001). Misoprostol induction of labor among women with a history of cesarean delivery. *Am J Obstet Gynecol*, Vol.184, No.6, (2001/05/12), pp. 1115-1117, ISSN 0002-9378 (Print)

Florica, M., O. Stephansson & L. Nordstrom (2006). Indications associated with increased cesarean section rates in a Swedish hospital. *Int J Gynaecol Obstet*, Vol.92, No.2, (2005/12/21), pp. 181-185, ISSN 0020-7292 (Print)

Gonzalez, C. H., M. J. Marques-Dias, C. A. Kim, S. M. Sugayama, J. A. Da Paz, S. M. Huson & L. B. Holmes (1998). Congenital abnormalities in Brazilian children associated with misoprostol misuse in first trimester of pregnancy. *Lancet*, Vol.351, No.9116, (1998/06/10), pp. 1624-1627, ISSN 0140-6736 (Print) 0140-6736 (Linking)

Graber, D. J. & K. H. Meier (1991). Acute misoprostol toxicity. *Ann Emerg Med*, Vol.20, No.5, (1991/05/01), pp. 549-551, ISSN 0196-0644 (Print)

Ho, M., S. Y. Cheng & T. C. Li (2010). Titrated oral misoprostol solution compared with intravenous oxytocin for labor augmentation: a randomized controlled trial. *Obstet Gynecol*, Vol.116, No.3, (2010/08/25), pp. 612-618, ISSN 1873-233X (Electronic) 0029-7844 (Linking)

Hofmeyr, G. J. & A. M. Gulmezoglu (2001). Vaginal misoprostol for cervical ripening and induction of labour. *Cochrane Database Syst Rev*, No.3, (2001/11/01), pp. CD000941, ISSN 1469-493X (Electronic)

Hofmeyr, G. J., A. M. Gulmezoglu & Z. Alfirevic (1999). Misoprostol for induction of labour: a systematic review. *Br J Obstet Gynaecol*, Vol.106, No.8, (1999/08/24), pp. 798-803, ISSN 0306-5456 (Print)

Keirse, M. J. (1993). Prostaglandins in preinduction cervical ripening. Meta-analysis of worldwide clinical experience. *J Reprod Med*, Vol.38, No.1 Suppl, (1993/01/01), pp. 89-100, ISSN 0024-7758 (Print)

Khabbaz, A. Y., I. M. Usta, M. I. El-Hajj, A. Abu-Musa, M. Seoud & A. H. Nassar (2001). Rupture of an unscarred uterus with misoprostol induction: case report and review of the literature. *J Matern Fetal Med*, Vol.10, No.2, (2001/06/08), pp. 141-145, ISSN 1057-0802 (Print) 1057-0802 (Linking)

Kolderup, L., L. McLean, K. Grullon, K. Safford & S. J. Kilpatrick (1999). Misoprostol is more efficacious for labor induction than prostaglandin E2, but is it associated with more risk? *Am J Obstet Gynecol*, Vol.180, No.6 Pt 1, (1999/06/16), pp. 1543-1550, ISSN 0002-9378 (Print)

Nystedt, A., U. Hogberg & B. Lundman (2006). Some Swedish women's experiences of prolonged labour. *Midwifery*, Vol.22, No.1, (2006/02/21), pp. 56-65, ISSN 0266-6138 (Print)

O'Driscoll, K., M. Foley & D. MacDonald (1984). Active management of labor as an alternative to cesarean section for dystocia. *Obstet Gynecol*, Vol.63, No.4, (1984/04/01), pp. 485-490, ISSN 0029-7844 (Print)

Orioli, I. M. & E. E. Castilla (2000). Epidemiological assessment of misoprostol teratogenicity. *BJOG*, Vol.107, No.4, (2000/04/12), pp. 519-523, ISSN 1470-0328 (Print) 1470-0328 (Linking)

Pastuszak, A. L., L. Schuler, C. E. Speck-Martins, K. E. Coelho, S. M. Cordello, F. Vargas, D. Brunoni, I. V. Schwarz, M. Larrandaburu, H. Safattle, V. F. Meloni & G. Koren (1998). Use of misoprostol during pregnancy and Mobius' syndrome in infants. *N Engl J Med*, Vol.338, No.26, (1998/06/25), pp. 1881-1885, ISSN 0028-4793 (Print) 0028-4793 (Linking)

Sanchez-Ramos, L., A. M. Kaunitz, G. O. Del Valle, I. Delke, P. A. Schroeder & D. K. Briones (1993). Labor induction with the prostaglandin E1 methyl analogue misoprostol versus oxytocin: a randomized trial. *Obstet Gynecol*, Vol.81, No.3, (1993/03/01), pp. 332-336, ISSN 0029-7844 (Print)

Shetty, A., P. Danielian & A. Templeton (2001). A comparison of oral and vaginal misoprostol tablets in induction of labour at term. *BJOG*, Vol.108, No.3, (2001/04/03), pp. 238-243, ISSN 1470-0328 (Print)

Shetty, A., P. Danielian & A. Templeton (2002a). Sublingual misoprostol for the induction of labor at term. *Am J Obstet Gynecol*, Vol.186, No.1, (2002/01/26), pp. 72-76, ISSN 0002-9378 (Print)

Shetty, A., R. Martin, P. Danielian & A. Templeton (2002b). A comparison of two dosage regimens of oral misoprostol for labor induction at term. *Acta Obstet Gynecol Scand*, Vol.81, No.4, (2002/04/16), pp. 337-342, ISSN 0001-6349 (Print)

Thomas, A., R. Jophy, A. Maskhar & R. K. Thomas (2003). Uterine rupture in a primigravida with misoprostol used for induction of labour. *BJOG*, Vol.110, No.2, (2003/03/06), pp. 217-218, ISSN 1470-0328 (Print) 1470-0328 (Linking)

Vargas, F. R., L. Schuler-Faccini, D. Brunoni, C. Kim, V. F. Meloni, S. M. Sugayama, L. Albano, J. C. Llerena, Jr., J. C. Almeida, A. Duarte, D. P. Cavalcanti, E. Goloni-

Bertollo, A. Conte, G. Koren & A. Addis (2000). Prenatal exposure to misoprostol and vascular disruption defects: a case-control study. *Am J Med Genet*, Vol.95, No.4, (2001/02/24), pp. 302-306, ISSN 0148-7299 (Print) 0148-7299 (Linking)

Waldenstrom, U., I. Hildingsson, C. Rubertsson & I. Radestad (2004). A negative birth experience: prevalence and risk factors in a national sample. *Birth*, Vol.31, No.1, (2004/03/16), pp. 17-27, ISSN 0730-7659 (Print)

Weeks, A. & Z. Alfirevic (2006). Oral misoprostol administration for labor induction. *Clin Obstet Gynecol*, Vol.49, No.3, (2006/08/04), pp. 658-671, ISSN 0009-9201 (Print)

Wing, D. A. (1999). Labor induction with misoprostol. *Am J Obstet Gynecol*, Vol.181, No.2, (1999/08/24), pp. 339-345, ISSN 0002-9378 (Print)

Wing, D. A., K. Lovett & R. H. Paul (1998). Disruption of prior uterine incision following misoprostol for labor induction in women with previous cesarean delivery. *Obstet Gynecol*, Vol.91, No.5 Pt 2, (1998/05/08), pp. 828-830, ISSN 0029-7844 (Print)

Zieman, M., S. K. Fong, N. L. Benowitz, D. Banskter & P. D. Darney (1997). Absorption kinetics of misoprostol with oral or vaginal administration. *Obstet Gynecol*, Vol.90, No.1, (1997/07/01), pp. 88-92, ISSN 0029-7844 (Print)

2

Timing of Elective Cesarean Delivery at Term

Raed Salim
*Department of Obstetrics and Gynecology, Emek Medical Center, Afula,
Rappaport Faculty of Medicine, Technion, Haifa,
Israel*

1. Introduction

The rate of cesarean delivery is constantly increasing for mothers of all ages, races, and ethnic groups (Martin et al., 2005). In view of that, timing of elective cesarean delivery at term has an essential public health implication. Term gestation, by definition, is a gestation of 37 weeks to 42 weeks from the day of the last menstrual period. Though infants born by elective cesarean delivery within this range are considered term infants, risk of serious perinatal morbidity and mortality may still occur and may differ according to the gestational age within this range.

Delaying delivery until 41 weeks or more will increase significantly the proportion of women who may go into spontaneous labor and consequently deliver by non-elective cesarean delivery rather than an elective one. In addition it has been reported that stillbirth, is almost doubled at 41 weeks of gestation and increase by a factor of up to 5 at 42 weeks as compared with 39 weeks (Meikle et al., 2005; Wood et al., 2008). Accordingly, performing elective cesarean before 41 weeks, if possible, is desirable.

In the other hand, as compared with births at 39 to 40 weeks, births at 37 weeks have been reported to be associated with an increased risk of neonatal morbidity. Compared with newborns delivered vaginally, a significantly increased risk of respiratory morbidity was found among infants delivered by an elective cesarean section at 37 compared to 39 weeks (Hansen et al., 2008). Lack of hormones associated with labor could explain this association. Labor and rupture of membranes may stimulate secretion of catecholamines in the fetus. As a result, a decrease in secretion of fetal lung liquids and an increase in their absorption have been reported. When cesarean sections are carried out before labor, this catecholamine surge is absent (Brown et al., 1983). In view of that, scheduling elective cesarean at 37 weeks is also undesirable.

Since neonatal respiratory morbidity at 38 weeks is still slightly higher compared to 39 weeks, the literature is nearly unanimous in recommending elective cesarean delivery at 39 weeks of gestation. However, delaying elective cesarean delivery from 38 to 39 weeks may have maternal and other fetal consequences that are not always addressed in studies that recommend delaying delivery to 39 weeks (Salim et al., 2009; Salim & Shalev, 2011).

Delaying delivery for an additional week increases the time that the woman and her fetus is vulnerable to a number of unexpected complications and increases the proportion of women who will deliver by non-elective cesarean delivery rather than an elective one. It has been reported that 10% to 14% of women may go into spontaneous labor between 38 and 39 weeks of gestation (Salim & Shalev, 2010; Thomas & Paranjothy, 2001). The meaning of these numbers is that over 10% of elective cesarean deliveries scheduled to 39 weeks will likely convert to non-elective ones between 38 to 39 weeks. The incidence may be even greater in public medical centers where the number of elective cesarean deliveries per week is initially limited by the availability of the operating theater. If scheduling starts from 39 weeks, an over booking in a certain week may result in delaying the timing of the scheduled cesarean delivery for some women to 40 weeks or more which may result in even a greater proportion of women presenting in labor before their scheduled cesarean delivery date.

The outcome of this particular group of women is less addressed in the literature when discussing the advantages of elective cesarean deliveries, since the majority of published studies on elective cesarean delivery exclude from statistical analysis women who delivered non-electively before the scheduled date of delivery. Other studies combined this cohort of women with those that delivered electively so that it is impossible to isolate the contribution of non-elective delivery to the outcome. A design centered on the actual delivery route will allow investigators to distinguish between labored and unlabored cesarean deliveries. In studies limited to unlabored cesareans, women who present in labor before their scheduled date of delivery are, by definition, excluded. Excluding these women may overestimate potential benefits and also potential harms because the studies then cannot account for any effect that labor has on outcomes of interest.

A search of PubMed, MEDLINE, EMBASE, and Cochrane Library databases up to February, 2012, did not detect any randomized controlled trial that compared the timing of elective cesarean delivery at 38 or 39 weeks and which investigated both perinatal and maternal outcomes.

In this chapter, I will present in details the perinatal and maternal benefits as well as the consequences resulting from scheduling elective cesarean delivery at 39 weeks compared to 38 weeks.

2. Perinatal and maternal benefits and consequences

2.1 Perinatal benefits

The main impact of delivery at 39 weeks as compared to 38 weeks is the reduction in neonatal respiratory morbidity.

Newborn and adult lungs function most effectively when almost devoid of liquid in the alveoli and airways, whereas to grow normally the fetal lungs must be distended by a volume of liquid that equals or exceeds the functional residual capacity of newborn and adult lungs (Berger et al., 1998). To create the liquid present in the fetal lungs, the pulmonary epithelium actively pumps Cl- ions into the future air-spaces (Olver & Strang, 1974). As a result, the fetal lung secretes a liquid which distends the future air-spaces and plays a crucial role in promoting lung growth.

Though liquid is essential for normal fetal lungs development, both experimental (Berger et al., 1996) and clinical (Hales et al., 1993) evidences support the view that prenatal clearance of lung liquid before birth is critical for the establishment of normal respiratory function immediately after delivery.

Infants delivered by cesarean section take longer than those born vaginally to increase their arterial oxygen levels (Oliver et al., 1961) and to establish adequate pulmonary gas exchange (Palme-Kilander et al., 193). The difference is evident clinically as an excess of respiratory illnesses such as transient tachypnoea of the newborn (Mikner et al., 1987; Hales et al., 1993) or respiratory distress syndrome and hyaline membrane disease (Brice et al., 1977).

Circulating epinephrine, which is known to increase during labor, has been shown to convert the lung of the late-gestation fetal lamb from liquid-secreting to liquid-absorbing through beta2-receptor activation of a Na+ pump located on the apical surface of the pulmonary epithelium (Brown et al., 1983). Na+ channels on the apical (luminal) side of the pulmonary epithelium increase in number with the approach of delivery (Baines et al., 2000). Maturation of this mechanism appears to be under the control of cortisol and thyroid hormone, both of which increase over the last days of gestation (Barker et al., 1991; Wallace et al,. 1996).

The view that Na^+ transport plays a vital role in respiratory adaptation at birth is supported by the finding of transient tachypnea of the newborn or other respiratory failure in babies in which the pump has not been activated or genetically abnormal (Gowen et al., 1988).

The timetable, with which lung liquid volume and secretion decline before term delivery, underlines the importance of the last days of gestation in adapting the fetus for the postnatal life. Lung liquid volume begins to fall before labor (Dickson et al., 1986). In addition the rate of flow of liquid out of the fetal trachea also begins to decline before labor ((Dickson et al., 1986; Olver et al., 1986; Kitterman et al., 1979). A more rapid fall between early and advanced labor then took place (Pfister et al., 2001). This final step in the clearance of lung liquid involves active reabsorption, a process that has been shown to be stimulated by the catecholamine surge which occurs just before the end of labor (Brown et al., 1983). Reabsorption of liquid from the lung is driven by active Na+ transport which then continues to play a dominant role in keeping the air space dry throughout postnatal life. In addition the larynx acts as a one-way valve allowing only liquid outflow under normal circumstances and prevents the entry of amniotic fluid (Brown et al., 1983) probably by a negative intra-pulmonary pressure produced near the end of labor (Pfister et al., 2001).

Existing evidence starkly demonstrates that late gestation and labor are beneficial to the baby for additional reasons. Surfactant synthesis and release are increased during labor (Ballard, 1986). The increasing concentration of cortisol (Bassett & Thorburn, 1969) and thyroid hormones (Fraser & Liggins, 1988) in the last days of gestation and during labor itself may accelerate maturation of the lung (Liggins et al., 1988) and play a key role in lung liquid reabsorption (Barker et al., 1991).

The mechanisms that adapt the lung for postnatal life can be seen to include a prolonged and gradual clearance of lung liquid beginning well before the onset of labor, together with an acceleration of clearance once labor is established. The respiratory vulnerability that elective cesarean delivery represents may therefore, not simply be attributable to the absence of labor, but also to the newborn missing out on a process that clears liquid from the lung over a period of days leading up to labor.

According to Bland et al the lungs of rabbits, delivered either vaginally or by cesarean section after a period in labor, contain less water than the lungs of rabbits delivered by cesarean section before the onset of labor (Bland et al., 1979). In human babies, Chiswick & Milner, from measurements of crying vital capacity, and Milner et al, from measurements of thoracic gas volume, concluded that lung aeration is established more slowly after cesarean than after vaginal delivery; and according to Bonn et al, the relative delay in aeration is greater when delivery is by cesarean section before the onset of labor (elective section) than when it is by section after some hours of labor. Obviously, these differences probably have nothing to do with squeezing the fetal thorax in the birth canal (Chiswick & Milner, 1976; Milner et al., 1978; Bonn et al., 1981).

These observations may explain the results of several studies that have described an increased risk of respiratory morbidity within each gestational week from 37 to 39 weeks among infants delivered by elective cesarean section. In a retrospective study of 1,284 elective cesarean deliveries, Zanardo et al reported that respiratory distress syndrome was diagnosed at a rate of 25 per 1,000 live births when cesarean delivery occurred between 37 0/7 weeks and 38 6/7 weeks of gestation, versus a significantly lower rate of respiratory distress syndrome, 7 per 1,000, with cesarean delivery after 39 0/7 weeks of gestation. Neonatal respiratory distress syndrome with vaginal deliveries did not vary (3 - 4/1000) across these gestational ages (Zanardo et al., 2004). Hansen et al assessed the association between elective cesarean sections and neonatal respiratory morbidity and the timing of elective cesarean sections. This was a prospective cohort study that included 2687 infants, without malformations, delivered by elective cesarean section in Denmark. Main outcome measures were respiratory morbidity (transitory tachypnoea of the newborn, respiratory distress syndrome, persistent pulmonary hypertension of the newborn) and serious respiratory morbidity (oxygen therapy for more than two days, nasal continuous positive airway pressure, or need for mechanical ventilation). Compared with newborns intended for vaginal delivery, an increased risk of respiratory morbidity within each gestational week from 37 to 39 weeks was found for infants delivered by elective cesarean section. At 37 weeks' gestation the odds ratio was about 4 folds (95% confidence interval 2.4 to 6.5), 3 folds at 38 weeks' gestation (95% confidence interval 2.1 to 4.3), and 1.9 folds at 39 weeks' gestation (95% confidence interval 1.2 to 3.0). The increased risks of serious respiratory morbidity showed the same pattern, with 5 folds increase for infants delivered at 37 weeks' gestation, 4 folds increase for infants delivered at 38 weeks, and more than 2 folds increase for infants delivered at 39 weeks, although the increased risk at 39 weeks was not statistically significant. These results remained essentially unchanged after exclusion of pregnancies complicated by diabetes, pre-eclampsia, and intrauterine growth retardation, or by breech presentation (Hansen et al., 2008).

Tita et al studied a cohort of consecutive women undergoing repeat cesarean sections performed at 19 centers of the Eunice Kennedy Shriver National Institute of Child Health and Human Development Maternal–Fetal Medicine Units Network from 1999 through 2002. Women with viable singleton pregnancies delivered electively were included. The primary outcome was the composite of neonatal death and any of several adverse events, including respiratory complications, treated hypoglycemia, newborn sepsis, and admission to the neonatal intensive care unit. The study included 13,258 cesarean deliveries performed electively. As compared with births at 39 weeks, births at 37 weeks were associated with a 2.1 folds increase in the risk of the primary outcome (95% confidence interval 1.7 to 2.5) and 1.5 folds for births at 38 weeks (95% confidence interval 1.3 to 1.7). The rates of adverse respiratory outcomes, mechanical ventilation, newborn sepsis, hypoglycemia, admission to the neonatal intensive care unit, and hospitalization for 5 days or more were increased by a factor of 1.8 to 4.2 for births at 37 weeks and 1.3 to 2.1 for births at 38 weeks (Tita et al., 2009).

The results of the above studies were confirmed by other studies that demonstrated consistently an increased neonatal respiratory morbidity with elective cesarean delivery performed earlier than 39 weeks.

2.2 Maternal benefits

A secondary analysis of the Cesarean Section Registry of the Eunice Kennedy Shriver National Institute of Child Health and Human Development Maternal Fetal-Medicine Units (NICHD MFMU) Network, reported maternal outcomes with regard to gestational age at delivery. The study included women with live singleton pregnancies delivered by prelabor elective repeat cesarean delivery from 1999 through 2002 at 19 U.S. academic centers. Gestational age was examined by completed weeks. Maternal outcomes included a primary composite of death, hysterectomy, uterine rupture or dehiscence, blood transfusion, uterine atony, thromboembolic complications, anesthetic complications, surgical injury or need for arterial ligation, intensive care unit admission, wound complications, or endometritis. The results demonstrated a comparable maternal outcome at 37, 38 and 39 weeks of gestation. In view of that, combined with the fact that neonatal morbidity is higher at births before 39 weeks, the authors recommended scheduling elective cesarean to 39 weeks (Tita et al., 20110). Nonetheless, the results of the above study were soon after challenged, and a letter to the editor was later published (Salim and Shalev, 2011).

2.3 Fetal and neonatal consequences related to delaying cesarean to 39 weeks

Women assigned to an elective cesarean delivery may go into labor prior to the scheduled date of surgery. About 10% to 14% of women may go into spontaneous labor between 38 and 39 weeks of gestation (Salim & Shalev, 2010; Thomas & Paranjothy, 2001). Hansen et al reported that up to 25% of women may enter labor before 39 weeks (Hansen et al., 2008). Laboring women might present during the early stages of labor, with or without membrane ruptures, or alternatively they may present during advanced stages of labor. Maternal and neonatal outcomes may be adversely affected when cesarean delivery is preceded by labor, even if labor is not advanced.

2.3.1 Fetal and neonatal morbidity

The implication of scheduling delivery to 39 weeks is that a proportion of elective cesarean deliveries will convert to non-elective ones, which may increase the risk of traumatic injury to the fetus/newborn (Hankins et al., 2006). The reported incidence of iatrogenic fetal trauma during cesarean delivery is 0.1% to 1.9% of births (Aburezq et al., 2005). Several risk factors for fetal injury at the time of the cesarean delivery have been identified through various case reports. These include lack of surgical experience, labor with thinning of the lower uterine segment exposing the fetus to injury with the scalpel, and a lack of amniotic fluid secondary to rupture of the membranes making the underlying fetal parts more accessible (Haas & Ayres, 2002; Puza et al., 1998). Fetal lacerations, finger injuries and amputations, penetrating brain injuries, skull fractures and long bone fractures have all been reported from the use of the scalpel or scissors at the time of cesarean delivery [3]. Although traumatic delivery is still associated with cesarean delivery, it is uncommon with elective, compared to non-elective cesarean delivery of the vertex fetus at term (Hankins et al., 2006).

In the term breech trial, 6% of women who were assigned to a planned cesarean delivery, delivered vaginally because cesarean delivery was not possible due to imminent vaginal delivery (Hannah et al., 2000). Perinatal mortality and serious neonatal morbidity of the breech presenting fetus are significantly lower in planned cesarean delivery than for vaginal birth according to the term breech trail. Delaying an elective cesarean delivery scheduled for breech presentation may expose some of the fetuses to preventable morbidity and mortality associated with vaginal breech delivery in cases where vaginal delivery is imminent at admission.

Delaying delivery until 39 weeks increases the time that the woman and her fetus is vulnerable to a number of unexpected complications and increases the proportion of women who may present in labor. The incidence of meconium staining of amniotic fluid has been reported to increase with increasing gestational age above 37 weeks of gestation (Saunders & Paterson, 1991). In addition, it is acknowledged that the process of labor may itself produce an encephalopathic response in infants who were previously injured and who are simply unable to make the usual compensatory responses to the stresses of labor (Hankins et al., 2006). This issue is crucial if women present during the advanced stages of labor before the scheduled cesarean.

2.3.2 Intrauterine fetal demise

An accumulative increased risk of intrauterine fetal death has been reported with increasing gestational age. Copper et al reported that the timing of fetal death for stillborn infants born between 23 and 40 weeks is evenly distributed with nearly 5% of all stillbirths occurring per week of gestation (Copper et al., 1994). This is important when considering all stillborn infants at 38 weeks and beyond, where significant complications of prematurity would be very rare if only these fetuses had simply been delivered earlier. Furthermore, it has been reported that a fairly stable rate of fetal death of 0.6 per 1000 live births occurs from 33 weeks to 39 weeks of gestation. However, at 39 weeks, the rate increases significantly to 1.9 per 1000 live births (Yudkin et al., 1987).

Others reported a fetal death rate per 1000 live births at weekly intervals from 37 to 41 weeks increasing from 1.3 at 37 weeks to 2.0 at 38 weeks, 2.9 at 39 weeks, 3.8 at 40 weeks, and 4.6 at 41 weeks of gestation (Fretts et al., 2004). It is clear that delivery at 38 weeks compared to 39 weeks or more would reduce intrauterine fetal deaths.

Ehrenthal et al evaluated the association of a new institutional policy limiting elective delivery before 39 weeks of gestation with neonatal outcome (Ehrenthal et al., 2011). This was a retrospective cohort study that was conducted to estimate the effect of the policy on neonatal outcome using a before and after design. All term singleton deliveries 2 years before and 2 years after policy enforcement were included. The results confirmed that a policy limiting elective delivery before 39 weeks of gestation was accompanied by a significant increase in the incidence of still birth (RR 3.67, 95% CI 1.02–13.15, P=.032).

De la Vega and coworkers in a mixed risk population with unrestricted access to testing for fetal wellbeing and sonographic evaluations concluded that, despite intensive surveillance, they were still unable to reduce the rate of fetal death. The investigators suggested that this is probably due to occurrence of acute placental and cord accidents that cannot be detected through antenatal fetal surveillance and are simply unavoidable (de la Vega et al,. 2002).

The sudden death of a fetus in utero has medical, social and economic implications. It is particularly tragic when it occurs shortly before the expected date of delivery.

2.4 Maternal consequences

As mentioned earlier women assigned to elective cesarean delivery and go into spontaneous labor, may present in early stages of labor with or without ruptured membranes or alternatively they may present at advanced stages of labor. As a result, maternal outcome may be affected due to the advance labor that preceded the scheduled cesarean delivery. In other precise situations, even when early stages of labor with or without ruptured membranes precede the scheduled cesarean delivery, maternal outcome may still be affected.

2.4.1 Perioperative complications

The rate of severe maternal morbidity caused by different modes of delivery among all singleton deliveries was studied in Finland in 1997 and 2002. Main outcome measures were deep venous thromboembolism, amniotic fluid embolism, major puerperal infection, severe hemorrhage, uterine rupture or inversion and intestinal obstruction. Severe maternal morbidity was significantly more frequent in non-elective than in elective operations. Moreover, operative interventions after the delivery was significantly more frequent after non-elective cesarean delivery than after elective cesarean delivery. There were more severe complications in the group of women older than 35 years than in the younger women (Pallasmaa et al., 2008). In another retrospective study, the prevalence and risk factors for bladder injury during cesarean delivery were investigated. Operator experience and the emergency nature of the cesarean delivery were both considered risk factors for bladder injury (Rahman et al., 2009).

2.4.2 Uterine rupture

The overall risk of uterine rupture for women with a prior cesarean delivery is higher among women undergoing a subsequent trial of labor as compared to elective cesarean delivery. Other than maternal morbidity, a ruptured uterus carries a greater risk for hypoxic-ischemic encephalopathy and perinatal deaths (Landon et al., 2004). The risk of rupture is greater among women after higher order repeated cesarean delivery and it had been reported to occur five times greater among women with 2 prior cesarean scars compared to women with only 1 prior cesarean scar (3.7% vs 0.8%, respectively) (Caughey et al,. 1999).

The risk of rupture is probably greater among parous women with multiple repeated cesarean deliveries, a situation commonly encountered in some regions. Patients with prior classical hysterotomies have been reported to have an even higher incidence of uterine rupture. Rupture has been reported to occur in many of these women even before the onset of labor (Halperin et al., 1988). Although the incidence of uterine rupture mentioned above has been reported to occur among women after a trial of labor, still, it's not rare to encounter women assigned to elective cesarean delivery, to present in advance stages of labor.

2.4.3 Anesthesia related complications

Failed intubation and pulmonary aspiration are the leading causes of anesthesia-related maternal morbidity and mortality. Fasting for a period of 6 to 8 hours is recommended before elective cesarean delivery (American College of Obstetrics and Gynecology [ACOG], 2002). Women scheduled for an elective cesarean delivery and who go into spontaneous labor may present while not in the fasting state. Performing an immediate cesarean delivery because the woman is in labor increases maternal morbidity and mortality. Alternatively, delaying the procedure 6 to 8 hours may increase the risk of converting early stages of labor to advance stages which may complicate the procedure. Furthermore, women whose indication for cesarean delivery human immunodeficiency virus infection or genital herpes, the risk of neonatal infection may increase if abdominal delivery is delayed.

2.4.4 Non surgical complications

Delaying delivery until 39 weeks has other non-surgical consequences. The rates of gestational hypertension, preeclampsia, and eclampsia increase from 37 to 42 weeks when calculated according to ongoing pregnancy (Caughey et al., 2003).

2.4.5 Urinary incontinence

Women with severe urinary incontinence have a marked deterioration in their quality of life, most substantially curtail activities, many become homebound, and for some, urinary incontinence is the defining event that prompts nursing home admission. In the United States each year, an estimated 135,000 women undergo surgery for urinary incontinence (Waetjen et al., 2003). An estimate of direct costs for urinary incontinence in the United States has been reported to be $16 billion per year (Wilson et al., 2001). Given the substantial public health burden of pelvic floor disorders, much research attention has been focused on identifying risk factors, especially modifiable risk factors, for the development of pelvic floor disorders. Many retrospective and cross-sectional studies implicate childbirth as a major risk factor for urinary incontinence in younger women. Whether, and to what degree, cesarean delivery may protect child-bearing women from developing urinary incontinence is an unresolved issue. Several prospective studies evaluated the risk of postpartum urinary incontinence by delivery type, grouping all cesarean deliveries together and reported inconsistent results.

The best data to investigate in order to evaluate the impact of cesarean delivery is that which separates out cesarean deliveries done before and after the onset of labor. Farrell et al assessed the incidence of urinary incontinence, 6 weeks postpartum according to the mode of delivery. After forceps delivery, the incidence was 35%, 23% after spontaneous vaginal delivery, 9% after cesarean during labor and 4% after cesarean before labor. By 6 months, these prevalence figures were 33%, 22% 12%, and 5%, respectively (Farrell et al., 2001).

Chin et al assessed the impact of delivery on the pelvic floor and to what degree could cesarean delivery prevent pelvic floor injury. Five hundred thirty nine women were divided into three groups according to the delivery method adopted: elective cesarean delivery, emergent cesarean delivery, and vaginal delivery. Only elective cesarean delivery was protective. They concluded that the key to the best protection against postpartum urinary incontinence seems to lie in the timing of the cesarean delivery; that is, the cesarean delivery has to be performed before labor or uterine contractions have commenced. In view of that, not all cesarean deliveries can be considered as a superior alternative for pelvic floor protection that would decrease the likelihood of postpartum urinary incontinence according to the authors (Chin et al., 2006).

2.4.6 Maternal mortality

In 1990, the results of a retrospective review of 108 maternal deaths occurring between 1975 and 1986 in Cape Town, South Africa Lilford were published (Lilford et al., 1990). The data suggested an increased risk of maternal mortality with non-elective intrapartum cesarean deliveries as compared with elective procedures. Another publication reporting on deliveries in Israel between 1984 and 1992 compared maternal mortality among vaginal deliveries, emergency cesarean deliveries, and elective cesarean deliveries. Fifty five cases were reported with an overall mortality rate of 6 per 100,000. Rates of maternal mortality were 2.8, 3.6, and 30 per 100,000 deliveries for elective cesarean deliveries, vaginal delivery, and emergency cesarean deliveries, respectively (Yoles & Maschiach, 1998).

The Report on Confidential Enquiries into Maternal Deaths, 1997 to 1999, reported the estimated maternal mortality rates and relative risk of direct deaths based on method of delivery. A significant higher maternal mortality rate was observed with emergency and urgent cesarean deliveries (Royal College of Obstetricians and Gynaecologists, 2001).

2.4.7 Special issue – Advance maternal age

More women are postponing pregnancy into the forth and fifth decades of life for a variety of reasons. In Finland the reported proportion of women giving birth at age 35 years or more was increased from 16.7% in 1997 to 19.2% in 2002 (Pallasmaa et al., 2008). Advanced maternal age, traditionally defined as age over 35 years, has been associated with increased obstetric morbidity and interventions. In addition, perinatal complications are reported to be higher in this patient population (Usta & Nassar, 2008).

Older women are more likely to have cesarean delivery without labor (Ecker et al., 2001). The risk for severe complications during emergency cesarean delivery in the group of women older than 35 years is higher than in the younger ones (Pallasmaa et al., 2008). Furthermore, intrauterine fetal death and perinatal mortality are significantly higher in older women even after excluding deaths due to congenital malformations and adjusting for existing illnesses or pregnancy complications (Jacobsson et al., 2004; Joseph et al., 2005). The highest rate of stillbirth was reported to occur among older women after 38 weeks of gestation (Smith, 2001).

2.5 Health care provider type and professional resources

The availability of resources, such as operating rooms and staff, may influence a health care provider's decision regarding when to schedule the date of the elective cesarean delivery. Non-elective cesarean deliveries, which by definition are poorly timed, may result in a patient that presents in the non fasting state, at a time that the hospital is staffed with less experienced surgeons and anesthetists whose skills are further compromised due to demanding working hours. All these factors present additional challenges to the patients' safety. One of the advantages of scheduled operations is the greater ease of balancing staffing levels with clinical volume. Inadequate levels of staffing, as well as fatigue among health care providers, may contribute to increased patient morbidity (Minkoff & Chervenak, 2003; Tucker, 2002).

3. Conclusion

Because of increased rates of neonatal respiratory complications, the literature is almost unanimously in favor of delaying elective cesarean delivery until 39 weeks of gestation unless there is evidence of fetal lung maturity. However, multiple chance events may influence outcome. For example, an elective cesarean delivery at 38 weeks may result in the delivery of an iatrogenically premature infant at risk for respiratory morbidity. On the other hand, delaying delivery to 39 weeks may result in an unexplained stillbirth, or spontaneous onset of labor with intrapartum complications that may compromise maternal and neonatal well-being. Decision analysis is a quantitative methodology for evaluating competing strategies under conditions of uncertainty.

About 14% of all women booked for an elective cesarean delivery at exactly 39 weeks and 0 days, would be expected to go into spontaneous labor between 38 to 39 weeks. For an average hospital with 4500 births a year, and a 10% elective cesarean delivery rate, scheduling delivery at 38 weeks rather than 39 weeks will result in an additional 10 neonates with respiratory morbidity a year, assuming an additional 2% neonatal morbidity for those delivered at 38 weeks as compared to 39 weeks (Tita et al., 2009). On the other hand, 63 non-elective cesarean deliveries would be prevented. In fact, since it is not feasible to book all women to exactly 39 weeks and 0 days, particularly in public medical centers, the number of non-elective operations that would be prevented may actually be higher. Other than decreasing the risk of non-elective cesareans, scheduling elective cesarean deliveries to 38 weeks may prevent cases of fetal death especially among older women.

Until prospective randomized trials are conducted, it is not easy to precisely answer all risk:benefit questions as to the best timing of when to schedule elective cesarean delivery; 38 or 39 weeks. Since several studies indicated that neonatal outcomes are improved by delaying cesarean until 39 weeks of gestation, the American College of Obstetricians and Gynecologists as well, recommended delaying cesarean delivery until 39 weeks of gestation in the absence of obstetric or medical indications for early delivery.

However, if dating is confirmed with an ultrasound study prior to 20 weeks of gestation, scheduling cesarean delivery at 38 0/7 weeks to 38 6/7 weeks may be, in my opinion, another reasonable and alternative option to 39 weeks. This is particularly true among a selected group of women, namely older women and women where a complicated cesarean delivery is anticipated. It is reasonable to inform women of the risks entailed with each of the above options. The clinician's role should be to provide the best evidence-based counseling possible to the woman, and to respect her autonomy and decision-making.

4. References

Aburezq, H., Chakrabarty, KH., & Zuker, RM. (2005). Iatrogenic fetal injury. *Obstetrics and Gynecology,* Vol.106, No.5 Pt 2, (November 2005), pp. 1720-1174, ISSN 0029-7844.

American College of Obstetrics and Gynecology. (2002). ACOG practice bulletin. Obstetric analgesia and anesthesia. Number 36, July 2002. American College of Obstetrics and Gynecology. *International Journal of Gynecology & Obstetrics,* Vol.78, No.3, (September 2002), pp. 321–335, ISSN 1879-3479.

Ballard, PL. (1986). Hormones and Lung Maturation. Springer-Verlag, Berlin, Heidelberg.

Baines, DL., Folkesson, HG., Norlin, A., Bingle, CD., Yuan, HT., & Olver, RE. (2000). The influence of mode of delivery, hormonal status and postnatal O2 environment on epithelial sodium channel (ENaC) expression in perinatal guinea-pig lung. *Journal of Physiology,* Vol.522, No. Pt1, (January 2000), pp. 147-157, ISSN 1469-7793.

Bassett, JM., & Thorburn, GD. (1969). Foetal plasma corticosteroids and the initiation of parturition in sheep. Journal of Endocrinology, Vol.44, No.2, (June 1969), pp. 285-286, ISSN 1479-6805.

Barker, PM., Walters, DV., Markiewicz, M., & Strang, LB. (1991). Development of the lung liquid reabsorptive mechanism in fetal sheep: synergism of triiodothyronine and hydrocortisone. *Journal of Physiology,* Vol.433, (February 1991), pp. 435-449, ISSN 1469-7793.

Berger, PJ., Smolich, JJ., Ramsden, CA., & Walker, AM. (1996). Effect of lung liquid volume on respiratory performance after Caesarean delivery in the lamb. *Journal of Physiology,* Vol.492, No.Pt3, (May 1996), pp. 905-912, ISSN 1469-7793.

Berger PJ, Kyriakides MA, Smolich JJ, Ramsden CA, Walker AM. (1998). Massive decline in lung liquid before vaginal delivery at term in the fetal lamb. *American Journal of Obstetrics and Gynecology,* Vol.178, No.2, (February 1998), pp. 223-227, ISSN 1097-6868.

Bland, RD., Mcmillan, DD., & Bressack, MA. (1979). Labor decreases lung water content of newborn rabbits. *American Journal of Obstetrics and Gynecology,* Vol.134, No.3, (October 1979), pp. 364-367, ISSN 1097-6868.

Bonn, AW., Milner, AD. & Hopkin, JG. (1981). Lung volumes and lung mechanics in babies born vaginally and by elective and emergency Caesarean section. *The Journal of pediatrics,* Vol.98, No.5, (May 1978), pp. 812-815, ISSN 1097-6833.

Brice, JEH., & Wailker, CHM. (1977). Changing pattern of respiratory distress in newborn. *Lancet,* Vol.2, No.8041, (October 1977), pp. 752-754, ISSN 1476-547X.

Brown, MJ., Olver, RE., Ramsden, CA., Strang, LB., & Walters, DV. (1983). Effects of adrenaline and of spontaneous labor on the secretion and absorption of lung liquid in the fetal lamb. *Journal of Physiology,* Vol.344, (November 1983), pp. 137-152, ISSN 1469-7793.

Caughey, AB., Stotland, NE., & Escobar, GJ. (2003). What is the best measure of maternal complications of term pregnancy: ongoing pregnancies or pregnancies delivered? *American Journal of Obstetrics and Gynecology,* Vol.189, No.4, (October 2003), pp. 1047-1052, ISSN 1097-6868.

Caughey, AB., Shipp, TD., Repke, JT., Zelop, CM., Cohen, A., & Lieberman, E. (1999). Rate of uterine rupture during a trial of labor in women with one or two prior cesarean deliveries. *American Journal of Obstetrics and Gynecology,* Vol.181, No.4, (October 1999), pp. 872-876, ISSN 1097-6868.

Chin, HY., Chen, MC., Liu, YH., & Wang, KH. (2006). Postpartum urinary incontinence: a comparison of vaginal delivery, elective, and emergent cesarean section.

International Urogynecology Journal and Pelvic Floor Dysfunction, Vol.17, No.6, (November 2006), pp. 631-635, ISSN 1433-3023.

Chiswick, M., & Milner, RDG. (1976). Crying vital capacity. Measurement of neonatal lung function. *Archives of disease in childhood,* Vol.51, No.1, (January 1976), pp. 22-27, ISSN 1468-2044.

Copper, RL., Goldenberg, RL., Dubard, MB., & Davis, RO. (1994). Risk factors for fetal death in white, black, and Hispanic women. Collaborative Group on Preterm Birth Prevention. *Obstetrics and Gynecology,* Vol.84, No.4, (October 1994), pp. 490-495, ISSN 0029-7844.

de la Vega, A., & Verdiales, M. (2002). Failure of intensive fetal monitoring and ultrasound in reducing the stillbirth rate. *Puerto Rico health sciences journal,* Vol.21, No.2, (June 2002), pp. 123-125, ISSN 0738-0658.

Department of Health, Scottish Executive Health Department, and Department of Health, Social Services and Public Safety, Northern Ireland. Why Mothers Die. Fifth Report on Confidential Enquiries into Maternal Deaths in the United Kingdom, 1997-1999. 2001 London, RCOG Press.

Dickson, KA., Maloney, JE., & Berger, PJ. (1986). Decline in lung liquid volume before labor in fetal lambs. *Journal of Applied Physiology,* Vol.61, No.6, (December 1986), pp. 2266-2272, ISSN 1522-1601.

Ecker, JL., Chen, KT., Cohen, AP., Riley, LE.,& Lieberman, ES. (2001). Increased risk of cesarean delivery with advancing maternal age: indications and associated factors in nulliparous women. *American Journal of Obstetrics and Gynecology,* Vol.185, No.4, (October 2003), pp. 883-887, ISSN 1097-6868.

Ehrenthal DB, Hoffman MK, Jiang X, Ostrum G. (2011). Neonatal outcomes after implementation of guidelines limiting elective delivery before 39 weeks of gestation. *Obstetrics and Gynecology,* Vol.118, No. 5, (November 2011), pp.1047-1055, ISSN 0029-7844.

Farrell, SA., Allen, VM., & Baskett, TF. (2001). Parturition and urinary incontinence in primiparas. *Obstetrics and Gynecology,* Vol.97, No.3, (March 2001), pp. 350-356, ISSN 0029-7844.

Fraser, M., & Liggins, GC. (1988). Thyroid hormone kinetics during late pregnancy in the ovine fetus. *Journal of Developmental Physiology,* Vol.10, No.5, (October 1969), pp. 461-471, ISSN 0141-9846.

Fretts, RC., Elkin, EB., Myers, ER., & Heffner, LJ. (2004). Should older women have antepartum testing to prevent unexplained stillbirth? *Obstetrics and Gynecology,* Vol.104, No.1, (July 2004), pp. 56-64, ISSN 0029-7844.

Gowen CW Jr, Lawson EE, Gingras J, Boucher RC, Gatzy JT, Knowles MR. (1988). Electrical potential difference and ion transport across nasal epithelium of term neonates: correlation with mode of delivery, transient tachypnea of the newborn, and respiratory rate. *The Journal of pediatrics,* Vol.113, No.1Pt1, (July 1988), pp. 121-127, ISSN 0022-6833.

Haas, DM., & Ayres, AW. (2002). Laceration injury at cesarean section. *Journal of Maternal-Fetal and Neonatal Medicine,* Vol.11, No.3, (March 2002), pp. 196-198, ISSN 1476-4954.

Hales, KA., Morgan, MlA., & Thurnau, GR. (1993). Influence of labor and route of delivery on the frequency of respiratory morbidity in term neonates. *International Journal of Gynecology and Obstetrics,* Vol.43, No. 1, (October 1993), pp. 35-40, ISSN 0020-7292.

Halperin, ME., Moore, DC., & Hannah, WJ. (1988). Classical versus low-segment transverse incision for preterm cesarean section: maternal complications and outcome of subsequent pregnancies. *British Journal of Obstetrics and Gynecology,* Vol.95, No.10, (October 1998), pp. 990–996, ISSN 0528-1471.

Hankins, GD., Clark, SM., & Munn, MB. (2006). Cesarean section on request at 39 weeks: impact on shoulder dystocia, fetal trauma, neonatal encephalopathy, and intrauterine fetal demise. *Seminars in Perinatology,* Vol.30, No.5, (October 2006), pp. 276-287, ISSN 0146-0005.

Hannah, ME., Hannah, WJ., Hewson, SA., Hodnett, ED., Saigal, S., & Willan, AR. (2000). Planned caesarean section versus planned vaginal birth for breech presentation at term: a randomised multicentre trial. Term Breech Trial Collaborative Group. *Lancet,* Vol.356, No.9239, (October 2000), pp. 1375-1383, ISSN 1476-547X.

Hansen, AK., Wisborg, K., Uldbjerg, N., & Henriksen, TB. (2008). Risk of respiratory morbidity in term infants delivered by elective caesarean section: cohort study. *British Medical Journal,* Vol.336, No.7635, (January 2008), pp. 85–87, ISSN 0007-1447.

Jacobsson, B., Ladfors, L., Milsom I. (2004). Advanced maternal age and adverse perinatal outcome. Obstet Gynecol 2004;104:727-33. *Obstetrics and Gynecology,* Vol.104, No.4, (October 2004), pp. 727-733, ISSN 0029-7844.

Joseph, KS., Allen, AC., Dodds, L., Turner, LA., Scott, H., & Liston, R. (2005). The perinatal effects of delayed childbearing. Obstetrics and Gynecology, Vol.105, No.6, (June 2005), pp. 1410-1418, ISSN 0029-7844.

Kitterman, JA., Ballard, PL., Clements, JA., Mescher, EJ., & Tooley, WH. (1979). Tracheal fluid in fetal lambs: spontaneous decrease prior to birth. *Journal of Applied Physiology,* Vol.47, No.5, (November 1979), pp. 985-989, ISSN 1522-1601.

Landon, MB., Hauth, JC., Leveno, KJ., Spong, CY., Leindecker, S., Varner, MW., Moawad, AH., Caritis, SN., Harper, M., Wapner, RJ., Sorokin, Y., Miodovnik, M., Carpenter, M., Peaceman, AM., O'Sullivan, MJ., Sibai, B., Langer, O., Thorp, JM., Ramin, SM., Mercer, BM., & Gabbe, SG. National Institute of Child Health and Human Development Maternal-Fetal Medicine Units Network. (2004). Maternal and perinatal outcomes associated with a trial of labor after prior cesarean delivery. *New England Journal of Medicine,* Vol.351, No.25, (December 2004), pp. 2581–2589, ISSN 0028-4793.

Liggins, GC., Schellenberg, JC., Mianzai, M., Kitterman, JA., & Lee, CCH. (1988). Synergism of cortisol and thyrotropinreleasing hormone in lung maturation in fetal sheep. *Journal of Applied Physiology,* Vol.65, No.4, (October 1988), pp. 1880-1884, ISSN 1522-1601.

Lilford, RJ., van Coeverden de Groot, HA., Moore, PJ., & Bingham, P. (1990). The relative risks of caesarean delivery (intrapartum and elective) and vaginal delivery: a detailed analysis to exclude the effects of medical disorder and other acute pre-existing physiological disturbances. *British Journal of Obstetrics and Gynecology,* Vol.97, No.10, (October 1990), pp. 883–892, ISSN 0528-1471.

Martin, JA., Hamilton, BE., Sutton, PD., Ventura, SJ., Menacker, F., & Munson, ML. (2005). Births: Final data for 2003. *National vital statistics reports;* vol.54, No.2, Hyattsville, MD: National Center for Health Statistics.

Meikle, SF., Steiner, CA., Zhang, J., & Lawrence, WL. (2005). A national estimate of the elective primary cesarean delivery rate. *Obstetrics and Gynecology,* Vol.115, No.4, (April 2005), pp. 751–756, ISSN 0029-7844.

Mikner, AD., Saunders, RA. & Hopkin, IE. (1978). Effects of delivery by caesarean section on lung mechanics and lung volume in the human neonate. *Archives of Disease in Childhood,* Vol.53, No. 7, (July 1978), pp. 545-548, ISSN 1468-2044.

Milner, AD., Saunders, RA., & Hopkin, IE. (1978). Effects of delivery by Caesarean section on lung mechanics and lung volume in the human neonate. *Archives of disease in childhood,* Vol.53, No.7, (July 1978), pp. 545-548, ISSN 1468-2044.

Minkoff, H., & Chervenak, FA. (2003). Elective primary cesarean delivery. *New England Journal of Medicine,* Vol.348, No.10, (March 2003), pp. 946–950, ISSN 0028-4793.

Oliver, T K Jr., Demis, JA., & Bates, GD. (1961). Serial bloodgas tensions and acid-base balance during the first hour of life in hutman infants. *Acta Paediatrica,* Vol.50, (July 1961), pp. 346-360, ISSN 1651-2227.

Olver, RE., & Strang, LB. (1974). Ion fluxes across the pulmonary epithelium and the secretion of lung liquid in the foetal lamb. *Journal of Physiology,* Vol.241, No.2, (September 1974), pp. 327-357, ISSN 1469-7793.

Olver, RE., Ramsden, CA., Strang, LB., & Walters, DV. (1986). The role of amiloride-blockade sodium transport in adrenaline-induced lung liquid reabsorption in the fetal lamb. *Journal of Physiology,* Vol.376, (July 1986), pp. 321-340, ISSN 1469-7793.

Pallasmaa, N., Ekblad, U., Gissler, M. (2008). Severe maternal morbidity and the mode of delivery. *Acta obstetricia et gynecologica Scandinavica,* Vol.87, No.6, (June 2008), pp. 662-668, ISSN 1600-0412.

Palme-Kilander, C., Tunell, R., & Chiwel, Y. (1993). Pulmonary gas exchange immediately after birth in spontaneously breathing infants. *Archives of Disease in Childhood,* Vol.68, No. 1, (January 1993), pp. 6-10, ISSN 1468-2044.

Pfister, RE., Ramsden, CA., Neil, HL., Kyriakides, MA., & Berger, PJ. (2001). Volume and secretion rate of lung liquid in the final days of gestation and labor in the fetal sheep. *Journal of Physiology,* Vol.535, No.Pt3, (September 2001), pp. 889-899, ISSN 1469-7793.

Puza, S., Roth, N., Macones, GA., Mennuti, MT., & Morgan, MA. (1998). Does cesarean section decrease the incidence of major birth trauma? *J Perinatol* 1998, 18:9–12. *Journal of Perinatology,* Vol.18, No.1, (January-February 1998), pp. 9-12, ISSN 1476-5543.

Rahman, MS., Gasem, T., Al Suleiman, SA., Al Jama, FE., ,Burshaid S., & Rahman, J. (2009). Bladder injuries during cesarean section in a University Hospital: a 25-year review. *Archives of Gynecology and Obstetrics,* Vol.279, No.3, (March 2009), pp. 349-352, ISSN 1432-0711.

Salim, R., Zafran, N., & Shalev, E. (2009) Timing of elective repeat cesarean delivery at term [letter]. *New England Journal of Medicine,* Vol.360, No.15, (April 2009), pp. 1570, ISSN 0028-4793.

Salim, R., & Shalev, E. (2010). Health implications resulting from the timing of elective cesarean delivery. *Reproductive Biology and Endocrinolgy,* Vol.8, (June 2010), pp. 68, ISSN 1477-7827.

Salim, R., & Shalev, E. (2011). Timing of Elective Repeat Cesarean Delivery at Term and Maternal Perioperative Outcomes [letter]. *Obstetrics and Gynecology,* Vol.117, No.6, (June 2011), pp. 1437, ISSN 0029-7844.

Saunders, N., & Paterson, C. (1991). Effect of gestational age on obstetric performance: when is "term" over? *Lancet,* Vol.338, No.8776, (November 2000), pp. 1190-1192, ISSN 1476-547X.

Smith, GC. (2001). Life-table analysis of the risk of perinatal death at term and post term in singleton pregnancies. *American Journal of Obstetrics and Gynecology,* Vol.184, No.3, (February 2001), pp. 489-496, ISSN 1097-6868.

Thomas, J., & Paranjothy, S. (2001). Royal College of Obstetricians and Gynaecologists Clinical Effectiveness Support Unit. The national sentinel caesarean section audit report. London: RCOG Press; 2001.

Tita, AT., Landon, MB., Spong, CY., Lai, Y., Leveno, KJ., Varner, MW., Moawad, AH., Caritis, SN., Meis, PJ., Wapner, RJ., Sorokin, Y., Miodovnik, M., Carpenter, M., Peaceman, AM., O'Sullivan, MJ., Sibai, BM., Langer, O., Thorp, JM., Ramin, SM., & Mercer, BM.. Eunice Kennedy Shriver NICHD Maternal-Fetal Medicine Units Network. (2009). Timing of elective repeat cesarean delivery at term and neonatal outcomes. *New England Journal of Medicine,* Vol.360, No.2, (January 2009), pp. 111-120, ISSN 0028-4793.

Tita, AT., Lai, Y., Landon, MB., Spong, CY., Leveno, KJ., Varner, MW., Caritis, SN., Meis, PJ., Wapner, RJ., Sorokin, Y., Peaceman, AM., O'Sullivan, MJ., Sibai, BM., Thorp, JM., Ramin, SM., & Mercer, BM. Eunice Kennedy Shriver National Institute of Child Health and Human Development (NICHD) Maternal-Fetal Medicine Units Network (MFMU). (2011). Timing of elective repeat cesarean delivery at term and maternal perioperative outcomes. *Obstetrics and Gynecology,* Vol.117, No.2 Pt 1, (February 2011), pp. 280-286, ISSN 0029-7844.

Tucker, J. (2002). UK Neonatal Staffing Study Group: Patient volume, staffing, and workload in relation to risk-adjusted outcomes in a random stratified sample of UK neonatal intensive care units: a prospective evaluation. *Lancet,* Vol.359, No.9301, (January 2002), pp. 99-107, ISSN 1476-547X.

Usta, IM., & Nassar, AH. (2008). Advanced maternal age. Part I: obstetric complications. *American Journal of Perinatology,* Vol.25, No.8, (September 2008), pp. 521-534, ISSN 0735-1631.

Waetjen, LE., Subak, LL., Shenm H., Lin, F., Wang, TH., Vittinghoff, E., & Brown, JS. (2003). Stress urinary incontinence surgery in the United States. *Obstetrics and Gynecology,* Vol.101, No.4, (April 2003), pp. 671-676, ISSN 0029-7844.

Wallace, MJ., Hooper, SB., & Harding, R. (1996). Role of the adrenal glands in the maturation of lung liquid secretory mechanisms in fetal sheep. *American Journal of Physiology,* Vol.270, No.1Pt2, (January 1996), pp. R33-R40, ISSN 1522-1539.

Wilson L, Brown JS, Shin GP, Luc K, Subak LL. (2001). Annual direct cost of urinary incontinence. *Obstetrics and Gynecology,* Vol.98, No.3, (September 2001), pp. 398-406, ISSN 0029-7844.

Wood, SL., Chen, S., Ross, S., & Sauve, R. (2008). The risk of unexplained antepartum stillbirth in second pregnancies following caesarean section in the first pregnancy. *British Journal of Obstetrics and Gynecology,* Vol.115, No.6, (May 2008), pp. 726–731, ISSN 0528-1471.

Yoles, I., & Maschiach, S. (1998). Increased maternal mortality in cesarean delivery as compared to vaginal delivery? *American Journal of Obstetrics and Gynecology,* Vol.178, (1998), pp. S78, ISSN 1097-6868.

Yudkin, PL., Wood, L., & Redman, CWG. (1987). Risk of unexplained stillbirth at different gestational ages. *Lancet*, Vol.1, No.8543, (May 1987), pp. 1192-1194, ISSN 1476-547X.

Zanardo, V., Simbi, AK., Franzoi, M., Solda, G., Salvadori, A., & Trevisanuto, D. (2004). Neonatal respiratory morbidity risk and mode of delivery at term: influence of timing of elective caesarean delivery. *Acta Paediatrica,* Vol.93, No.5, (May 2004), pp. 643-647, ISSN 1651-2227.

3

Anesthesia for Cesarean Section

Sotonye Fyneface-Ogan
*Department of Anesthesiology, Faculty of Clinical Sciences,
College of Health Sciences, University of Port Harcourt,
Nigeria*

1. Introduction

Cesarean section is frequently becoming a popular mode of child delivery world-wide. The rate of Cesarean section could be as high as 18/100 in Africa (Aisien et al, 2002) to 32/100 deliveries in the United States (Declercq et al, 2011). The use of anesthesia makes a Cesarean delivery possible. Various forms of anesthesia have been used to perform this surgery. However, the use of general anesthesia has fallen dramatically in the past few decades and now accounts for only about 5 percent of Cesarean deliveries in the United States and United Kingdom. In the sub-saharan Africa, 80 -90% of the Cesarean sections are performed under spinal anesthesia (Fyneface-Ogan et al, 2005). Although spinal analgesia is now the mainstay of anesthesia in countries like India and parts of Africa, excluding the major centres, current usage of this technique is waning in the developed world, with epidural analgesia or combined spinal-epidural anesthesia emerging as the techniques of choice where the cost of the disposable 'kit' is not a challenge.

This chapter endeavors to take an in-depth review of anesthesia for Cesarean section. Although the trend for anesthesia for Cesarean section is towards the use of a combined spinal-epidural technique (Rawal et al, 2000), other options of anesthesia will be reviewed with the intent to highlight the importance of safety during the procedure.

2. Preoperative evaluation and management

The essence of preoperative evaluation of the pregnant woman is in order to delineate the potential difficulties in the line of the anesthetic management and; allay any anxiety associated with the procedure. The paradigm of preoperative assessment is now shifting from predicting risk or anticipated difficulty to actively managing it.

2.1 Preoperative visit

Preoperative evaluation of parturients undergoing Cesarean section is well regarded as a vital part of their care (Garcia-Migel et al 2003). This evaluation forms part of the clinical investigation carried out before anesthesia for Cesarean section and it is the sole responsibility of the attending Anesthetist. It is well known that preoperative visit and proper evaluation create trust and confidence in parturients (Association of Anesthetists of Great Britain and Ireland [AAGBI], 2001).

The aims of preoperative visit and assessment include:

- to reduce the risk associated with Cesarean section and anesthesia
- to increase the quality (thus reducing the cost) of peroperative care (AAGBI, 2001)
- to restore the parturient to the desired functional level
- to obtain the parturient's informed consent for anesthetic procedure

Preoperative Evaluation and Management

Generally, parturients are very apprehensive and becoming more sophisticated particularly as they now have access to clinical information. Therefore, high quality clinical information is now a clear requirement as shared decision-making is frequently encouraged. For parturients, both written and verbal information should be provided as regards how it affects them and their babies. In the United Kingdom (Department of Health, 2001), it is not acceptable for parturients to be denied any information about anesthesia until the time of preoperative visit; at such stage the parturient will not be in a position genuinely to make a decision. Every information made available to parturients should be clearly understood explaining every technical detail. Such information should address the side effects and complications associated. Evidence supports the shift in trend of practice towards shared decision-making, where patients are encouraged to express their views and participate in making clinical decisions (Frosch and Kaplan, 1999). Patients are also becoming more informed about the various options available in anesthetic care and their participatory role in treatment outcome. With this rising trend of patients' involvement, the preferred anesthetic care maybe the sole decision of the parturient (Fyneface-Ogan et al, 2009).

A proper preoperative evaluation of the parturient before anesthesia and Cesarean section is aimed at;

- improving outcome
- identifying potential anesthetic difficulties
- identifying existing medical conditions
- improving safety by assessing and quantifying risk
- allowing planning of preoperative care
- providing the opportunity for explanation and discussion
- allaying anxiety and fear

An interaction with the pregnant patient during the preoperative visit and evaluation may reveal allergies, undesirable side effects of medications or other agents, known medical problems, surgical history, major psychological/physical traumas and current medications. A focused evaluation of the patient may also reveal depleted cardiopulmonary function, poor homeostatic status, personal or family history of anesthetic problems, smoking and alcohol habits.

Questionnaires aimed at generating basic background information have been developed (AAGBI, 2001). These have been found to improve efficiency in the preoperative clinics. Options are available to patients to fill the questionnaires immediately or at the end of last antenatal visit. This questionnaire does not serve as a substitute to proper history taking and clinical evaluation of the patient.

A complete physical examination of the pregnant woman is required to ascertain the possibilities of an existing potential difficulty. Such difficulty could present special challenge during procedures like airway manipulation, establishing a neuraxial block, venous access etc. The presence of any of these potential difficulties might persuade the attending Anesthetist to favor either general or regional anesthesia.

Airway difficulties associated with failed intubation are very common in obstetric patients (approximately 1:238 compared with 1:2220 in non-pregnant population) (Rahman and Jenkin, 2005). Failed intubation reflects the relatively high incidence in the pregnant population. This high incidence among parturients could be due to changes in soft tissues of the airway mucosa, swollen and engorged breasts along with full dentition. Therefore it is imperative to try and identify beforehand airway that is likely to prove difficult. Some bedside assessments are carried out to identify potential airway problems but unfortunately these tests have very low predictive values amongst obstetric patients. Generally, difficult intubation is frequently common in parturients with the following physical characteristics:

- inability to see the uvula or soft palate when the patient is asked to open her mouth and protrude her tongue in a sitting position (Mallampati class III and IV) (Mallampati et al, 1985)
- receding mandible
- protruding maxillary incisors
- a short neck (Rocke et al, 1992)
- keeping a packed African hair style (Famewo, 1982)

Nevertheless, the management of the airway is the responsibility of the attending Anesthetist. It is important to note that a difficult airway exists when the attending Anesthetist has difficulties with mask ventilation, tracheal intubation or both. The incidence of mask ventilation is 5% (CI: 3.9-6.1) (Langeron et al 2000). However, a poorly managed airway may be associated with airway trauma or cardiac or neurological hypoxic injury.

Except in the presence of intercurrent medical disease(s), the routine laboratory investigations preceding anesthesia and Cesarean section are few. The requested laboratory investigations are requested for on clinical grounds. Routine investigations carried out include hemoglobin check, grouping and cross-matching of blood, platelet count. However cross-matching of blood that is not transfused consumes blood bank resource unnecessarily increases the blood inventory that must be maintained, and increases the number of units that become outdated. Occasionally, for example, if a massive hemorrhage is anticipated following Cesarean section, this may be a deliberate policy. Therefore the maximum surgical blood order schedule suggests that, for patients with a high likelihood of blood transfusion, the number of units cross-matched be twice the median requirement for that surgical procedure (crossmatch-to-transfusion ratio of 2:1) (Friedman et al 1976). However a recent study suggests that the crossmatch-to-transfusion ratio may be reduced with the introduction of a Patient-Specific Blood Ordering System that estimates a postoperative hematocrit using the patients' blood volume, the surgeon-defined expected blood loss and preoperative hematocrit (Palmer et al, 2003).

2.2 Premedication

Premedication may be an important component of obstetric anesthesia practice. It may allay the parturient's anxiety (Leigh et al, 1977), alleviate preoperative pain, reduce the pain of vascular canulation or regional anesthesia, reduce nausea and vomiting, minimize risk of aspiration, act as an antisialogogue or facilitate a smooth anesthetic induction. Therefore where these effects are desired, premedication should be prescribed, be correctly given and be effective.

Premedication is known to block the preoperative stress response and lowers beta-endorphin levels in these parturients (Walsh et al, 1987). Following premedication, anesthesia induction is aided by concomitant sedative premedication. However, it is common to withhold premedication from patients having Cesarean section on the grounds that the agents including opioids cause depression of the newborn. The effects of most of the agents used for premedication are readily reversible; therefore there is no scientific evidence in support of withdrawal of premedicants.

2.3 Fasting and prophylaxis against acid aspiration

Parturients are at risk of gastric aspiration under general anesthesia. A high incidence of aspiration of 1:900 during Cesarean section and 1:9200 parturients, with no fatalities, have been reported (Soriede et al, 1996). The altered physiological state in pregnancy is associated with alterations in the rate of gastric emptying and the competence of the gastro-esophageal barrier. The reduction in competence of the barrier is worse in parturients under general anesthesia leading to increased risk of regurgitation and pulmonary aspiration due to retention of gastric contents. The presence of severe pain, and inadequate starvation could result in reduced gastric emptying. The physiological mechanisms that prevent regurgitation and aspiration include the lower esophageal sphincter (LES), and the upper esophageal sphincter (UES) tones, and depressed laryngeal reflexes. It is important to appreciate how these mechanisms may be impaired so that the risk of aspiration pneumonitis can be minimized.

The LES forms the border between the stomach and the esophagus. At this point, the left margin of the lower esophagus makes an acute angle with the gastric fundus and contraction of the right crus of the diaphragm forms a sling around the abdominal esophagus.

Fasting before the administration of anesthetics in parturients aims to reduce the volume and acidity of the stomach contents during surgery, thus reducing the risk of regurgitation and pulmonary aspiration. The former two involve adequate fasting, a decrease in gastric acidity, facilitation of gastric drainage, and maintenance of a competent LES, although the latter two factors may require tracheal intubation or the use of other airway devices and application of cricoid pressure. With the exception of ketamine, most anesthetic techniques are likely to reduce UES tone and increase the likelihood of regurgitation of material from esophagus into the hypopharynx.

Recent guidelines recommended a shift in the fasting policy from the standard "nil by mouth from midnight" approach to a more relaxed policy which permits a period of restricted intake up to a few hours before surgery (Brady et al 2003). Liberal preoperating fasting routines are now frequently implemented world-wide. In general, clear fluids are allowed up to two hours before anesthesia, and light meals up to six hours. Although parturients have traditionally been denied food and drink for 6 hours before induction of general anesthesia, where this "time-line" originated from is not clear. In addition, there is insufficient evidence to address the safety of preoperative fasting for solids although a conscious opinion of a fasting period of 6 hours for a light meal, such as tea and toast is well established (ASA Task Force, 1999).

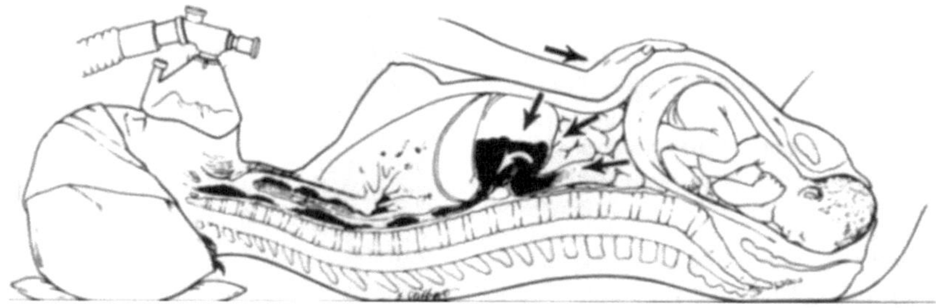

Fig. 1. Regurgitation of stomach content under general anesthesia

All pregnant women from the second trimester develop an increased risk of regurgitation of stomach contents. At the time of delivery there is a chance of requiring general anesthesia, which may often be required in a non-starved woman, and therefore a risk of pulmonary aspiration. Aspiration of gastric contents is a rare but potentially serious adverse event. It is much commoner in the pregnant population undergoing general anesthesia for Cesarean section. Emphasis should be to deliver the safest anesthetic care to the pregnant woman while balancing all relevant risks.

The identification of predisposing factors for pulmonary aspiration is paramount in its prevention. Risk factors include increased gastric pressure, increased tendency to regurgitate, and laryngeal incompetence (Engelhardt & Webster, 1999). Contrary to vomiting, which is an active process, regurgitation is passive in nature. Pulmonary consequences of gastric aspiration fall into three groups:

i. particle-related
ii. acid-related
iii. bacterial

Particle-related complications may result in acute airway obstruction leading to arterial hypoxemia and may cause immediate death. The harmful effects of acid aspiration may occur in two phases:

i. immediate direct tissue injury
ii. subsequent inflammatory response (Knight et al, 1992).

Gastric contents are not sterile and infection with bacteria following aspiration may result in pneumonia (Johanson & Harris).

In the management and prevention of gastric aspiration, all parturients should be considered to be at high risk of requiring anesthetic intervention. Outcomes recorded in birth centres caring for even low risk pregnancies, where all women were allowed to eat and drink as they desired, have shown 15.4% required transfer to another hospital and 4.4 % required Cesarean delivery (Rooks et al 1989). Risk of aspiration is a function of those factors which influence gastric volume and pH, opioid effects, the experience and expertise of the anesthetist managing the airway, as well as maternal obesity (Lewis 2007; McClure & Cooper 2005).

Although the incidence of aspiration in pregnant women has changed over recent decades, it now occurs less frequently. This reduced frequency could be due to the high rates of use of regional anesthesia for Cesarean section. The tendency for this gastro-respiratory accident is more in the parturients due to both hormonal and mechanical factors. Significant risk factors for aspiration include the presence of food and opioid analgesia in labor (Murphy et al 1984; Wright 1992,). Loss of consciousness and sedation contribute to these risks.

The diagnosis of gastric aspiration is seldom a problem, the clinical features being those described by Mendelson (Mendelson 1946), namely progressive dyspnea, hypoxia, bronchial wheeze and patchy consolidation and collapse in the lungs, all following the inhalation of gastric contents during the course of general anesthesia. Although the disease manifests in the same way all through the years, the prognosis has improved over the years in the developed world.

Aspiration when it occurs remains an important cause of death and morbidity. Aspiration pneumonitis carries a 30-percent mortality rate and accounts for up to 20 percent of all deaths attributable to anesthesia. In the US between 1979 and 1990, 23% of maternal deaths were found to be due to aspiration (Hawkins et al 1997). Over the years, the introduction of several measures designed to reduce the risk of aspiration in pregnant women have been associated with a profound effect in reducing mortality from aspiration. Popularization of regional anesthesia, fasting in labor, use of antacid premedication, prokinetics, H2-blockers, mechanical factors such as cricoid pressure, intubation with cuffed tracheal tubes and have all been identified as contributing to the dramatic fall in maternal mortality (Cooper et al 2002).

Gastric content values of volume and pH, and competence of lower esophageal tone play major role in the occurrence of aspiration. Risk of pneumonitis is said to occur when there is a combination of pH less than 2.5 and a volume greater than 25 ml of stomach contents. For the pregnant woman, the critical values of gastric contents are a pH value of <2.5 and a volume of >0.4 ml/kg.

Certain factors contribute to the risk of aspiration in parturients. Although it has been contentious as to whether gastric emptying and gastric pH are decreased throughout pregnancy, it is well known that gastric emptying is delayed during labor and delivery. In addition, anatomic changes resulting from displacement of the stomach by the pregnant uterus and decreased lower esophageal sphincter tone, caused by increased progesterone levels, produce an increased incidence of gastroesophageal reflux in the pregnant woman.

Weight gain in pregnancy contributes immensely towards difficulty in airway management and in addition, is associated with a significantly higher gastric volume in labor (Roberts & Shirley 1974). Another major key player in causing a delay in the gastric emptying follows the administration of parenteral opioids during late pregnancy and labor (Nimmo et al 1975). Opioids administered epidurally or intrathecally in labor may also have this effect, although it would appear to be dose-dependent. It has been shown that gastric emptying could be delayed in parturients who had received a high dose of fentanyl by epidural infusion (Porter et al 1997).

Following the severe morbidity and mortality associated with aspiration pneumonitis, its preventative strategies should aim at increasing the pH and/or reduce intragastric volume. Many preparations such as antacids, prokinetic, mechanically emptying the stomach using a naso-gastric tube are in use either alone or in combination (Paranjothy et al 2011).

It is, therefore, suggested that oral ranitidine 150 mg should be administered 2 hours before an elective Cesarean section and preferably 150 mg the previous evening. As part of the preparation for an emergency Cesarean section an intravenous ranitidine 150 mg with 30 ml of freshly prepared 0.3 molar solution of sodium citrate should be given 30-60 minutes before surgery. Other usual precautions to avoid acid aspiration should also be taken.

2.3.1 Mechanical suctioning

Medical suction is an essential part of clinical practice. Since the 1920s, it has been used to empty the stomach, and in the 1950s, airway suction levels were first regulated for safety. Ideally, clinicians need the best flow rate out of a vacuum system at the lowest negative pressure. Three main factors affect the flow rate of a suction system:

- The amount of negative pressure (vacuum)
- The resistance of the suction system
- The viscosity of the matter being removed

The negative pressure used establishes the pressure gradient that will move air, fluid, or secretions. Material will move from an area of higher pressure in the patient to an area of lower pressure in the suction apparatus. A naso-gastric tube is passed into the parturient with the aim of the tube tip reaching the base of the stomach. A negative pressure is applied to empty the stomach of recently ingested materials and fluid. The advantage in removing particulate material and fluid can speed airway management and reduce the risk or minimize the complications from aspiration (Vandenberg et al, 1998).

2.3.2 Antacids

Antacids are of two types - particulate and non-particulate antacid. The use of antacids is now being restricted to non-particulate sub-type such as sodium citrate. Particulate antacids such as those containing magnesium or aluminium are likely to be associated with more severe pneumonitis should aspiration occur (Eyler et al 1982; Gibbs et al 1979).

2.3.3 Sodium citrate

Sodium citrate is the most effective agent for immediate neutralization of acidic gastric contents (Gibbs et al 1982). A 0.3 mol/l (8.8%) in a volume of 30 ml has pH of 8.4 and causes mean pH to increase to more than 6 for one hour. Molar solution of sodium citrate has been found to be equally effective in emergency and elective cases and with either general or regional anesthesia (Lin et al 1996, Stuart et al 1996). A rebound decrease in gastric pH below 2.5 can occur therefore sodium citrate 0.3 mol/l is recommended as a regular 2-4 hourly regimen for women in labor (Robert & Shirley, 1976).

2.3.4 H_2 receptor antagonists

The H_2 antagonists are competitive antagonists of histamine at the parietal cell H_2 receptor decreasing the production of acid by these cells. In this group agents include cimetidine, ranitidine, and famotidine. They suppress the normal secretion of acid by parietal cells and the meal-stimulated secretion of acid. They accomplish this by two mechanisms: Histamine released by enterochromaffin-like cells in the stomach is blocked from binding on parietal cell H_2 receptors, which stimulate acid secretion; therefore, other substances that promote acid secretion (such as gastrin and acetylcholine) have a reduced effect on parietal cells when the H_2 receptors are blocked.

One of the commonest H2 receptor antagonists in use is ranitidine. It is a histamine H_2-receptor antagonist that inhibits stomach acid production. It is commonly used in treatment of peptic ulcer disease (PUD) and gastro esophageal reflux disease (GERD). It has been demonstrated that 150 mg of oral ranitidine when given two to three hours before surgery resulted in a mean gastric pH of 5.86 within 60 minutes (Escolano 1996). It has also been shown that there is no significant difference between 150 mg and 300 mg, with both taking around 60 minutes to achieve a sustained increase in pH which then lasts for approximately five hours. When used in obstetric patients, these effects may be less predictable particularly in the context of active labor or concurrent opioid use (Murphy et al 1984,), or in the presence of particulate material in the stomach of non-fasted patients (Rout et al 1993), or with emergency as compared to elective surgery (Lim & Elegbe 1992).

The intravenous ranitidine have a faster rate of onset. An intravenous route of administration of 50 mg ranitidine during elective or emergent cesarean section achieves a gastric pH >2.5 and volume <25 ml within 45 minutes (Tripathi et al 1995).

2.3.5 Prokinetics

Prokinetics include the drugs, domperidone, metoclopramide and cisapride. Prokinetics claim to restore gastric motility and to increase the tone in the lower esophageal sphincter by enhancing acetylcholine release in the group of nerves that control upper gastrointestinal motility. These actions are said to speed up gastric emptying and reduce reflux into the esophagus. Metoclopramide, the most frequently used increases the rate of gastric emptying, has an antiemetic and increases lower esophageal sphincter tone. It has been shown that in combination with other agents in obstetric patients at a dose of 10 mg intravenous (Stuart et al 1996)

2.3.6 Proton Pump Inhibitors

Proton pump inhibitors (PPIs) are a group of drugs whose main action is a pronounced and long-lasting reduction of gastric acid production. PPIs act by irreversibly blocking the hydrogen/potassium adenosine triphosphatase enzyme system (the H +/K+ ATPase or more common gastric proton pump) of the gastric parietal cells. The proton pump is the terminal stage in gastric acid secretion, being directly responsible for secreting H^+ ions into the gastric lumen, making it an ideal target for inhibiting acid secretion.

Omeprazole has been the agent most extensively studied amongst PPIs. It can be given orally or by intravenous injection and has been studied at doses of 40 mg and 80 mg. The onset of effect after IV administration is similar to that of ranitidine and should be considered to be at least 40 minutes (Tripathi et al 1995). In the setting of emergency Cesarean section, a single intravenous dose of omeprazole 40 mg results in the same percentage of patients with the combination of pH <2.5 and volume > 25 ml as ranitidine 50 mg IV when combined with sodium citrate (Tripathi et al 1995, Stuart et al 1996,).

3. Immediate preanesthetic preparation

Following proper preoperative evaluation, consent for anesthesia and surgery obtained and possible premedicant administered, and the parturient is transferred to the operating theatre while maintaining a 15-20° lateral uterine displacement (to prevent aorto-caval compression). Maternal hypotension from caval compression is a common problem during Cesarean section under anesthesia more so during spinal anesthesia. The possible explanation for this is combined aorto-caval compression by gravid uterus in parturient in addition to reduced systemic vascular resistance by spinal anesthesia. It was first reported in 1952 as "supine hypotension in late pregnancy" (Howard et al). This describes the hypotension which occurs in parturients upon assuming the supine position, and resolves with lateral positioning.

Some factors such as late pregnancy, the supine, and to a lesser extent, the sitting position, and more frequently in those with varicose veins have associated with this grave state. This form of hypotension occurs following compression of the inferior vena cava (IVC) by the gravid uterus with a consequent reduction in venous return. About five minutes are generally required for significant hypotension to become manifest (Howard et al 1953). Supine hypotension is most severe in non-laboring patients undergoing Cesarean section than those who are laboring (Brizgys et al, 1987). Supine hypotension is cured by delivery.

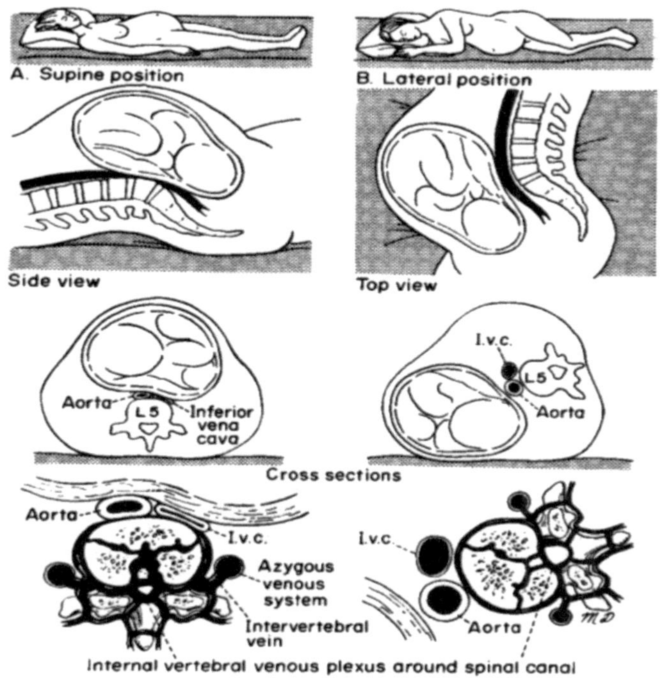

Fig. 2. Position of Gravid uterus on Inferior Vena Cava

Two compensatory mechanisms have been described for reducing the degree of hypotension which occurs as a result of impairment of venous return. Firstly, there may be a generalized increase in sympathetic tone and, secondly, the internal vertebral venous plexus and the azygos vein can act as a collateral conduit for blood returning from the lower part of the body. It was subsequently recognized that aortic compression could be as important as caval compression in the generation of decreased utero-placetal perfusion and fetal distress.

Maternal hypotension as measured by a reduction in brachial artery blood pressure occurs as a result of a reduction in venous return. It is most pronounced in hypovolemic states, either actual, as occurs with hemorrhage, or relative, as occurs following sympathetic blockade. Acute fetal distress can be caused by:

- hypoperfusion of the uteroplacental unit secondary to maternal hypotension, or
- occult aortic compression (in the presence of a normal maternal brachial arterial blood pressure) causing a reduction in iliac arterial flow.

Full left or right lateral position completely relieves aorto-caval compression. Elevating the mother's right hip 10-15cm completely relieves aorto-caval compression in 58% of term parturients (Kinsella et al, 1990). Lateral uterine displacement therefore, remains an all important technique in the prevention of supine hypotension and in the management of hypotension in all women during pregnancy.

4. Modes of anesthesia for cesarean section

General goals in choosing anesthesia are:

- the safety of the mother
- the safety of the baby
- the comfort of the mother
- the ability to perform the surgery under that anesthetic technique.

There are two general categories of anesthesia for Cesarean section - general anesthesia and regional anesthesia. Regional anesthesia includes both spinal and epidural techniques. General anesthesia is usually reserved for patients that must have anesthesia "right away" because their surgery is being done for a true emergency. In these situations, regional techniques may take too long to perform. It is also performed when contraindications for regional anesthesia are present.

However, there are some risks associated with general anesthesia that can be avoided with regional anesthesia. Therefore, regional anesthesia is almost universally preferred when time is not as much of a factor. Internationally, obstetric anesthesia guidelines recommend spinal and epidural over general anesthesia (GA) for most Cesarean sections (Cyna & Dodd, 2007). The primary reason for recommending regional blocks is the risk of failed tracheal intubation and aspiration of gastric contents in pregnant women who undergo GA (Bloom et al, 2005). While there is evidence that GA is associated with an increased need for neonatal resuscitation (Gordon et al, 2005), evidence about specific delivery indications and about neonatal outcomes subsequent to resuscitation is limited.

4.1 Regional anesthesia for cesarean section

Obstetric anesthesia has evolved substantially in the last two decades, with regional techniques becoming increasingly popular for Cesarean section. The method of choice may be a spinal, an epidural or a combination of the two (combined spinal epidural anesthesia). Spinal anesthesia has evolved as the preferred anesthetic technique for most cases of Cesarean section.

Although regional anesthesia has several advantages such as preservation of consciousness, avoidance of neonatal depression that occurs with general anesthesia, and avoidance of airway manipulation, it is contraindicated in conditions of hypovolemia, coagulopathies, infection at the site of injection and when the patient rejects the procedure. Some complications have been associated hypotension, post dural puncture headache (if spinal anesthesia is used) local anesthetic toxicity (involving central nervous system, cardiovascular system), high spinal, total spinal anesthesia (if inadvertent injection occurs during epidural injection), bradycardia and failed block.

4.2 Preparation for regional anesthesia

The administrator of the regional anesthetic should be aware of the potential complications associated with this technique and also be knowledgeable to manage them. Complications such as hypotension, respiratory arrest following excessive cephalad spread, seizures from central nervous system toxicity, cardiovascular collapse could occur. Therefore, the anesthetic machine should be checked and made ready, tracheal tubes of appropriate sizes, laryngoscope with appropriate blade sizes, suction machine, monitoring equipment, vasopressor agent like ephedrine, drugs for possible conversion to general anesthesia be made available for possible use and oxygen source.

Neuraxial block can impair respiratory function by paralysis of the intercostals muscles due to a high block. A satisfactory regional anesthesia for Cesarean delivery requires a block level to at least the T5 dermatome and this can alter respiratory performance (Kelly et al, 1996). Therefore, many anesthetists will administer supplementary oxygen to mothers undergoing regional anesthesia for Cesarean section to obviate the effect of an excessive cephalad spread of the local anesthetic. It has been found that administering supplemental oxygen during emergency Cesarean section increases fetal oxygenation without increasing lipid peroxidation in both the compromised and uncompromised fetuses (Khaw et al, 2002; Ogunbiyi et al, 2003),

4.3 Spinal anesthesia

Spinal anesthesia also called spinal analgesia or sub-arachnoid block (SAB), is a form of regional anesthesia involving injection of a local anesthetic agent into the subarachnoid space, generally through a fine needle, usually 9 cm long (3.5 inches). For extremely obese patients, some anesthesiologists prefer spinal needles which are 12.7 cm long (5 inches). The tip of the spinal needle has a point or small bevel. Recently, pencil point needles have been made available (Hart & Whitacre, 1951; Sprotte et al, 1987). Regardless of the anesthetic agent (drug) used, the desired effect is to block the transmission of afferent nerve signals from peripheral nociceptors. Sensory signals from the site are blocked, thereby eliminating pain. The degree of neuronal blockade depends on the amount and concentration of local anesthetic used and the properties of the axon. Thin unmylenated C-fibres associated with pain are blocked first, while thick, heavily mylenated A-alpha motor neurons are blocked last. The desired result is total numbness of the area. A pressure sensation is permissible and often occurs due to incomplete blockade of the thicker A-beta mechanoreceptors. This allows surgical procedures to be performed with no painful sensation to the person undergoing the procedure.

Spinal anesthesia for Cesarean section is gradually gaining popularity and substituting the general anesthesia. The use of spinal anesthesia for Cesarean delivery was facilitated by the popularization of pencil-point needles, which dramatically reduced the incidence of postdural puncture headache.

The International goal for protection of future mothers is 80-90% of all Cesarean section to be carried out under spinal anesthesia. This is a simple and reliable regional anesthetic technique that provides a high quality sensory and motor blockade immediately following the subarachnoid administration of the local anesthetic agent (Gogarten & Van Aken, 2005). It offers some advantages over general anesthesia in many ways such as minimal exposure of fetus to medications, parturient remaining conscious throughout the anesthesia and surgery. The preservation of airway protective reflexes becomes a desirable quality in abolishing the risk of aspiration.

Maternal hypotension is one of the commonest challenges that may accompany spinal anesthesia for Cesarean section. The incidence of hypotension could be as high as 80% (Rout & Rocke, 1994) and it could compromise the wellbeing of both mother and fetus (Vorke et al, 1982). Hypotension following spinal anesthesia for Cesarean section may be associated with associated symptoms such as nausea and vomiting which still persist, despite many efforts to improve their treatment and prevention. Rapid administration of crystalloid solutions before spinal anesthesia has been recommended by many anesthesiologists to prevent hypotension (Clark et al, 1976)). Although controversy still exists, there is accumulating evidence that crystalloid solutions are particularly ineffective in preventing hypotension after extensive sympathetic blockade associated with spinal anesthesia (Jackson et al, 1995).

Preloading is routinely carried before the institution of neuraxial block. About 500 – 1000 ml of fluid (10-15 ml/kg crystalloid over 20 minutes) or colloid (such as 6% hydroxyethyl starch, 4% succinylated gelatin (Turker et al, 2011)) is used. Crystalloid rapidly moves into the interstitial space and therefore, the increase in central blood volume garnered from an intravenous bolus of crystalloid (no matter how much) is fleeting. Colloids remain within the intravascular space for a prolonged period, therefore, are more effective at both increasing cardiac output and reducing the incidence of hypotension. Unfortunately, colloids are less available, more expensive and have a low risk of severe allergic reaction. One method that has shown promise is to delay the preload until after the spinal block or concomitant to induction of the spinal anesthetic (co-hydration or co-load). One study which compared preload and co-load using lactated ringer found that cardiac output remained elevated above baseline for 30 min after induction of anesthesia in the co-load group (Kamenik & Payer-Erzen, 2001). Another study also showed that rapid crystalloid infusion during or at the time of spinal induction was more effective at preventing hypotension than a preload of the same volume of crystalloid prior to Cesarean section (Dryer et al, 2004).

Most spinal anesthetics are conducted with the parturient on the operating table in order to reduce tendency of multiple patient transfers from one trolley/bed to the other. It is of the essence to ensure asepsis during the performance of the procedure, equipment check, intravenous fluids, and source of oxygen and means of delivering it, monitors to check blood pressure, oximetry, electrocardiogram and the availability of vasopressor. In addition, the anesthetic machine must be prepared and cart should have tracheal tubes of appropriate sizes, laryngoscopes and drugs for possible administration of general anesthesia.

Proper positioning is essential for a successful conduction of spinal anesthesia. This is often done either while the patient is in sitting or the lateral position. In the lateral, the patient is positioned with their back parallel with the side of the operating table. Thighs are flexed up, and neck is flexed forward (see Fig. 3a) Patient should be positioned to take advantage of the baricity of the spinal local anesthetic.

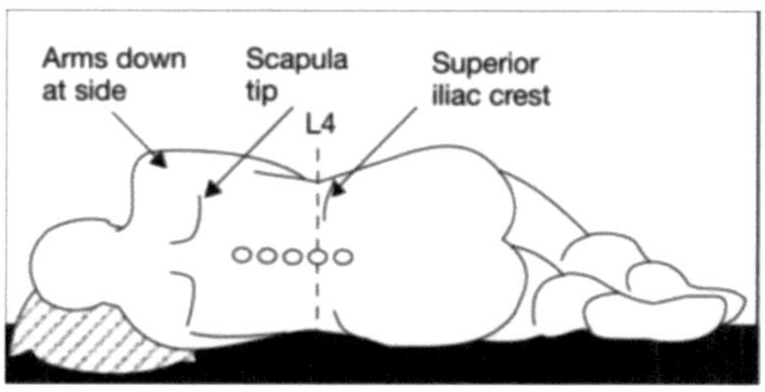

Fig. 3a. Lateral position for spinal block

In the sitting position, the patient's feet are placed on a stool while she sits up straight, her head flexed, arms hugging a pillow (see Fig. 3b).

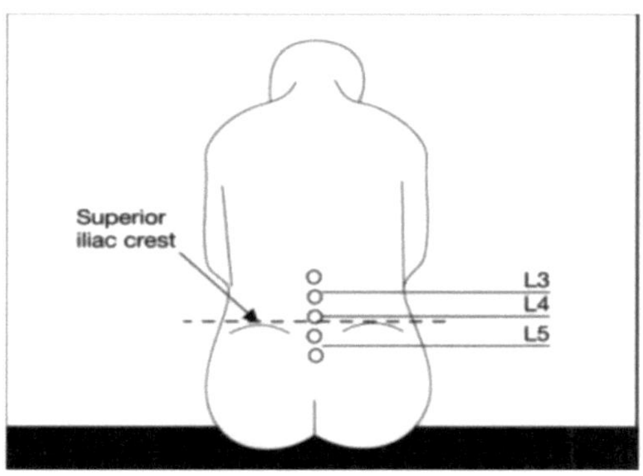

Fig. 3b. Sitting position for spinal block

In the administration of the local anesthetic for subarachnoid block, the size and type of needle are of vital importance. The most frequently used needle is the pencil tip. The Quincke needle inflicts more damage to the dural sheath at the point of entry and leads to post-dural puncture headache. Following aseptic protocols, the predetermined dose of the local anesthetic for the subarachnoid injection is drawn up and tagged. Also drawn up is the local anesthetic to be used for skin infiltration into the 2ml syringe. The patient is positioned and the back cleaned with antiseptic. The interspinous space is located after draping of the back of the parturient. A skin wheal of local anesthetic is raised at the intended interspinous space. An introducer is inserted as 25 gauge needles are often used. The introducer is advanced into the ligamentum flavum while avoiding accidental dural puncture. The 25 gauge spinal needle is then passed through the introducer with the bevel directed laterally (if Quincke tip needle is used). While advancing the needle, an increased resistance is felt as the needle enters the ligamentum flavum, followed by a loss of resistance as the epidural space is entered. Another loss of resistance is usually felt as the dura is pierced and CSF back flow occurs through the needle when the stylet is removed.

The local anesthetic is injected through the needle as soon as the stylet is removed. The spinal needle, introducer and syringe are withdrawn as one immediately after the injection is complete, and a sticking plaster is applied to the puncture site. The parturient is quickly returned supine while ensuring left lateral uterine displacement to avoid aorto-caval compression. It is important to assess the height of the block before commencement of any surgical stimulation. It is unnecessary to test sensation with a sharp needle and leave the patient with a series of bleeding puncture wounds. It is better to test for a loss of temperature sensation using a swab soaked in alcohol.

The addition of opioids to local anesthetics has been widely used in clinical practice for over 30 years; however, the efficacy and safety of this method are still in dispute. It is a common practice to use 2.0 – 2.5 ml hyperbaric bupivacaine 0.5% alone or in combination with opioid to improve the quality of the block without producing a higher level of analgesia to pinprick (Russell, 1995) and, provide some postoperative analgesia. In order to limit the adverse effects, local anesthetic agents are combined with low doses of opioids. Administered subarachnoidally, they reduce the dose of bupivacaine; improve the quality of intraoperative analgesia and their analgesic effects last in the postoperative period (Hamber & Viscomi, 1999; Chung et al, 2002).

Some anesthesiologists prefer lipophilic opioids highlighting their quick onset of action (intraoperative), analgesic effects in the early postoperative period (6 h) and minor adverse side effects (Hunt et al, 1989). Fentanyl is recommended in the dose of 20-30 µg (Hamber & Viscomi, 1999). In the case of morphine, 50 µg does not provide analgesic effects while the dose of 200 µg induces too strong adverse effects (pruritus, nausea and vomiting) and symptoms of late respiratory depression (Milner et al, 1996).

All agents injected into the subarachnoid space must be preservative-free solution. The height of block appropriate for Cesarean section is T6 bilaterally. Hypotension is very common following spinal anesthesia for Cesarean section. The extensive pharmacologic sympathectomy causes arteriolar dilatation, venodilatation and suppression of the ionotropy and chronotropy of the heart. This in combination with the aorto-caval compression leads rapidly to hypotension, bradycardia and low cardiac output. Arterial hypotension is a dangerous complication for both the parturient and the fetus. The hypotension manifests with clinical signs on the parturients side as nausea, vomiting and yawning. The long-lasting profound hypotension causes fetal acidosis and neonatal depression.

In clinical practice, the hypotension is treated promptly with vasopressors such as ephedrine and phenylephrine in boluses or as infusion. Ephedrine, most frequently used, is a directly acting beta-1 and indirectly acting alpha-1 adrenergic agonist. One part of its vasoconstricting capacity is as a result of elevated production of angiotensin-2. Ephedrine is administered in boluses of 3-5 mg while phenylephrine is given as 0.05-0.1 mg blouses. Monitoring of the patient under anesthesia and surgery cannot be over-emphasized. During the intraoperative period, pain or discomfort could arise. In such cases, a mixture of 50% oxygen in nitrous oxide could be administered along with intravenous opioid like low doses of fentanyl.

Following the delivery of the baby, 5-10 units of oxytocin are normally administered to aid myometrial contraction. Routine postoperative procedures are carried out at the end of the anesthesia and surgery.

4.4 Epidural anesthesia

This is a form of regional analgesia involving injection of drugs through a catheter placed into the epidural space. The injection can cause both a loss of sensation (anesthesia) and a loss of pain (analgesia), by blocking the transmission of signals through nerves in or near the spinal cord.

Epidural anesthesia is a form of neuraxial block technique for Cesarean section. Its use in humans was first described in 1921 (Pages, 1921). Later, the Tuohy needle which is still most commonly used for epidural anesthesia was introduced (Tuohy, 1937). Improvements in equipment, drugs and technique have made it a popular and versatile anesthetic technique, with applications in obstetrics and pain control. Both single injection and catheter techniques can be used. Its versatility means it can be used as an anesthetic, as an analgesic adjuvant to general anesthesia, and for postoperative analgesia following Cesarean section.

Epidural anesthesia can be used as the sole anesthetic for labor and Cesarean section. The advantage of epidural over spinal anesthesia is the ability to maintain continuous anesthesia after placement of an epidural catheter, thus making it suitable for procedures of long duration such as labor and delivery. This feature also enables the use of this technique into the postoperative period for analgesia, using lower concentrations of local anesthetic drugs or in combination with different agents.

The disadvantages of epidural anesthesia are that the onset of the block takes a longer time than spinal anesthesia and the spread of block could be uneven, often resulting to poor anesthesia of the sacral roots. Cardiovascular stability is one of its advantages implying that this technique could be tolerated by parturients with cardiac diseases. Following the insertion of the epidural catheter, the duration of anesthesia/analgesia can be prolonged from repeated top-ups with local anesthetic agents or a combination of such agents and opioids.

4.4.1 Technique of epidural anesthesia

The standard procedure for the administration of epidural anesthesia is essentially the same for subarachnoid block. Asepsis must be maintained throughout the procedure.

Following the cleaning draping of the parturients' back, a subcutaneous wheal at the midpoint (at the planned puncture site) between two adjacent vertebrae is raised using a local anesthetic. This area is infiltrated deeper in the midline and paraspinously to anesthetize the posterior structures. A puncture at the site is done using a 19G needle. The epidural needle is inserted in to the skin at this point, and advanced through the supraspinous ligament, with the needle pointing in a slightly cephalad direction. It is then advanced into the interspinous ligament until distinct sensation of increased resistance is felt as the needle passes into the ligamentum flavum.

The end point of the procedure is the loss of resistance to either air or fluid (saline or local anesthetic). Other methods of identifying the epidural space include the use of Epidural balloon (Fyneface-Ogan & Mato, 2008), Episure syringe (Riley & Carvalho, 2007) and the Bi-digital pressure method (Carden & Ori, 2006). Occasionally, false loss of resistance may cause some difficulty with placing an epidural. Once the needle enters the ligamentum flavum, there is usually a distinctive sensation of increased resistance, as this is a dense ligament with a leathery consistency.

The agents and doses used for epidural anesthesia for Cesarean section include

- Bupivacaine 0.5% 15-20 ml with 1 in 200, 000 epinephrine
- Lidocaine 2% 15-20 ml with 1 in 200, 000 epinephrine
- Fentanyl 50 microgram or diamorphine 2.5 mg may be added to the local anesthetic to improve the quality of anesthesia.

4.5 Combined spinal epidural anesthesia

The combined spinal-epidural (CSE) technique has gained increasing popularity for patients undergoing major surgery below the umbilical level who require prolonged and effective postoperative analgesia. Although the CSE technique has become increasingly popular over the past two decades, it is a more complex technique that requires comprehensive understanding of epidural and spinal physiology and pharmacology. It combines the rapidity, density, and reliability of a subarachnoid anesthetic with the flexibility of continuous epidural anesthesia to extend the duration of analgesia (Rawal et al, 2000). The technique is particularly popular in obstetric anesthesia and analgesia. A modification of the conventional CSE is the sequential CSE technique, in which spinal anesthesia is induced with a small-dose intrathecal local anesthetic and opioids to produce a limited anesthetic that can be extended with epidural top-ups of local anesthetic or saline. This epidural volume extension (EVE) may be due to several mechanisms including the 'volume effect' in which the dura is compressed by epidural saline, resulting in 'squeezing' of cerebrospinal fluid and more extensive spread of subarachnoidal local anesthetic (Lew et al, 2004). The volume effect appears to be time-dependent; beyond 30 min or after two-segment regression has begun, any epidural top-up of saline would have no effect on block extension and may even accelerate regression of the spinal anesthetic.

There are four main varieties of combined spinal epidural anesthesia. These are:

- Single Needle - Single Interspace method
- Double Needle - Double Interspace method
- Double Needle - Single Interspace method
- Needle Beside Needle - single interspace method

The detailed description of these techniques is beyond the scope of this chapter. It is important to note that the "needle through needle" technique is the most popular variety of CSE techniques (Cousins MJ, 1988). This results in high success rates and obviates a separate second needle placement in the majority of cases, minimizing patient discomfort. It is also simple and quick, requiring approximately 30 seconds longer than the time needed for routine lumbar epidural catheter placement. Technical performance of this technique is improved when properly matched epidural and spinal needles are used. The reason for its popularity is the ability of extra-dural needle to guide the fine spinal needle to the dura mater. In addition, patients prefer a single skin puncture (Lyons et al, 1992).

In the CSE technique, the subarachnoid block is performed using the same dose of local anesthetic described for spinal anesthesia. The epidural catheter is placed to allow top-ups of local anesthetics during prolonged surgery or for the administration of analgesic in the postoperative period.

Combined spinal epidural anesthesia especially in elective Cesarean section, which affords time to perfect the analgesia with the epidural if necessary, provide exceptional standards of analgesia. There is no standard CSE or epidural technique. Compared with epidural, CSE provides faster onset of effective pain relief from time of injection, and increases incidence of maternal satisfaction (Hughes et al, 2003). Combined spinal epidural anesthesia appears to be safe as an anesthetic technique for severe pre-eclampsia/eclampsia (Vande Velde, 2004).

4.6 Local infiltrative anesthesia

Local infiltrative anesthesia is not a common technique of anesthesia for Cesarean section. This form of anesthesia is often practiced in poor resource settings. It is frequently carried out by the surgeon. The use of local infiltrative anesthesia has been used in very poor clinical state such as eclampsia (Fyneface-Ogan & Uzoigwe, 2008). It is safe and is beneficial for the mother and child in the following ways:

- Can be a life saving procedure
- Recovering time is less
- None or very little side effects
- Economical (for both mother & Government)
- Post operative care is relatively easy
- Fetus will be in a good condition
- Makes surgical intervention easily available, accessible and affordable.

A hand on experience is essential. It is contraindicated in the following:

- Two previous Cesarean sections
- Associated adnexial pathology
- Obese patient
- Placenta previa
- Apprehensive cases

5. General anesthesia for cesarean section

The use of general anesthesia for Cesarean section is declining world-wide. Although there are few, if any, absolute contraindications to general anesthesia, regional anesthesia appears to be the preferred method in order to avoid the risk of airway challenges. As early bonding immediately after delivery is being encouraged, increasingly parturients are choosing to remain awake to witness the birth of their babies. General anesthesia requires the production of unconsciousness, provision of adequate analgesia and muscle relaxation. The administration of this form of anesthesia offers some advantages such as uterine relaxation for extracting difficult breech presentation, removing retained placentas and conduct utero-fetal surgeries. Other advantages of this form of anesthesia include rapid induction, less hypotension (appropriate in settings of acute maternal hypovolemic state), better cardiovascular stability, better control of the parturient's airway, and found to be useful in patients with coagulopathies, pre-existing neurologic or lumbar disc disease or infections.

A detailed preoperative evaluation cannot be over-emphasized if general anesthesia will be used for Cesarean section. The leading causes of maternal mortality such as failed tracheal intubation, failed ventilation and oxygenation, and/or pulmonary aspiration of gastric contents are linked to poor airway management (Ross BK, 2003). Therefore anticipation of a difficult tracheal intubation may reduce the incidence of failed intubations. A thorough examination of the neck, mandible, dentition, and oropharynx often helps predict which patients may have such problems. Difficult airway predictors found to be useful include Mallampati classification, short neck, receding mandible, and prominent maxillary incisors. It has been shown that higher incidence of failed intubation is more amongst parturients than the non-pregnant women. This is frequently attributed to airway edema, full dentition, and large breasts can obstruct the handle of the laryngoscope in pregnant women with short neck.

5.1 Failed intubation drill

Airway evaluation is not perfect and problems may arise even if the patient is evaluated as not presenting airway difficulties. Failed intubation occurs more in the pregnant population (*vide supra*). If it occurs, management is geared towards maintaining oxygenation and preventing aspiration of gastric contents. The failed intubation drill is a guideline that represents the default strategy for tracheal intubation when this is not predicted to be difficult. This strategy must cope with the unexpected difficult direct laryngoscopy. It is widely practiced for Cesarean section under general anesthesia.

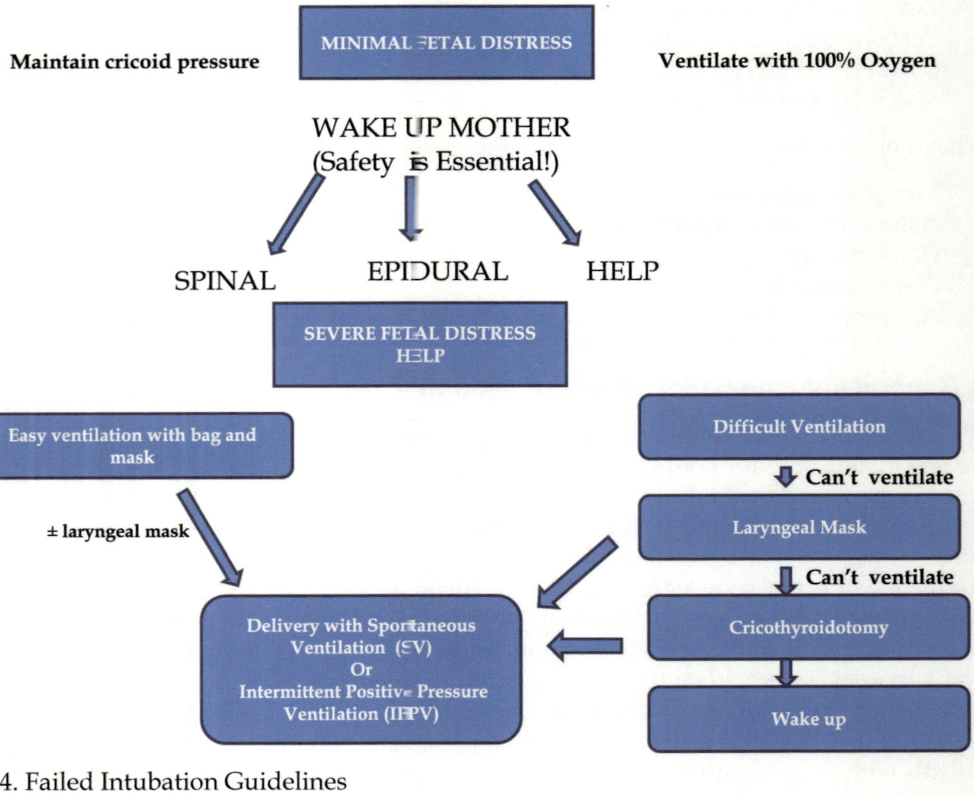

Fig. 4. Failed Intubation Guidelines

Early recognition of failure is of vital importance and assistance sought immediately while maintaining the cricoids pressure. During the failed intubation drill, the left lateral uterine displacement should be ensured. Oxygenation of the patient should continue through the face mask using 100% oxygen by an assistant squeezing the reservoir bag if both hands are needed to stabilize the mask. If the Cesarean section is an elective, the patient is allowed to wake up and alternative technique planned. Such intended general anesthesia can be converted into regional technique. In emergency, the surgery may continue with mask ventilation and application of cricoids pressure throughout the duration. In this situation, the patient's stomach must be emptied using a wide bore tube while maintaining a left lateral displacement of the uterus. The surgical field can also be infiltrated with local anesthetic to reduce the need for volatile anesthetic. However, should ventilation by face mask, laryngeal mask airway or any other device fails, cricothyrotomy is performed immediately and the patient made to wake up. The use of fibreoptic bronchoscope is gaining attention following failed tracheal intubation in the airway management of obese pregnant women undergoing Cesarean section (Dhonneur et al, 2007). However, this has not been extensively studied in the pregnant population.

5.2 Anesthetic management

Following proper preoperative assessment, the conduction of general anesthesia for Cesarean section commences with administration of non-particulate antacid within an hour of induction. An intravenous ranitidine 150 mg or 30 ml 0.3M sodium citrate is administered. A wide-bore intravenous canula (preferably, size 16 G or 18 G) is placed for intravenous fluid administration. The patient is placed supine with a wedge under the right hip for left uterine displacement. Preoxygenation is commenced with 100% oxygen for about 5 minutes while monitors are applied. The parturient is prepared and draped for surgery. Before the commencement of surgery, a rapid sequence induction with cricoid pressure applied and maintained (by an assistant until position of the tracheal tube is verified and cuff inflated) using thiopental 4-6 mg/kg (propofol 2 mg/kg) or ketamine 1.5 mg/kg (if patient is asthmatic) and suxamethonium 1.5 mg/kg. Surgery commences after tube placement is confirmed by capnography. Fifty percent nitrous oxide in oxygen with low dose halothane (0.5%) or 1% sevoflurane or 0.75% isoflurane or 3% desflurane is used for maintenance. These low doses of the halogenated agents do not produce excessive uterine relaxation but play a significant role in ensuring amnesia during anesthesia and surgery. Intermediate acting muscle relaxant such as atracurium, mivacurium, rocuronium or cis-atracurium is required to maintain muscle relaxation.

Excessive ventilation during anesthesia should be avoided. Maternal hyperventilation (arterial carbon dioxide pressure < 20 mm Hg) during general anesthesia may be harmful to the unborn fetus. Uterine blood flow is reduced during the institution of positive-pressure ventilation, and hyperventilation causes a leftward shift in the maternal oxygen-hemoglobin dissociation curve and decreases oxygen availability to the fetus (Levinson et al, 1974). Hypocarbia may also cause decreased umbilical blood flow from vasoconstriction (Motoyama et al, 1966).

Following the delivery of the baby and the placenta, 20 units of oxytocin is added into each litre of intravenous fluid and titrated slowly. Oxytocin should be used with caution as it has been associated with severe hypotension and tachycardia (Hendricks & Brenner, 1970).

Although the exact mechanism is unknown, the preservative, chlorobutanol, has been suggested as the cause of these hemodynamic changes (Rosaeg & Cicutti, 1998). The nitrous concentration may then be increased to 70% and an opioid may also be given to augment the analgesic effect of the nitrous and also to ensure amnesia. Methylergonovine 0.2 mg may be administered intramuscularly should the uterus fail to contract. Poor uterine contraction may lead more blood loss during surgery. Prior to the end of the surgery the gastric content is aspirated via oro-gastric tube to reduce the tendency for pulmonary aspiration during emergence from anesthesia.

5.3 Reversal and recovery

At the end of the surgery, the effect of the muscle relaxant is reversed and the oro-gastric tube removed. The hypopharynx is suctioned dry and trachea is extubated when patient is fully awake to prevent the risk of regurgitation and aspiration (Asai et al, 1998).

6. Anesthesia for emergency cesarean section

Emergency Cesarean section is done to avert potential loss of life of the mother, newborn or both. Good multidisciplinary communication is pivotal in the management of an emergency Cesarean section for good feto-maternal outcome. A four-point classification (see Table 1a below) of urgency of Cesarean section, similar to that used by the National Confidential Enquiry into Perioperative Deaths, has been validated and accepted by anesthetists and obstetricians based on theoretical and actual scenarios (Lucas et al, 2000). Categories 1 and 2 are considered as emergency Cesarean section is while Category 3 case (e.g. a woman who has booked for an elective Cesarean section but goes into labor ahead of her scheduled operation date) is no longer elective, but neither is this a true 'emergency' scenario.

Grade	Definition (at time of decision to operate)
Category 1	Immediate threat to life of woman or fetus
Category 2	Maternal or fetal compromise, not immediately life-threatening
Category 3	Needing early delivery but no maternal or fetal compromise
Category 4	At a time to suit the woman and maternity team

(Lucas et al, 2000)

Table 1a. Categorization of urgency of Cesarean Section

Anesthesia for emergency Cesarean section can pose many challenges to the attending anesthetist. One of the greatest challenges for an unprepared attending is to be compelled to administer general anesthesia under less than ideal conditions to an unfasted parturient. This predicament can often be avoided if anesthetist is informed earlier about the existence of such 'high-risk' cases before the rapid deterioration of the maternal–fetal clinical state and the decision for Cesarean section is finally made. This would serve to enhance the preparedness of the attending and operating theatre staff in the eventuality of Cesarean section.

Most often, emergency Cesarean section is carried out on account of a deteriorating fetal or maternal clinical state. Table 1b, shows some feto-maternal indications that require or may require emergency Cesarean section.

Fetal scalp pH <7.20
Category III fetal heart rate tracings (Macones et al, 2008)
Cord prolapsed
Uterine rupture
Cepahlo-pelvic disproportion diagnosed during labor
Pre-eclampsia/eclampsia
Antepartum hemorrhage
Failure of labour to progress

Table 1b. Feto-Maternal Indications

Being a complex multidisciplinary procedure, it has been recommended that Caesarean section should be ready to be performed within 30 minutes of decision-to-operate is made. It has been suggested that most of the emergency Cesarean sections can be performed under regional anesthesia (Royal College of Anaesthetists, 2006). For the parturient with epidural catheter in labor, the anesthetic technique of choice will be to top-up the epidural. If this is contra-indicated, a single shot spinal anesthesia will be appropriate for most of the women laboring without labor epidural catheter. Whether the top-up should be administered in delivery room or theatre is controversial (Moore & Russell, 2004) Topping-up in the delivery room might gain time, but maternal monitoring is suboptimal when the risk of high block or systemic local anesthetic toxicity is greatest. Waiting until arrival in theatre before starting to top-up can invoke obstetrician impatience and a call for general anesthesia. A compromise is to administer a small initial dose in the delivery room (e.g. 10 ml plain bupivacaine 0.5%) and further 5-ml increments as required in theatre.

Single-shot spinal anesthesia can be administered to laboring women without epidural catheter. However, active bleeding, cardiac disease, uncorrected coagulopathy and a high suspicion of bacteremia are contraindications to single-shot spinal anesthesia. Most often hyperbaric bupivacaine 0.5%, 2 ml is appropriate for most women; the addition of fentanyl 20 μg enhances blockade of visceral pain. Preload (administration of fluid before spinal anesthesia) has been superseded by 'co-load' – a fluid bolus coinciding with the sympathetic blockade. Timing of the administration of vasopressors is important in the event of hypotension. Phenylephrine or ephedrine should be available for possible use. Reflex bradycardia (heart rate 45– 50 beat/min) is to be expected after an alpha-adrenergic agonist, and an anticholinergic agent (atropine) should be immediately available, although administration is rarely necessary.

The rapid sequence induction (using thiopental, succinylcholine, cricoid pressure, tracheal intubation) appears to be the safest approach to general anesthesia for emergency Cesarean section (Levy, 2006). The use of muscle relaxant and end-tidal vapor concentrations >0.75% in nitrous have been recommended. There is no justification for administration of low inspired vapor concentrations that risk awareness. In the event of severe hypovolemia, anesthesia can be induced and maintained with intravenous ketamine (1.5 mg/kg), which has a useful sympathomimetic effect.

In all the options of anesthesia for emergency Cesarean section, the need for adequate monitoring of the parturients, both intraoperative and postoperative analgesia and maintenance of proper fluid therapy cannot be over-emphasized. Fluid input and output must be charted meticulously. No study has shown that crystalloid or colloid is superior. Crystalloid infusion may reduce plasma colloid oncotic pressure, but the longer half-life of colloid infusions may contribute to circulatory overload during the period of postpartum mobilization of the increased extracellular fluid volume of pregnancy. In the event of a continued synthetic oxytocin after surgery, administration should be in small doses either by syringe pump or gravimetric method via an intravenous infusion. Blood transfusion should be carried out with caution. Administration of blood and blood products seems to be a risk factor for the development of pulmonary edema (Tuffnell et al, 2005).

The general approach to pain after Cesarean section is changing, shifting away from traditional opioid-based therapy toward a "multimodal" or "balanced" approach. Multimodal pain therapy involves the use of a potent opioid regimen, such as patient-controlled analgesia or neuraxial opioids, in combination with other classes of analgesic drugs. Theoretically, the use of analgesic drugs in combination allows for additive or even synergistic effects in reducing pain while decreasing the side effects produced by each class of drug because smaller drug doses are required. Typical analgesic regimens include opioids; non-opioid analgesics, such as acetaminophen; and non-steroidal anti-inflammatory drugs, with the variable addition of local anesthetic techniques. Despite current advances in postoperative pain therapy, pain relief may still be inadequate for a substantial number of women. This may be particularly true as they make the transition from relative dependency on potent opioid regimens to full dependency on oral analgesics on the second postoperative day (Angle & Walsh, 2001).

7. Conclusion

Anesthesia for Cesarean section continues to be one of the most commonly performed world-wide. Regional anesthesia has become the preferred technique for Cesarean delivery. Compared to general anesthesia, regional anesthesia is associated with reduced maternal mortality, the need for fewer drugs, and more direct experience of childbirth, faster neonatal-maternal bonding, decreased blood loss and excellent postoperative pain control through the use of neuraxial opioid. However, it is important to prevent aorto-caval compression and promptly treat hypotension during regional anesthesia for Cesarean section. The advantages of general over regional anesthesia are well known to include a more rapid induction, less hypotension, less maternal anxiety and its application in situations where there is a contraindication to regional anesthesia. Although literatures available indicate that both techniques are safe. Loss of airway control has been associated with severe morbidity and mortality during general anesthesia. The need for proper preoperative evaluation and airway assessment, the availability of an assistant, a backup plan for failed tracheal intubation, quick airway access and adequate oxygenation during general anesthesia for Cesarean section cannot be overemphasized.

8. Acknowledgement

I wish to thank Gloria Sotonye-Ogan for typing and patiently proof-reading this manuscript.

9. References

Aisien AO, Lawson JO & Adebayo AA. (2002). A five year appraisal of caesarean section in a northern Nigerian University Teaching Hospital. *Niger Postgrad Med J*, Vol. 9, pp. (146-150)

American Society of Anesthesiologists Task Force on Preoperative Fasting. (1999). Practice guidelines for preoperative fasting and the use of pharmacologic agents to reduce the risk of pulmonary aspiration: application to healthy patients undergoing elective procedures: a report by the American Society of Anesthesiologist Task Force on Preoperative Fasting. *Anesthesiology*, Vol. 90, pp. (896-905)

Angle P & Walsh V. (2001). Pain relief after Cesarean section. *Tech Reg Anesth Pain Mgt*, 5, 36-40

Association of Anaesthetists of Great Britain and Ireland. (2001) Pre-operative assessment: the role of the anaesthetist. *AAGBI*, London (see: www.aagbi.org/pdf/pre-operative_ass.pdf)

Asai T, Koga K, & Vaughan RS. (1998). Respiratory complications associated with tracheal intubation and extubation. *Br J Anaesthesia*, Vol. 80, pp. (767-775)

Bloom SL, Spong CY, Weiner SJ, Landon MB, Rouse DJ, Varner MW, Moawad AH, Caritis SN, Harper M, Wapner RJ, Sorokin Y, Miodovnik M, O'Sullivan MJ, Sibai B, Langer O & Gabbe SG. (2005). Complications of anesthesia for cesarean delivery. Obstet Gynecol, Vol. 106, pp. (281-287)

Brady M, Kinn S & Stuart P . (2003) Preoperative fasting for adults to prevent perioperative complications. *Cochrane Database Syst Rev*, (4), CD004423

Brizgys RV, Dailey PA, Schnider SM, Kotelko DM & Levinson G. (1987). The incidence and neonatal effects of maternal hypotension during epidural anesthesia for cesarean section. *Anesthesiology*, Vol. 67, pp. (782-786)

Carden E & Ori A. (2006).The BiP Test: a modified loss of resistance technique for confirming epidural needle placement. *Pain Physician*, Vol. 9, pp. (323-325)

Chung CJ, Yun SH, Hwang GB, Park JS & Chin YJ. (2002). Intrathecal fentanyl added to hyperbaric ropivacaine for cesarean delivery. *Reg Anesth Pain Med*, Vol. 6, pp. (600-603)

Clark RB, Thompson DS & Thompson CH. (1976). Prevention of spinal hypotension associated with Cesarean section. *Anesthesiology*, Vol. 45, pp. (670-674)

Cooper GM, Lewis G & Neilson J. (2002). Confidential enquiries into maternal deaths, 1997-1999. (Editorial). *Br J Anaesth*, Vol. 89, pp. (369-372)

Corke BC, Datta S, Ostheimer GW, Weiss JB & Alper MH. (1982). Spinal anaesthesia for ceasarean section. The influence of hypotension on neonatal outcome. *Anaesthesia*, Vol. 37, pp. (658-662)

Cousins MJ. (1988). The spinal route of analgesia. Acta Anaesthesiol Beig, Vol. 39, pp. (71-82)

Cyna AM & Dodd J. (2007). Clinical update: obstetric anesthesia. Lancet, Vol. 370, pp. (640-642)

Declercq E, Young R, Cabral H & Ecker J. (2011). Is a rising cesarean delivery rate inevitable? Trends in industrialized countries, 1987 to 2007. *Birth*, Vol. 38, pp. (99-104)

Department of Health. (2001). Reference guide to consent for examination or treatment. *DH, London* (see: www.dh.gov.uk/assetRoot/04/01/90/79/04019079.pdf)

Dhonneur G, Ndoko S, Amathieu R, el Housseini L, Poncelet C & Tual L. (2007). Tracheal intubation using the Airtraqs in morbid obese patients undergoing emergency cesarean delivery. *Anesthesiology*, Vol. 106, pp. (629–630)

Dyer RA, Farina Z, Joubert IA, Du Toit P, Meyer M, Torr G, Wells K & James MFM. (2004). Crystalloid preload versus rapid crystalloid administration after induction of spinal anesthesia (co-load) for elective cesarean section. *Anaesth Intensive Care,* Vol. 32, pp. (351-357)

Engelhardt T & Webster NR. (1999). Pulmonary aspiration of gastric contents in anaesthesia. *Br J Anaesth,* Vol. 83, pp. (453-460)

Escolano F, Sierra P, Ortiz JC, Cabrera JC & Castaño J. (1996). The efficacy and optimum time of administration of ranitidine in the prevention of the acid aspiration syndrome. *Anaesthesia,* Vol. 51, pp. (182-184)

Eyler SW, Cullen BF, Murphy ME & Welch WD. (1982). Antacid aspiration in rabbits: a comparison of Mylanta and Bicitra. *Anesth Analg,* Vol. 61, pp. (288-292)

Famewo CE . (1983). Difficult intubation due to a patient's hair style. *Anaesthesia* Vol. 38, pp. (165-166)

Friedman BA, Oberman HA, Chadwick AR & Kingon KI. (1976).The maximum surgical blood order schedule and surgical blood use in the United States. *Transfusion,* Vol. 16, pp. (380-387)

Frosch DL & Kaplan RM. (1999). Shared decision making in clinical medicine: past research and future directions. *Am J Preventive Med,* Vol. 17, pp. (285-294)

Fyneface-Ogan, Mato CN & Odagme MT. (2005). Anaesthesia for Caesarean section: a ten year review. *World Anaesth,* Vol. 8, pp. (18-21)

Fyneface-Ogan S, Mato CN & Ogunbiyi OA. (2009). Comparison of maternal satisfaction following epidural and general anaesthesia for repeat caesarean section. *East Afr Med J,* Vol. 86, pp. (557-563)

Fyneface-Ogan S & Mato CN. (2008). A clinical experience with epidural balloon in the localisation of the epidural space in labouring parturients. *Nig Q J Hosp Med,* Vol. 18, pp. (166-169)

Fyneface-Ogan S & Uzoigwe SA. (2008)Caesarean section outcome in eclamptic patients: a comparison of infiltration and general anaesthesia. *West Afr J Med,* Vol. 27, pp. (250-254)

García-Miguel F J, Serrano-Aguilar P & López-Bastida J. (2003). Preoperative assessment. *Lancet,* Vol. 362, pp. (1749–1757)

Gibbs CP, Spohr L & Schmidt D. (1982). The effectiveness of sodium citrate as an antacid. *Anesthesiology,* Vol. 57, pp. (44-46)

Gogarten W & Van Aken H. (2005). Regional anaesthesie in der Geburtshilfeneue Entwiklungen. *Zentralbl Gynakol,* Vol. 127, pp. (361-367)

Gordon A, McKechnie EJ & Jeffery H. (2005). Pediatric presence at cesarean section: justified or not? *Am J Obst Gynecol,* Vol. 193, pp. (599-605)

Hamber EA & Viscomi CM. (1999). Intrathecal lipophilic opioids as adjuncts to surgical spinal anesthesia. *Reg Anesth Pain Med,* Vol. 24, pp. (255-263)

Hart JR & Whitacre RG. (1951). Pencil point needle in the prevention of post spinal headache. *JAMA,* Vol. 147, pp. (657-658)

Hawkins J, Koonin LM, Palmer SK & Gibbs CP. (1997). Anaesthesia related deaths during obstetric delivery in the United States 1979-1990. *Anesthesiology,* Vol. 86, pp. (277-284)

Hendricks CH & Brenner WE. (1970). Cardiovascular effects of oxytocic drugs used post partum. *Am J Obstet Gynecol,* Vol. 108, pp. (751-60)

Howard BK, Goodson JH & Mengert WF. (1953). Supine hypotensive syndrome in late pregnancy. *Obstet Gynecol,* Vol. 1, pp. (371-377).

Hughes D, Simmons SW, Brown J & Cyna AM. (2003). Combined spinal epidural versus epidural analgesia in labor. *Cochranes Database Syst Rev;* Vol. 4: CD.003401.

Hunt CO, Naulty JS, Bader AM, Hauch MA, Vartikar JV, Datta S, Hertwig LM & Ostheimer GW. (1989). Perioperative analgesia with subarachnoid fentanyl-bupivacaine for cesarean delivery. *Anesthesiology* ,Vol. 71, pp. (535-540)

Jackson R, Reid JA & Thorburn J. (1995). Volume preloading is not essential to prevent spinal induced hypotension at caesarean section. *Br J Anaesth,* Vol. 75, pp. (262-265)

Johanson WG jr, & Harris GD. (1980). Aspiration pneumonia, anaerobic infections and lung abscess. *Med Clin North Am, Vol.*64, pp. (385-394)

Kamenik M, & Paver-Erzen V. (2001). The effects of lactated ringer's solution infusion on cardiac output changes after spinal anesthesia. *Anesth Analg,* Vol. 92, pp. (710-714)

Kelly MC, Fitzpatrick KTJ & Hill DA. (1996). Respiratory effects of spinal anesthesia for Caesarean section. *Anaesthesia,* Vol. 51, pp. (1120–1122)

Khaw KS, Wang CC, Ngan Kee WD, Pang CP & Rogers MS. (2002). Effects of high inspired oxygen fraction during elective Caesarean section under spinal anesthesia on maternal and fetal oxygenation and lipid peroxidation. *Br J Anaesth,* Vol. 88, pp. (18–23)

Kinsella SM, Whitwam JG, & Spencer JAD. (1990). Aortic compression by the uterus: Identification with the Finapress digital artery pressure instrument. *Br J Obstet Gynaecol,* Vol. 97, pp. (700-705)

Knight PR, Druskovich G, Tait AR & Johnson KJ. (1992). The role of neutrophils, oxidants and proteases in the pathogenesis of acid pulmonary injury. *Anesthesiology,* Vol. 77, pp. (772-778)

Langeron O, Masso E, Huraux C, Guggiar, M, Bianchi A, Coriat P & Riou B. (2000). Prediction of Difficult Mask Ventilation. *Anesthesiology,* Vol. 92, pp. (1229–1136)

Leigh JM, Walker J & Janaganathan P. (1977). Effect of preoperative anaesthetic visit on anxiety. *Br Med J,* Vol. 2, pp. (987- 989)

Levinson G, Shnider SM, deLorimier AA & Steffenson JL. (1974). Effects of maternal hyperventilation on uterine blood flow and fetal oxygenation and acid-base status. *Anesthesiology,* Vol. 40, pp. (340-347)

Levy DM. (2006). Traditional rapid sequence induction is an outmoded technique for caesarean section and should be modified. Proposed. *Int J Obstet Anaesth,*Vol. 15: pp. (227-229)

Lew E, Yeo SW & Thomas E. (2004). Combined spinal–epidural anesthesia using epidural volume extension leads to faster motor recovery after elective cesarean delivery: A prospective, randomized, double-blind study. *Anesth Analg,* Vol. 98, pp. 810–814.

Lewis G. (2007). The Confidential Enquiry into Maternal and Child Health (CEMACH). Saving Mothers' Lives: reviewing maternal deaths to make motherhood safer –

2003-2005. The Seventh Report on Confidential Enquiries into Maternal Deaths in the United Kingdom, CEMACH, London.

Lim SK & Elegbe EO (1992). Ranitidine and sodium citrate as prophylaxis against acid aspiration syndrome in obstetric patients undergoing caesarean section. *Singapore Med J,* Vol. 33, pp. (608-610)

Lin CJ, Huang CL, Hsu HW & Chen TL. (1996). Prophylaxis against acid aspiration in regional anesthesia for elective cesarean section: a comparison between oral single-dose ranitidine, famotidine and omeprazole assessed with fiberoptic gastric aspiration. *Acta Anaesthesiol Sin,* Vol. 34, pp. (179-184)

Lucas DN, Yentis SM, Kinsella SM, Holdcroft A, May AE, Wee M & Robinson PN. (2000). Urgency of caesarean section: a new classification. *J R Soc Med*, Vol. 93, pp. (346–350)

Lyons G, Macdonald R & Miki B. (1992). Combined epidural/spinal anesthesia for Cesarean section. Through the needle or in separate spaces? *Anaesthesia,* Vol. 47, pp. (199-201)

Macones GA, Hankins GD, Spong CY, Hauth J, & Moore T. (2008). The 2008 National Institute of Child Health and Human Development workshop report on electronic fetal monitoring: update on definitions, interpretation, and research guidelines. *Obstet Gynecol,* Vol. 112, pp. (661-666)

Mallampati SR, Gatt SP, Gugino LD, Desai SP, Waraksa B, Freiberger D & Liu PL. (1985). A clinical sign to predict difficult tracheal intubation: A prospective study. *Can Anaesth Soc J*, Vol. 32, pp. (429-434)

McClure J & Cooper G. (2005). Fifty years of confidential enquiries into maternal deaths in the United Kingdom: should anaesthesia celebrate or not? (editorial). *Int J Obstet Anesth,* Vol. 14, pp. (87-89)

Mendelson CL. (1946). Aspiration of stomach contents into the lungs during obstetric anesthesia. *Am J Obstet Gynecol,* Vol. 52, pp. (191-205)

Milner AR, Bogod DG & Harwood RJ. (1996). Intrathecal administration of morphine for elective Caesarean section. A comparison between 0.1 mg and 0.2 mg. *Anaesthesia,* Vol. 51, pp. (871-873)

Moore P & Russell IF. (2004). Epidural top-ups for category I / II emergency caesarean section should be given only in the operating theatre. *Int J Obstet Anesth,* Vol. 13, pp. (257–265)

Motoyama EK, Rivard G, Acheson F & Cook CD. (1966). Adverse effect of maternal hyperventilation on the foetus. *Lancet* Vol. 1, pp. (286-288)

Murphy DF, Nally B, Gardiner J & Unwin A. (1984). Effect of metoclopramide on gastric emptying before elective and emergency caesarean section. *Br J Anaesth,* Vol. 56, pp. (1113-1116)

Nimmo WS, Wilson J & Prescott LF. (1975). Narcotic analgesics and delayed gastric emptying during labour. *Lancet,* Vol. 1, pp. (890-893)

Ogunbiyi OA, Mato CN & Isong EC. (2003). Oxygen saturation after spinal anesthesia. Any need for supplemental oxygen? *Afr J Anaesth Int Care,* Vol. 4, pp. (5 – 6.).

Page´s F. (1991). Metameric anesthesia. 1921. *Rev Esp Anestesiol Reanim,* Vol. 3, pp. (318–326)

Palmer T, Wahr JA, Reilly MO & Greenfield MLVH. (2003). Reducing unnecessary cross matching: A patient-specific blood ordering system is more accurate in predicting who will receive a blood transfusion than the maximum blood ordering system. *Anaesth Analg,* Vol. 96, pp. (369-375)

Paranjothy S, Griffiths JD, Broughton HK, Gyte GM, Brown HC & Thomas J. (2011). Interventions at caesarean section for reducing aspiration pneumonitis. *Int J Obstet Anesth,* Vol. 20, pp. 142-148

Porter JS, Bonello E & Reynolds F. (1997). The influence of epidural administration of fentanyl infusion on gastric emptying in labour. *Anaesthesia,* Vol. 52, pp. (1151-1156)

Rahman K & Jenkins JG. (2005). Failed tracheal intubation in obstetrics: no more frequent but still managed badly. Anaesthesia, Vol. 60, pp. (168-171)

Rawal N, Holmstrom B, Crowhurst JA & Van Zundert A. (2000). The combined spinal epidural technique. *Anesthesiol Clin North America,* Vol. 18, pp. (267–295)

Riley ET, Carvalho B. (2007). The Episure syringe: a novel loss of resistance syringe for locating the epidural space. Anesth Analg, Vol. 105, pp. (1164-1166)

Roberts RB & Shirley MA. (1974). Reducing the risk of acid aspiration during cesarean section. *Anesth Analg,* Vol. 53, pp. (859-868)

Rocke DA, Murray WB, Rout CC & Gowus E. (1992). Relative risk analysis of factors associated with difficult intubation in obstetric anesthesia. *Anesthesiology,* Vol. 77, pp. (67-73)

Rooks JP, Weatherby NL, Ernst EK, Stapleton S, Rosen D & Rosenfield A. (1989). Outcomes of care in birth centres; the national birth centre study. *N Engl J Med,* Vol. 321, pp. (1804-1811)

Rosaeg OP, Cicutti NJ, & Labow RS. (1998). The effect of oxytocin on the contractile force of human atrial trabeculae. *Anesth Analg,* Vol. 86, pp. (40-44)

Rout CC & Rocke DA. (1994). Prevention of hypotension following spinal anesthesia for Cesarean section. *Int Anesthesiol Clin,* Vol. 32, pp. (117-135)

Royal College of Anaesthetists UK. (2006). Raising the Standard: A compendium of audit recipes for the continuous quality improvement in anaesthesia. (2nd ed.) pp. 166-167: Technique of anaesthesia for Caesarean section.

Ross BK. (2003). ASA closed claims in obstetrics: lessons learned. *Anesthesiol Clin North America,* Vol. 21, pp. (183-197)

Russell IF. (1995). Levels of anesthesia and intraoperative pain at caesarean section under regional block. *Int J Obstet Anesth,* Vol. 4, pp. (71–77)

Soreide E, Bjornestad E & Steen PA. (1996). An audit of perioperative aspiration pneumonitis in gynecological and obstetric patients. *Acta Anaessthesiol Scand,* Vol. 40, pp. (14-19)

Sprotte G, Schedel R, Pajunk H & Pajunk H. (1987). An "atraumatic" universal needle for single-shot regional anesthesia: clinical results and a 6 year trial in over 30,000 regional anesthesias. *Reg Anaesth,* Vol. 10, pp. (104-10).

Stuart JC, Kan AF, Rowbottom SJ, Yau G & Gin T. (1996). Acid aspiration prophylaxis for emergency caesarean section. *Anaesthesia,* vol. 51, pp. (415-421)

Tripathi A, Somwanshi M, Singh B & Bajaj P. (1995). A comparison of intravenous ranitidine and omeprazole on gastric volume and pH in women undergoing emergency caesarean section. *Can J Anaesth,* Vol. 42, pp. (797-800)

Tuffnell DJ, Jankowicz D, Lindow SW, Lyons G, Mason GC, Russell IF & Walker JJ. (2005). Outcomes of severe pre-eclampsia/eclapmsia in Yorkshire 1999 /2003. *Br J Obstet Gynaecol,* Vol. 112, pp. (875–880)

Tuohy EB. (1937). Newer developments in anesthesia. *Minn Med,* Vol. 20, pp. (362- 368)
Turker G, Yilmazlar T, Mogol EB, Gurbet A, Dizman S & Gunay H. (2011). The effects of colloid pre-loading on thromboelastography prior to caesarean delivery: hydroxyethyl starch 130/0.4 versus succinylated gelatine. *J Int Med Res,* Vol. 39, pp. (143-149)
Vande Velde M, Berends N, Spitz B, Teukens A & Vanderneersen E. (2004). Low-dose combined spinal epidural anesthesia versus conventional epidural anesthesia for Caesarean Section in pre eclampsia: a retrospective analysis. *Eur J Anaesthesiol,* Vol. 21, pp. (454-459)
Vandenberg JT, Rudman NT, Burke TF & Ramos DE. (1998). Large-diameter suction tubing significantly improves evacuation time of simulated vomitus. Am J Emerg Med, Vol. 16, pp. (242-244)
Walsh J, Puig MM, Lovitz MA & Turndorf H. (1987). Premedication abolishes the increase in plasma beta-endorphin observed in the immediate preoperative period. *Anesthesiology,* Vol. 66, pp. (402-405)

4

Cesarean Delivery: Surgical Techniques – The Fifteen Minute Cesarean Section

Robert D. Dyson
*Gateway Women's Clinic
Portland, Oregon,
USA*

1. Introduction

There is more than one way to skin a cat.

I never liked that old saying because I am very fond of cats. Eventually, however, I learned that it referred not to felines but to catfish, which have no scales and are notoriously difficult to prepare for the frying pan. The point, of course, is that there are many ways to do a cesarean delivery and the vast majority of the time, the outcome is good. However, there can be great differences in the risk of febrile morbidity, in the risk of postoperative adhesions, and in the length of time that the patient is on the table. For example, in the very nice review of techniques published by Hofmeyr et al. (2009) mean operating times varied from 27.5 to 56.5 minutes, with the single exception being the Misgav Ladach technique (Darj & Nordstrom, 1999), where the mean was reported to be 12.5 minutes. However, this technique involves a good deal of finger dissection, which I find awkward, and uses only a single layer closure of the uterine incision, which may increase the risk of uterine rupture in future pregnancies (Bujold et al., 2010)

What I propose to do here is to summarize the technique on which I have settled after more than four thousand procedures done personally. In the absence of complications, operating time "skin to skin" is typically about fifteen minutes, including a two-layer uterine closure and a subcuticular skin closure. The shorter operating time means less tissue desiccation and with that, I believe, less postoperative pain and less risk of both febrile morbidity and postoperative adhesions. The way to shorten operating time is to move efficiently and to eliminate steps that are simply not needed. Emphasis here is on the latter.

2. Positioning the patient: Don't forget the tilt

The traditional position for a cesarean delivery is to have the woman supine but tilted to the left with a rolled towel or other wedge placed beneath the right side of the pelvis. The purpose is to shift the weight of the uterus (which is nearly always dextro-rotated) away from the compressible vena cava and onto the spine and aorta, thus preventing hypotension and the nausea and decreased fetal blood flow that might otherwise result. It is true that most women will do fine without the tilt but it is simple, logical and free and certainly sometimes useful.

Rather than leaving the woman supine, it is often useful to give her a bit of a head-down tilt (Trendelenburg). In heavier patients or with twins, it can be very useful and, if not too much, is very well tolerated. Of course, the spinal or epidural anesthesia needs to be well established first. Once that is done, a little tilt is often not noticed by the woman but may be very useful to the surgeon.

3. Do we need a retention catheter in the bladder?

No, not really, but it helps. A full bladder can make entry into the abdomen dangerous, but if the bladder is already relatively empty, a Foley catheter is not necessary. If an inadvertent cystotomy occurs, a simple purse string suture of a rapidly dissolving material (such as chromic) can be used for closure, followed by two or three days of drainage. That is all that is needed. These injuries on the dome of the bladder heal much quicker than injuries made near or through the trigone, such as might occur during a vaginal hysterectomy. If the bladder is full enough to be in the way, it can be drained with suction tubing and a number 14 needle.

An advantage of having a retention catheter is that if the extent of the bladder is not obvious, the catheter bulb can be pulled up to better define the margins. Did you ever wonder whether a stitch went into the bladder? That is the way to find out.

If general anesthesia is used for a cesarean delivery, the catheter can be removed as soon as the patient is awake. However, if epidural or spinal morphine is used for postoperative analgesia, it is best to leave the catheter for about 18 hours, as inability to void is common, putting the woman at risk of bladder over-distension. If the bladder accumulates more than about six hundred mL, the little actin and myosin fibers that form the smooth muscle of the bladder may be pulled apart and no longer able to find each other. Six to twelve hours of decompression may be needed before the bladder can function normally again.

4. Making the incision

When I first started practice, I habitually made my cesarean incision transversely and in the depths of the natural crease that usually is present a couple of finger breadths above the pubic symphysis. Then I went to a lecture where we were told to move it upward, out of the crease, to reduce the risk of infection. It took me a while to decide that the move created more problems than it solved. It meant going through a thicker layer of tissue; the incision was more visible and less cosmetically pleasing later; and the wound seemed to have a higher incidence of separation because gravity tended to pull it apart. Hence, I advocate following the natural crease. If the area is prepped adequately, allowed to dry a bit before the incision is made and then kept dry in the immediate postpartum days, wound infection and separation seem to be very rare. Women love it, as the incision tends to disappear. The only part of the surgery visible to them is the incision. No matter what happens underneath, if the incision looks good and there are no complications, patients tend to think they have had a great surgeon.

I mark the skin with a surgical marking pen before the area is draped so that I can confidently put the incision in the right spot when visibility is compromised by the drapes. I like the incision to extend about 7.5cm on either side of the midline, with the midline marked so that I can find it during closure. If the surgical incision is made boldly and rapidly with a scalpel, and carried down quickly to the fascia, there is no time for blood to obscure the working site and hence no need for cautery. I score the anterior rectus fascia with the scalpel in the midline and then quickly extend the fascial incision laterally on either side with scissors, though some people prefer to open the fascia laterally with finger dissection. If one is in a hurry, the medial fibers of the rectus muscles can be cut so that fingers can be used to expose the peritoneum more quickly. The muscles are then pulled apart laterally with no dissection of the rectus sheath. In most cases, however, I separate the rectus sheath from the muscles cephalad and caudad with scissors, staying near the midline to avoid injury to the nerves associated with the superficial branch of the inferior epigastric artery. (Cutting those nerves produces an annoying hypesthesia in a triangular area above the incision that can last for many months.)

5. The obese patient

Many tricks involving pulleys, Montgomery straps, and Elastoplast tape have been proposed to pull the pannus off the area of incision in the massively obese. I find this embarrassing to the woman and quite unnecessary. I believe in keeping things simple. First, a bit of Trendelenburg helps enormously and is well tolerated even when the woman is awake. Second, I make the incision transversely (and at least 15cm wide) in the depths of the sub-pannus crease, as described above. The subcutaneous tissue is thinnest there, which makes life easier for the surgeon and provides less room for postoperative seromas and hematomas to form and get infected. I believe that if the area is prepped adequately and then someone holds the pannus up while the area dries and gets draped, infection risk is minimal.

The third point is to use a disposable O-ring wound retractor such as the Alexis^R O made by Applied Medical Corp. It simply makes the procedure amazingly easier because it provides better visualization and the rigid external ring helps hold the pannus away from the incision.

As will be discussed later, closing the subcutaneous tissue with at least a few interrupted, rapidly dissolving sutures can reduce postoperative problems (Naumann et al., 1995) and closing the skin with a subcuticular stitch rather than staples also reduces infection and disruption according to a meta-analysis published by Tuuli et al. (2011). In these heavier women I also always seal the surface with one of the polyacrylic glues. The theory, unsupported by data as far as I know, is that germs simply cannot live in that stuff.

6. Preventing deep vein thrombosis

Prophylaxis for thromboembolism is important for all cesarean patients, but even more important for older women, for smokers, and for the obese. The least that should be done in every case is intermittent pneumatic compression devices for the first twenty four hours. In obese women, or those with other additional risk factors, consideration should be given to heparin or low molecular weight heparin (for example, 40mg of enoxaparin) subcutaneously. If general anesthesia is to be used, heparin can be given preoperatively but if a spinal or epidural is used, your anesthesia person should be consulted. They will probably want you to wait 12 to 24 hours before giving the heparin because of fear of an epidural hematoma.

7. Prophylactic antibiotics

Prophylactic antibiotics are routinely used for cesarean deliveries these days, typically cefazolin even in the penicillin allergic, given ideally 30 to 60 minutes before the incision (Sullivan et al., 2007). (The textbooks talk about a 15% cross-reaction between cefazolin and penicillin in the penicillin allergic patient but I have never seen it happen.) However, in the obese, usual doses of cefazolin may be inadequate. Pevzner et al.(2011), have demonstrated that the usual two grams of cefazolin, even when given at the ideal 30 to 60 minutes preoperatively, will often produce tissue levels in the wound that are inadequate to be bacteriocidal when the BMI is over 40. Although, as they point out, there are insufficient data to dose cefazolin specifically to BMI, it may be more appropriate to use three grams IV in the massively obese.

8. Transverse or vertical incision?

I cannot remember the last time I did a vertical skin incision except to remove and try to improve an old and ugly scar. Delivery through a low transverse incision, if entry is done as described above, should take two to three minutes or less. In an emergency, the scalpel can be used with just a few strokes to open the skin, the subcutaneous tissue, the fascia, and the rectus muscles in the midline. Lateral pull then exposes the peritoneum with the uterus immediately below. The bladder might be in the way, especially if there are adhesions from a previous surgery or if there has been a long and obstructed labor. If the peritoneum seems thicker than usual, think of bladder and move higher. Otherwise, a quick tenting of the peritoneum with forceps and a cut with the scissors provides rapid and clean entry that can be enlarged bluntly by just pulling laterally.

A vertical incision, in my hands at least, takes longer to make and much longer to close. The vertical scar often widens out and becomes unsightly, especially if there is an early next pregnancy. Incisional hernia is also a problem with vertical incisions and almost never happens with the low transverse incision. And then there is that same issue mentioned above, that women tend to rate the skill of their surgeon by how the incision looks when it heals. The low transverse incision is not only stronger and more comfortable than the vertical incision, it always looks better afterward.

9. To burn or not to burn: Electrocautery use

Several decades ago, where I was trained, we were not allowed to use electrocautery in a cesarean delivery. I cannot remember why, but I got used to doing without it and have done so ever since. I do not even place a grounding pad. (Which means I do not have to worry about setting an alcohol skin prep afire, nor is there any need to remove metal jewelry.) On rare occasions when I have a bleeding vessel that does not stop after a minute or so of being crushed with a hemostat, it can simply be tied off. When I am assisting a surgeon who is skeptical about the no-burn philosophy, I suggest that they forego cautery use until closure. By that time, all the little vessels that would have been burned on the way into the abdomen will have stopped bleeding and there is typically nothing left to burn.

I am not, of course, talking about someone with a coagulopathy such as happens with severe pre-eclampsia, von Willebrand's disease, etc. But in a normal person, vessels contract and blood clots within the vessels so rapidly that the electrocautery just destroys tissue without any benefit. Dead tissue increases inflammation and pain and increases the risk of infection. I could not find a controlled trial on the subject, but in my opinion, electrocautery use in the vast majority of cases just increases operating time, prolongs recovery, and increases postoperative pain. In the absence of good smoke evacuation, electrocautery use also puts the woman at risk of having to smell her own flesh cooking.

10. The uterine incision: Don't cut the baby!

Once in the peritoneal cavity, the lower uterine segment can be identified and entered. Development of a bladder flap before the uterine incision is made has been shown to be unnecessary (Hohlagschwandtner et al., 2001). It is simpler and faster to just transversely score the lower uterine segment at the upper edge of the bladder flap (in other words, at the upper edge of the visceral reflection of the bladder peritoneum --- however, see the warning about obstructed labors in the next section). The myometrium is scored transversely part way through the muscle and then, to avoid cutting the baby with the scalpel, I use a curved hemostat like a little shovel to go deeper until the membranes are encountered. The incision is then extended with finger tips (pulling vertically or horizontally) until adequate for delivery. Occasionally, the lower segment simply is not wide enough and a vertical incision in the uterus is chosen. However, in most cases where the incision is too small, one does not discover that until the head refuses to come through it, especially with a breech baby. At that point, the simplest and quickest way to get more room is to "T" the incision upward in the midline. The corners of the T become avascular and are at risk of not healing well, the solution to which is to cut a bit off of each corner before closing the uterus. This converts the upside down T to an upside down "V" and you will find that the incision can be closed transversely just as if no T had been made. There is a little more tension on the incision in the midline but a two-layer closure should take care of that.

It is, of course, useful to know ahead of time where the placenta is to be found. A low anterior placenta need not change the choice of incision. Just work fast to get through the placenta (mostly with blunt dissection) and expose the baby. A rarely needed trick is to deliver the placenta before the baby. A rapid manual extraction of the placenta creates a great deal of new space so the baby can usually be delivered in the next few seconds with less trauma to it and with no hypoxia. I have found this to be especially useful with very small babies.

11. Obstructed labors: That is the vagina, not the uterus

If a labor is allowed to go on long enough, nearly everyone will dilate to ten centimeters. However, it is not dilation that gets us a vaginal birth, it is descent of the baby through the pelvis. That point is often overlooked --- "she is making progress" we are told, meaning that the cervix is dilating, if ever so slowly. It is not progress, however, if the head is not descending, because if the head cannot come down, the uterus will be pulled by its own contractions up into the abdomen. When the cesarean delivery is finally done in such cases, feel around a bit. What you are apt to find is that the lower uterine segment is no longer in the pelvis but is now in the abdomen, leaving the bladder behind and no longer reflected onto the uterus. Cutting at the upper edge of the bladder flap can actually result in a vaginal incision, made below (caudad to) the cervix.

The problem with this error is that the vagina is very vascular and does not contract as does the uterus. We depend on contraction of the uterus to occlude vessels and to prevent excessive bleeding. It is very difficult to get hemostasis with a vaginal entry, even with electrocautery. And since the bladder is not where we expected to find it, injury is much more likely. So if you are doing a cesarean section for obstructed labor, check all the landmarks, including the round ligaments, to get oriented and then make the uterine incision higher than you might otherwise do.

12. Elevating the head

As we all know, elevating an impacted fetal head can be very hard. Serious injury to the baby's neck is a real risk. If that risk is anticipated, it is prudent to push the head out of the pelvis before the operation starts. However, usually the problem comes as a surprise.

The first thing that most of us try, when the head is truly impacted, is to get another person to push up through the vagina. He or she should use as many fingers as possible, or even an entire fist, to spread the forces. If that fails, the next simplest maneuver is to flex the hips by elevating the knees, one person reaching under the drapes from either side of the patient.

Sometimes, contraction of the uterus is a problem. One can get half a minute or so of uterine relaxation (a half minute that seems like hours) with sublingual nitroglycerin. If that is unavailable, 0.2mg of intravenous terbutaline can be tried. It takes a bit longer to have an effect and another twenty minutes to wear off.

An impacted head is very often the result of obstructed labor with an occiput posterior presentation. When the uterus is opened, the baby's chin or chest is the first thing seen. This makes a reverse breech extraction as described by Fong et al. (1997) straightforward. One simply pulls the feet out of the incision and then delivers the baby as one would do with a typical breech, being careful not to hyperextend the neck.

13. The transverse lie

I was taught that the uterine incision should be perpendicular to the baby. That would mean a vertical uterine incision if a transverse lie is encountered. However, a vertical incision would rule out vaginal birth in the future and put her at extra risk of uterine rupture even before the onset of her next labor. It is better, it seems to me, to convert the baby to breech or vertex after opening the abdomen but before opening the uterus. If there is difficulty in doing that, a little sublingual nitroglycerin or intravenous terbutaline as described above will relax the uterus and facilitate the maneuver. Of course, if the baby is back up and feet down, conversion is not needed.

14. Active or passive placental removal?

Once the baby is delivered, draining the placenta appears to result in less fetomaternal transfusion (Leavitt et al.,2007). In my opinion, it also makes delivery of the placenta quicker and easier. I prefer a rapid manual removal of the placenta after changing my dominant hand glove if it has been in the vagina. The uterine cavity can be explored at the same time. The literature supports spontaneous extraction of the placenta by cord traction and oxytocin, rather than manual removal, as providing less risk of infection and lower blood loss (Anorlu et al., 2008). And there are studies that suggest changing gloves is not important (Atkinson et al.,1996). My experience has been different. With prophylactic antibiotics, changes of the contaminated glove and rapid manual extraction of the placenta while oxytocin is running, I think the risk of endometritis is minimal. It has been a very long time since I have seen a postoperative fever.

15. Exteriorize the uterus? Why?

Exteriorizing the uterus is probably a useful procedure in a teaching institution, because everyone can see what is being done. Whether it has any other advantage or risk is controversial, and the literature is conflicting. I find it time consuming, awkward, abrasive to peritoneal surfaces (increasing the risk of adhesions --- a factor not addressed by the literature I found). If we leave it where it belongs, we do not need to struggle to get it back inside after closure of the hysterotomy, worry about clots forming in the huge and distended broad ligament veins, nor about air embolus.

16. Uterine closure: Two layers, one suture, one knot

The controversy over closure of the myometrium in one layer or two seems pretty well over. The one-layer closure simply has a higher failure rate in subsequent pregnancies (Bujold et al., 2002; Durnwald et al., 2003; Bujold et al., 2010). I have always preferred two layers, the first a full thickness layer to get hemostasis (with or without "locking" the stitches) and the second an imbricating layer to bring the cephalad and caudad peritoneum together and cover up the exposed myometrial edges that might otherwise adhere to tissue above it during healing. Theoretically, one should use a monofilament suture because a braided suture in an area so often contaminated would give bacteria more places to hide. And although most people use slowly dissolving suture material, in fact, the uterus shrinks so rapidly that by the next day the suture line must surely be very loose. Hence, I don't think the speed of suture dissolution is an important factor.

Whatever type of suture material I have, I prefer to use a single suture pack for both layers of the closure, sewing first away from myself with the full thickness layer (locked or not) and then bringing the same suture back to the starting point without cutting or tying until I get there (Dyson, 2010). To start, I pass the suture deep into the myometrium at the near edge of the hysterotomy, then "follow" myself as I sew the full thickness layer to and a bit beyond the distal edge of the hysterotomy. Without tying or cutting, I convert to a deep parallel Lambert type imbricating stitch to bring the suture back to me. I will have tagged the loose end with a hemostat when I started. Now I just tie the running end of the suture when it gets back to me to that tagged end. If the Lambert stitch is placed at the cut edge of the peritoneum above and below the incision, or even a little further away, the serosal edges will come together to hide raw edges of the myometrium and present a smooth surface for healing. The entire double layer closure takes only about two minutes and there is only one knot to tie (and to come untied).

17. Check the ovaries

Those of us who do not exteriorize the uterus should remember to take a look at the ovaries before closing the abdomen. I have found many ovarian tumors that way, mostly just cystic teratomas, of course, but it is a shame to leave them as they will one day likely need removal. It only takes a few minutes to shell one of these benign tumors out of the ovary and if done carefully, without rupture, there is often no bleeding and no need for suture. One purse string suture inside the ovary will approximate the surfaces enough to allow healing. I think we tend to forget that ovaries are very good at healing (they rupture and heal with every ovulation) so that sewing the ovarian surface is really counterproductive.

In addition to removing ovarian tumors, we have the opportunity to remove fibroids if they are subserosal, especially if on a stalk. Most of us have done that once, but if you are so tempted, be prepared to be late for dinner as getting hemostasis may be a major problem. Those vessels feeding the placenta on the endometrial side are as big as a small finger but stop bleeding as soon as the uterus contracts. The myometrium on the serosal surface is also very vascular but does not behave the same way. It is better to leave the fibroids for another day unless they are on a very narrow stalk that can simply be tied off.

18. Irrigate, but with what?

I am a big fan of irrigating. "The solution to pollution is dilution" I was told as a resident and it makes a lot of sense, though the literature is not as convincing (Harrigill et al., 2003). I prefer to irrigate a little at a time (the principle of serial dilution) using physiologic, isotonic solutions such as lactated Ringer's or "normal" saline. Some very good surgeons prefer water. One can see small bleeding vessels better with water, as the red blood cells burst from its hypotonicity, leaving a pink but clear liquid. My worry is that surface epithelial cells might similarly be destroyed. We know that injuring a serosal surface is the first step to getting adhesions, hence it makes sense to avoid epithelial damage from rubbing, blotting, burning, drying or (maybe) using hypotonic solutions to irrigate.

19. Peritoneal closure?

Since I do not create a bladder flap, I have no need to close the visceral peritoneum, except as it is re-approximated with the hysterotomy incision. However, closing the rectus muscles along with the underlying peritoneum is attractive to me. I once had a patient whose small bowel was coughed up through the gap in the rectus muscles and found the fascial suture line, where it stuck, requiring a return to the operating room. Therefore, I agree with Cheong et al. (2009) that some sort of closure of the parietal peritoneum can reduce adhesions. However, peritoneal surfaces seem to "flow" together rapidly if given the chance. Hence, I favor a simple mattress suture that incorporates a full-thickness bite through the rectus muscles and peritoneum near the midline, crosses the midline, comes to the surface on the other side and is then returned beneath the surface to near its starting point. The advantage of a mattress suture is that it tents up the midline away from the underlying uterus and may thus reduce the common problem of adhesion between the uterus and overlying tissue. This one suture also loosely re-approximates the rectus muscles. Actually closing the muscles has been shown to increase postoperative pain (Berghella et al., 2005) but this one stitch seems like a good compromise. Plastic surgeons charge a lot of money to repair a diastasis of these muscles, so there must be a problem here that we can help to prevent.

20. Fascial closure

A simple running closure using delayed absorbable suture is commonly used to re-approximate the cut edges of the anterior rectus sheath. A short stitch interval of a centimeter or so is advocated (unlike the closure of the uterine incision, which can be spaced more generously) with wide bites of a centimeter or more on either side of the cut. It is faster to use a single suture for the entire incision, though that means a "loop to strand" knot at the final end. Alternately, one can run the suture line from either end to the middle, tagging the first suture to reach the middle and tying it (strand to strand) to the mirror image suture when it in turn gets to the middle.

21. Subcutaneous closure

Some sort of closure of the subcutaneous tissue is advocated if the thickness is greater than two centimeters (Chelmow et al., 2004). A rapidly dissolving monofilament suture would be the theoretical ideal as the purpose is to prevent hematomas and seromas that may get infected. If infection of the area were to happen, a suture that disappears quickly would have an obvious advantage.

22. Skin closure

I prefer a subcuticular skin closure. It takes a minute or two longer than staples but the careful approximation of edges inherent in a subcuticular technique leads to rapid healing with a usually good cosmetic result. There are data (Tuuli et al., 2011) to suggest that a subcuticular closure results in fewer wound infections, which makes sense to me, since everything is beneath the surface. More importantly, women like it. Seeing staples in the skin is unpleasant for them, and they worry that removal will be painful (which, of course, it usually isn't).

I prefer to use a Keith needle with a fine, delayed absorbable suture. The Keith (straight) needle has a reputation for causing more needle-stick injuries, but I think that is because people tend to sew toward themselves with it, the way we do with almost all suture lines. If one pushes the needle away from oneself and picks up the needle with forceps instead of fingers, I do not see why needle injuries should occur. The Keith needle seems to me to be faster than a curved needle, and there is a tendency with it to keep the suture closer to the cut edge, avoiding some of the tension and puckering that can inhibit skin healing.

If I am especially worried about infection, I seal the surface of the skin with polyacrylic glue. I could find no data to prove that glue reduces wound infection but it seems logical. I also like to apply a moderate pressure dressing to inhibit seroma and hematoma formation. We also know from many studies that wounds heal more rapidly if the surface is made anaerobic, as it would be with either a pressure dressing or with glue.

23. Conclusion: Time is more than just money

The approach outlined here results in a cesarean section that, in the absence of complications, takes about fifteen minutes to perform, including a subcuticular skin closure and a double layer uterine closure. We are usually ready to close the skin at ten to twelve minutes from the start time. An additional advantage, though I have no formal statistics, seems to be a greatly reduced rate of febrile morbidity and postoperative adhesions.

Post cesarean febrile morbidity is reported in a Cochrane review to be typically about 20% (Smaill & Gyte, 2010). And adhesions are found at the first repeat surgery in roughly a third of women after one previous cesarean section and approximately half of those undergoing their third cesarean section (Tulandi et al., 2009). In contrast, of the more than four thousand cesarean deliveries I have personally performed, there have been many repeat surgeries, including high order repeats. Yet I cannot remember the last time we had febrile morbidity postoperatively and we virtually never find any kind of adhesions at subsequent surgeries.

The principles espoused here are simple and logical. We know that it takes blood and epithelial damage to create adhesions. Eliminating blood from a cesarean delivery is impossible, so protecting epithelial surfaces is the way to prevent adhesions. That means using suction instead of sponges to improve visualization, it means avoiding epithelial damage by drying (keep the uterus in the abdomen, irrigate as needed, eliminate unnecessary steps so that operating time is minimized), and it means avoiding where possible the tissue damage that is inherent in electrocautery use. Placing the incision in the thinnest part of the lower abdomen, closing the subcutaneous layer if it is over two centimeters, sealing the surface with a subcuticular stitch, and making the incision anaerobic for the first day at least with a pressure dressing and/or with glue, seem also to be logical steps that help with a rapid recovery and fever-free postoperative course.

The number of cesarean sections that we do has been increasing year by year in nearly every country of the world. This, in my opinion, has been driven largely by a decreasing tolerance for taking risks with the baby, but has been made possible by increases in safety of the mother when cesarean delivery is used. The principles outlined here seem like` a step further along that same road.

24. References

Anorlu, R., Maholwana, B. & Hofmeyr, G. (2008). Methods of Delivering the Placenta at Cesarean Section. *Cochrane Database Syst. Rev.; CD004737*

Atkinson, F., Owen, J. & Hauth, J. (1996). The Effect of Manual Removal of the Placenta on Post-Cesarean Endometritis. *Obstetrics & Gynecology*, Vol. 87, p. 99

Berghella, V., Baxter, J. & Chauhan, S. (2005). Evidence-Based Surgery for Cesarean Delivery. *American Journal of Obstetrics & Gynecology*, Vol. 193, p. 1607

Bujold, E., Bujold, C., Hamilton, E., et al. (2002). The Impact of a Single-Layer or Double-Layer Closure on Uterine Rupture. *American Journal of Obstetrics & Gynecology*, Vol. 186, p. 1326

Bujold, E., Goyet, M., Marcoux, S. et al. (2010). The Role of Uterine Closure on the Risk of Uterine Rupture. *Gynecology* Vol. 116, p. 43

Chelmow, D., Rodriguez, E. & Sabatini, M. (2004). Suture Closure of Subcutaneous Fat and Wound Disruption after Cesarean Delivery: A Meta-Analysis. *Obstetrics & Gynecology*. Vol. 103, p. 974

Cheong, Y., Premkumar, G., Metwally, M. et al. (2009) To Close or Not to Close? A Systematic Review and a Meta-Analysis of Peritoneal Non-Closure and Adhesion Formation after Caesarean Section. *European Journal of Obstetrics, Gynecology & Reproductive Biology*, Vol. 147, p. 3

Darj, E. & Nordstrom, M. (1999). The Misgav Ladach Method for Cesarean Section Compared to the Pfannenstiel Method. *Acta Obstetrics & Gynecology, Scandinavia*. Vol. 78, p. 37

Durnwald, C. & Mercer, G. (2003) Uterine Rupture, Perioperative and Perinatal Morbidity After Single-Layer and Double-Layer Closure at Cesarean Delivery. *American Journal of Obstetrics & Gynecology*, Vol. 189, p. 925

Dyson, R (2010). The Fifteen Minute Cesarean Delivery. *American Journal of Obstetrics & Gynecology*, Vol. 203(2), p. e18

Fong, Y. & Arulkumaran, S. (1997) Breech Extraction --- An Alternative Method of Delivering a Deeply Engaged Head at Cesarean Section. *International Journal of Gynecology & Obstetrics*. Vol. 56, p. 183

Harrigill, K., Miller, H. & Haynes, D. (2003) The Effect of Intraabdominal Irrigation at Cesarean Delivery on Maternal Morbidity: A Randomized Trial. *Obstetrics & Gynecology*, Vol. 101, p. 80

Hofmeyr, J., Novikova, N., Mathai, M. & Shah, A. (2009). Techniques for Cesarean Section. *American Journal of Obstetrics & Gynecology*, Vol. 201, p. 431

Hohlagschwandtner, M., Ruecklinger, E., Husslein, P. & Joura, E. (2001). Is the Formation of a Bladder Flap at Cesarean Necessary? A Randomized Trial. *Obstetrics & Gynecology*, Vol. 98, p. 1089

Leavitt, B., Huff, D., Bell, L. & Thurnau, G. (2007) Placental Drainage of Fetal Blood at Cesarean Delivery and Feto-Maternal Transfusion: A Randomized Controlled Trial. *Obstetrics & Gynecology*, Vol. 110, p. 608

Naumann, R., Hauth, J., Owen, J. et al. (1995). Subcutaneous Tissue Approximation in Relation to Wound Disruption After Cesarean Delivery in Obese Women. *Obstetrics & Gynecology*, Vol. 85, p. 412

Pevzner, L., Swank, M., Krepel, C. et al. (2011). Effects of Maternal Obesity on Tissue Concentrations of Prophylactic Cefazolin During Cesarean Delivery. *Obstetrics & Gynecology*, Vol. 117, p. 877

Smaill, F. & Gyte, G. (2010) Antibiotic Prophylaxis Versus No Prophylaxis for Preventing Infection after Cesarean Section. *Cochrane Database Syst. Rev. 20(1);* CD007482

Sullivan, S., Smith, T., Chang, E. et al. (2007) Administration of Cefazolin Prior to Skin Incision is Superior to Cefazolin at Cord Clamping in Preventing Postcesarean Infectious Morbidity: A Randomized, Controlled Trial. *American Journal of Obstetrics & Gynecology* Vol. 196, p. 455.e1

Tulandi, T., Agdi, M., Zarei, A. et al. (2009) Adhesion Development and Morbidity After Repeat Cesarean Delivery. *American Journal of Obstetrics & Gynecology*. Vol. 201, p. 56.e1

Tuuli, M, Rampersad, R., Carbone, J. et al. (2011) Subcuticular Suture for Skin Closure After Cesarean Delivery. A Systematic Review and Meta-Analysis. *Obstetrics & Gynecology* Vol. 117, p. 682

5

Evidence-Based Obstetric Anesthesia: An Update on Anesthesia for Cesarean Delivery

Andre P. Schmidt[1,2,3,4] and Jose Otavio C. Auler Jr.[1]
[1]Department of Anesthesia, Instituto Central, Hospital das Clinicas, Universidade de Sao Paulo, Sao Paulo,
[2]Department of Anesthesia and Perioperative Medicine, Hospital de Clinicas de Porto Alegre (HCPA), Porto Alegre,
[3]Department of Biochemistry, Federal University of Rio Grande do Sul (UFRGS), Porto Alegre,
[4]Department of Surgery, Federal University of Health Sciences of Porto Alegre (UFCSPA), Porto Alegre,
Brazil

1. Introduction

Severe hemorrhage and infection causing significant morbidity and mortality limited the use of cesarean section until the twentieth century, when important advances in aseptic, surgical, and anesthetic techniques improved the safety of this procedure for both woman and fetus [1-3].

The most common indications for cesarean delivery include dystocia, prior cesarean delivery, malpresentation, multiple gestation, fetal distress (nonreassuring fetal status), and maternal request [1-3]. Since late 70's, a progressive increase in the cesarean delivery rates has been observed worldwide and several factors are associated with this finding: maternal, obstetric, fetal, medicolegal, and social factors are pivotal for this increment. Actually, cesarean delivery rates have increased to around 30% in the last decade [1-3]. Notably, cesarean delivery rates are likely to increase further as women are requesting an elective cesarean delivery even for their first baby. Although controversial, the American College of Obstetricians and Gynecologists (ACOG) has suggested that it is ethical for an obstetrician to perform an elective cesarean delivery if the physician believes that the cesarean delivery promotes the health of the mother and fetus more than a vaginal delivery.

The selection of regional or general anesthesia for cesarean delivery depends on the experience of the anesthesiologist, past medical history of the patient, indications and urgency of the cesarean delivery, maternal status, and desires of the patient. Past medical, surgical, and obstetric history, presence or absence of labor, and available resources should also be considered by the anesthesiologist [4-6]. Considering these issues, the main aims of this chapter are to discuss the most important topics involved in anesthesia for cesarean delivery and the most recent scientific evidences regarding techniques and perioperative management of obstetric patients. We emphasize that this chapter is only a brief review focusing on main issues involved in anesthesia for cesarean delivery and more comprehensive reviews and recommendations are available elsewhere [4-6].

2. Perianesthetic evaluation of the obstetric patient

2.1 Preanesthetic evaluation

All women admitted for labor and delivery are potential candidates for the emergency administration of anesthesia. Considering this fact, the anesthesiologist ideally should evaluate every patient shortly after admission. The anesthesiologist should conduct a focused history and physical examination before providing anesthesia care. This should include, but should be not limited to, a maternal health and anesthetic history, a relevant obstetric history, a baseline blood pressure measurement, allergies, and performance of an airway, heart, and lung examination [7]. When a neuraxial anesthetic is planned, the patient's back should also be examined. Ideally, for high-risk women, preanesthetic evaluation should occur in the late second or early third trimester. This practice offers the opportunity to provide women with information, solicit further consultations, optimize medical conditions, and discuss plans and preparations for the upcoming delivery, perhaps in a multidisciplinary basis [8,9]. In some cases, the urgency or emergency of the situation allows limited time for evaluation before induction of anesthesia. Nevertheless, essential information must be obtained, and risks and benefits of anesthetic management decisions should be discussed on a case-by-case basis.

Usually, obtaining an informed consent is strongly recommended [10]. The ethical issues in obtaining consent from the obstetric patient can be challenging considering the potential clinical situations, such as the pain and stress of labor and sudden changes in maternal and fetal status, sometimes requiring emergency care. Nevertheless, there is general consensus that pregnant women appear to want more rather than less information regarding the risks of anesthetic interventions during a preanesthetic evaluation. Women usually should be aware of the following neuraxial anesthetic risks: the possibility of intraoperative discomfort and a failed/partial blockade, the potential need to convert to general anesthesia, the presence of weak legs, hypotension episodes associated to discomfort, and the occurrence of an unintentional dural puncture (whenever an epidural technique was used) [11]. Backache and urinary retention could be considered for discussion, but the risk for paraplegia should not to be routinely addressed unless the patient specifically asked about it [11]. Finally, and most important, anesthesiologists are encouraged to discussion of anesthetic risks and techniques and use informed consent as an opportunity to establish a closer patient-physician relationship rather than a simple tool to avoid litigation.

2.2 Fasting recommendations and aspiration prophylaxis

Although there is a lack of data regarding the relationship between recent food intake and subsequent aspiration pneumonitis, the patient should be always asked about oral intake and fasting period. Gastric emptying of clear liquids during pregnancy probably occurs relatively quickly since the residual content of the stomach does not appear to be different from baseline fasting levels in nonlaboring pregnant women [12,13]. The uncomplicated patient undergoing elective cesarean delivery may drink modest amounts of clear liquids (water, fruit juices without pulp, clear tea, etc) up to 2 hours before induction of anesthesia

[6]. The volume of liquid ingested is less important than the absence of particulate matter. Women with additional risk factors for aspiration (e.g., morbid obesity, diabetes, difficult airway), or laboring women at increased risk for cesarean delivery may have further restrictions of oral intake [6]. Routinely, ingestion of solid foods should be avoided during labor and in women undergoing elective cesarean delivery. A fasting period for solids of 6 to 8 hours is still recommended [6].

In women scheduled to cesarean section and considered to be in high-risk for aspiration, a pharmacological prophylaxis should be considered if time permits. The literature does not sufficiently examine the relationship between reduced gastric acidity and the frequency of emesis, pulmonary aspiration, morbidity, or mortality in obstetric patients who have aspirated gastric contents. Evidence supports the efficacy of preoperative nonparticulate antacids (0.3 M sodium citrate) in decreasing gastric acidity during the peripartum period, without affecting gastric volume [14]. Additionally, the literature suggests that H_2 receptor antagonists such as ranitidine or famotidine are effective in decreasing gastric acidity in obstetric patients and supports the efficacy of metoclopramide in reducing peripartum nausea and vomiting [15]. Notably, intravenously administered H_2 receptor antagonists and metoclopramide require at least 30 to 45 minutes to effectively reduce gastric acidity [15]. Proton pump inhibitors such as omeprazole can achieve a higher gastric pH than the H_2 receptor antagonist ranitidine [16], although ranitidine combined with sodium citrate is more cost effective [17].

2.3 Equipment and facilities in obstetric anesthesia

Labor and delivery units may be adjacent to or distant from the operating rooms. Nonetheless, equipment, monitoring material, facilities, and support personnel available in the obstetric operating room should be comparable to those available in the main operating room [6]. In addition, personnel and equipment should also be available to care for obstetric patients recovering from major neuraxial or general anesthesia and postoperative (post-cesarean) recovery unit should be completely equipped as well. Resources for the conduct and support of neuraxial anesthesia and general anesthesia should include those necessary for the basic delivery of anesthesia and airway management as well as those required to manage complications. The immediate availability of these resources is essential, given the frequency and urgency of the anesthesia care provided. Equipment and supplies should be checked on a frequent and regular basis and the necessary drugs, including vasopressors, emergency medications, and drugs used for general and neuraxial anesthesia should be promptly available [6].

Additionally, attention should be given to the availability and accurate functioning of monitors for anesthesia and the management of potential complications (e.g., failed intubation, cardiopulmonary arrest, inadequate analgesia, significant hypotension or bradycardia, respiratory depression, pruritus, vomiting, etc) [6]. Basic monitoring includes maternal pulse oximetry, electrocardiogram (ECG), noninvasive blood pressure monitoring and fetal heart rate (FHR) monitoring. Invasive hemodynamic monitoring should be considered in women with cardiovascular diseases, refractory hypertension, or other specific situations. Bispectral index monitors or other depth of anesthesia monitors have received only limited evaluation in women undergoing cesarean delivery but could be considered in some situations [18].

3. Anesthesia for cesarean delivery

3.1 Regional versus general anesthesia: what are the main evidences?

Neuraxial techniques (spinal, epidural, combined spinal-epidural – CSE) are the preferred methods of providing anesthesia for cesarean delivery as compared to general or local anesthesia. Notably, more recently, neuraxial anesthesia is administered to some women who would have received general anesthesia in the past. For example, umbilical cord prolapse, placenta previa, some cardiovascular diseases and severe preeclampsia are no longer considered absolute indications for general anesthesia. Several studies and surveys indicated a progressive increase in the use of neuraxial anesthesia, especially spinal anesthesia, for both elective and emergency cesarean deliveries and similar increases have been observed in both developed and developing countries [19]. Table 1 describes the main factors involved in the process of selection and indication of anesthetic techniques for cesarean delivery.

Regional (neuraxial) versus general anesthesia for cesarean delivery – main indications
Regional (neuraxial) anesthesia:
- Risk factors for difficult airway or aspiration
- Maternal desire to witness birth and/or avoid general anesthesia
- Improved postoperative analgesia (neuraxial opioids)
- Presence of comorbid conditions
- Reduced fetal drug exposure and blood loss
- Allows presence of husband or support person
General anesthesia:
- Presence of comorbid conditions that contraindicate a neuraxial technique
- Insufficient time to induce neuraxial anesthesia for urgent delivery
- Failure of neuraxial technique
- Maternal refusal or failure to cooperate with neuraxial technique
- Planned of more complex surgical procedures during cesarean delivery (e.g. ex-utero intrapartum treatment (EXIT) procedure)

Table 1. Main factors involved in the selection of anesthetic techniques for cesarean delivery

The greater use of neuraxial anesthesia for cesarean delivery has been attributed to several factors, such as the growing use of epidural techniques for labor analgesia, improvement in the quality of neuraxial anesthesia with the addition of an opioid or other adjuvants to the local anesthetic, the risks of airway complications during general anesthesia in obstetric patients, the need for limited neonatal drug transfer, the ability of the mother to remain awake to experience childbirth, presence of a support person in the operating room, lack of experience of the anesthesiologists to provide general anesthesia in the obstetric setting and several others [20-23].

When choosing regional or general anesthesia for cesarean delivery, we should always consider both maternal and neonatal outcomes. Maternal outcome studies have primarily focused on maternal morbidity and mortality, and neonatal outcome studies have focused essentially on umbilical cord pH, Apgar score, the need for ventilatory assistance at birth, and neurobehavioral scores.

Maternal mortality following general anesthesia has been a primary factor for the transition toward greater use of neuraxial anesthesia for cesarean delivery in the last few decades. Notably, maternal outcome seems to be better with regional anesthesia than with general anesthesia. Hawkins and colleagues compared the anesthesia-related maternal mortality rate from 1979 to 1984 with that for the period from 1985 to 1990 in the United States and found that the case-fatality risk ratio for general versus neuraxial anesthesia was as high as 16.7 in the years 1985 to 1990 [24]. The reason for this difference is primarily related to the respiratory system of the parturient since difficult tracheal intubation is 10 times higher in the parturient than in the general population and hypoxemia develops faster during periods of apnea. Of interest, these data may overstate the relative risk of general anesthesia, because this form of anesthesia is used principally when neuraxial anesthetic techniques are contraindicated for medical reasons and/or may reflect the growing acceptance of performing neuraxial techniques in parturients with significant comorbidities [21,22]. Importantly, although general anesthesia is still correlated with higher incidence of maternal deaths as compared to regional anesthesia, a recent report suggests that a significant reduction in general anesthesia-related deaths occurred in the recent years [25].

Of note, airway management experience is decreasing in the obstetric setting. Hawthorne and colleagues found that the incidence of failed tracheal intubation increased from 1 in 250 in 1984 to 1 in 300 in 1994 [26]. In a recent review of maternal mortality causes, Mhyre and colleagues found that "airway problems" is still a leading cause of maternal mortality, but that the problems occurred mostly during emergence or tracheal extubation [27].

Maternal morbidity is also lower with the use of neuraxial anesthesia techniques than with general anesthesia. In a systematic review of controlled trials comparing major maternal and neonatal outcomes with the use of neuraxial anesthesia and general anesthesia for cesarean delivery, Afolabi and colleagues found less maternal blood loss and shivering but more nausea in the neuraxial group [20]. Prospective audits of post-cesarean delivery outcomes have indicated that in the first postoperative week, women who received neuraxial anesthesia had less pain, gastrointestinal stasis, coughing, fever, and depression and were able to breast-feed and ambulate more quickly than women who received general anesthesia [23].

Although neonatal outcome seems to be better when regional anesthesia is used, differences among diverse anesthetic techniques are not so clear. Apgar and neonatal neurobehavioral scores are relatively insensitive measures of neonatal well-being, and umbilical cord blood gas and pH measurements may reflect an obstetric bias (indication for the cesarean delivery rather than differences in anesthetic techniques). Some previous studies have found that umbilical artery pH was greater in the neonate delivered with general anesthesia, but clinical parameters (e.g., Apgar score and the need for assisted ventilation) were better when regional anesthesia was used [28]. The acidemia found following regional anesthesia seems to be increased after spinal as compared to epidural anesthesia, but has not been related to any clinically significant neonatal complication [20,28].

Therefore, the decision to use a particular anesthetic technique for cesarean delivery should be individualized and based on several factors. These should include anesthetic, obstetric, or fetal risk factors, urgency, the preferences of the patient, and the judgment of the anesthesiologist. Neuraxial techniques are usually recommended and preferred to general anesthesia for most cesarean deliveries. For these reasons, most elective cesarean deliveries are now performed under regional anesthesia [29].

3.2 Spinal, epidural, combined spinal-epidural or general anesthesia

Spinal anesthesia is commonly used rather than epidural anesthesia for elective cesarean delivery because with spinal anesthesia the speed of onset is quicker, the quality of anesthesia is considered to be superior and the failure rate is lower. Riley and colleagues found that spinal anesthesia leads to a more efficient utilization of operating room time than epidural anesthesia because time until skin incision is faster with spinal anesthesia [30]. The most common complication from spinal anesthesia is hypotension, which may explain the decreased umbilical artery pH as compared with both epidural and general anesthesia [31]. The spinal anesthesia is a simple and reliable technique that allows visual confirmation of correct needle placement (by visualization of cerebrospinal fluid leak) and is technically easier to perform than the epidural. Spinal anesthesia provides a rapid onset of dense blockade that is typically more profound than that provided with an epidural technique, resulting in a reduced need for supplemental intravenous analgesics or conversion to general anesthesia [30,32,33]. Considering that a smaller amount of local anesthetic is needed to establish a functional spinal blockade, spinal anesthesia is associated with negligible maternal risk for systemic local anesthetic toxicity and with minimal drug transfer to the fetus, as compared to epidural and general anesthesia [34]. Given these advantages, spinal anesthesia is now the most commonly used anesthetic technique for cesarean delivery worldwide [19,35].

As commonly used for other conventional surgical procedures, the spinal technique should be performed at the L_3 to L_4 interspace or below. These interspaces are used to avoid the potential for spinal cord trauma. Spinal anesthesia is usually administered as a single-injection procedure through a non-cutting, pencil-point needle that is usually 25-gauge or smaller. A number of different needle designs are available and the size and design of the needle tip affect the incidence and severity of post-dural puncture headache (PDPH). For that reason, if spinal anesthesia is chosen, small pencil-point spinal needles should be used instead of larger cutting-bevel spinal needles [36].

Continuous spinal anesthetic technique can be used in some circumstances, especially in the setting of an unintentional dural puncture with an epidural needle. Additionally, intentional continuous spinal anesthesia may also be desirable in certain settings, when the reliability of a spinal technique and the ability to precisely titrate the initiation and duration of anesthesia are recommended (e.g., morbidly obese patients or some cardiovascular diseases). However, technical difficulties, catheter failures, concerns about the risks for neurological complications and a higher incidence of post-dural puncture headache severely restrict this technique from a widespread use [37,38].

The overall use of epidural anesthesia for elective cesarean delivery has decreased, in part because the resulting block is less reliable than that provided by spinal anesthesia. Conversely, the use of epidural anesthesia for nonelective cesarean delivery has increased, primarily as a result of the greater use of epidural analgesia during labor [30]. Although medications used in the spinal and epidural spaces are identical, epidural local anesthetic and opioid doses are up to 10 times greater than doses given spinally leading to concerns regarding toxicity and efficacy. Contrariwise, advantages of the epidural technique include a slower onset of sympathetic blockade, which may allow compensatory mechanisms to attenuate the severity of hypotension episodes [30]. Furthermore, a catheter-based technique also allows titration of the level and duration of anesthesia and continuous post-cesarean delivery analgesia.

The CSE technique incorporates the rapid and predictable onset of a spinal blockade with the ability to augment anesthesia by injection of additional drug through the epidural catheter [39-41]. In 1981, Brownridge [39] reported the first use of the CSE technique for cesarean delivery through separate spinal and epidural needles introduced at different interspaces. Carrie and O'Sullivan [40] subsequently reported the needle-through-needle technique via a single interspace for cesarean delivery, which has become the most popular technique. More recently, Davies and colleagues compared CSE with epidural anesthesia alone for elective cesarean delivery and reported more rapid onset, greater motor blockade, and lower pain scores at delivery in the CSE group [41]. The main disadvantages of CSE techniques are an untested epidural catheter and hypotension [42]. Additionally, the CSE technique is certainly more time-consuming as compared to spinal anesthesia only.

An alternative CSE technique is the extradural volume extension (EVE) technique [43-45]. In this technique, spinal administration of a small dose of local anesthetic is followed by the administration of saline through the epidural catheter. Although there were conflicting findings, this technique has been related to a higher rostral spread of the blockade [43-45].

Table 2 demonstrates the main differences regarding the various neuraxial anesthetic techniques for cesarean delivery. With all neuraxial techniques, an adequate sensory level of anesthesia is essential to minimize maternal pain and avoid the urgent need for administration of general anesthesia. Because motor nerve fibers are typically larger and more difficult to block, the complete absence of hip flexion and ankle dorsiflexion most likely indicates that a functional sensory and sympathetic block is also present in a similar (primarily lumbosacral) distribution. However, because afferent nerves innervating abdominal and pelvic organs accompany sympathetic fibers that ascend and descend in the sympathetic trunk (T_5 to L_1), a sensory block that extends rostrally from the sacral dermatomes to T_4 should be the goal for cesarean delivery anesthesia [46-48]. The majority of anesthesiologists use the absence of cold temperature sensation to a T_4 level to indicate an adequate blockade height for cesarean delivery [46-48]. Alternatively, a T_6 blockade to touch may provide a pain-free cesarean delivery for most parturients and could be used as a reference. Because the undersurface of the diaphragm (C_3 to C_5) and the vagus nerve may be stimulated by surgical manipulation during cesarean delivery [49], maternal discomfort and other symptoms, particularly nausea and vomiting may occur despite a T_4 level of blockade. The use of systemic and especially neuraxial opioids are effective in preventing or alleviating these symptoms [49,50].

Technique	Advantages	Disadvantages
Spinal anesthesia	Technically simple	Limited duration
	Rapid onset and dense blockade	Limited level block titration
	Low doses of local anesthetic required	Increased incidence of hypotension
Epidural anesthesia	No dural puncture is required	Slow onset of surgical anesthesia
	Ability to titrate extent of sensory blockade	Higher incidence of failure
	Continuous perioperative anesthesia	High doses of local anesthetic required
CSE* anesthesia	Low doses of local anesthetic and opioid	Delayed verification of
	Rapid onset and dense blockade	functioning epidural catheter
	Ability to titrate extent of sensory blockade	Technique slightly more difficult
	Continuous perioperative anesthesia	Time consuming

*CSE = Combined spinal-epidural anesthesia.

Table 2. Main advantages and disadvantages regarding type of neuraxial anesthesia for Cesarean Delivery

The choice of local anesthetic agent (and adjuvants) used to provide spinal anesthesia depends on the expected duration of the surgery, the postoperative analgesia plan, and the preferences of the anesthesiologists. For cesarean delivery, the local anesthetic agent of choice is typically bupivacaine since its spinal administration usually results in a dense block of long duration. However, several different doses of bupivacaine have been described in the literature and the dose of spinal bupivacaine that has been successfully used for cesarean delivery ranges from 4.5 to 15 mg [40,46,49]. In general, pregnant women require smaller doses of spinal local anesthetic as compared to nonpregnant women. Reasons include a smaller CSF volume in pregnancy, rostral movement of hyperbaric local anesthetic in the supine pregnant patient, and the greater sensitivity of nerve fibers to the local anesthetic during pregnancy [51]. Overall, the mass of local anesthetic, rather than the concentration or volume, is thought to influence the spread of the resulting blockade [52]. However, the specific influence of the dose and baricity on the efficacy of the block is somewhat controversial and may be influenced by other factors, such as co-administration of neuraxial opioids.

More recent data suggest that lower anesthetic doses can be used, although there is some controversy regarding recommendations. The anesthesiologist should consider whether adjuvant drugs will be used and whether the risks of giving supplemental analgesia or conversion to general anesthesia that are associated with low doses of bupivacaine outweigh the potential benefits (i.e., less hypotension, faster recovery) [53-57]. For a single-shot spinal anesthesia for cesarean delivery, most anesthesiologists use a dose of bupivacaine between 10 and 15 mg, in combination with opioids, sufentanil or fentanyl and morphine.

Conventional doses of hyperbaric bupivacaine are most often used to provide CSE anesthesia for cesarean delivery. However, a satisfactory block has been reported with plain bupivacaine drug doses as low as 4.5 mg [57]. Nonetheless, the CSE technique may use a lower dose of spinal bupivacaine (7.5 to 10 mg) followed by incremental injection of local anesthetic through the epidural catheter to achieve a T4 level of anesthesia [43,44], a procedure called sequential CSE. The purported advantage of this approach is a lower incidence of hypotension. With the sequential CSE technique, Thoren and colleagues observed a more gradual onset of hypotension and a lower initial anesthesia level with the spinal dose [44]. However, all parturients in the CSE group required additional doses of local anesthetic through the epidural catheter. The sequential CSE technique may be of particular advantage in certain high-risk parturients (e.g., significant cardiac disease) in whom avoidance of severe hypotension is pivotal.

Finally, the most common local anesthetic used for the initiation and maintenance of epidural anesthesia for cesarean delivery is 2% lidocaine with epinephrine. The epidural administration of lidocaine in concentrations less than 2%, or without the addition of epinephrine (which independently augments the analgesia through alpha-adrenergic receptor blockade), may result in anesthesia that is inadequate for surgery [58]. Surgical anesthesia can also be produced with epidural administration of 0.5% bupivacaine. Nevertheless, the slow onset of blockade and the risk of cardiovascular toxicity from unintentional intravascular injection or systemic absorption limit the contemporary use of this agent. The single-isomer, levorotatory local anesthetics, 0.5% to 0.75% ropivacaine and 0.5% levobupivacaine, may be preferable to racemic bupivacaine because of their better safety profiles. Except for the safety profile, there are no significant clinical advantages to these single-isomer local anesthetics when equipotent doses are administered. Similarly to spinal anesthesia, opioids (sufentanil or fentanyl and morphine) are also usually administered in combination with local anesthetics.

Although neuraxial techniques are typically preferred when anesthesia is provided for cesarean delivery, there are some clinical situations in which the administration of general anesthesia is considered the most appropriate option. The basic elements for preparation and care of the obstetric patient undergoing cesarean delivery also apply to the patient undergoing general anesthesia. The preanesthetic evaluation should focus on assessment of physical characteristics, particularly airway features, and comorbidities. Pregnancy-induced changes in the upper airway may be exacerbated during labor [59]. Importantly, failed intubation, failed ventilation and oxygenation, and pulmonary aspiration of gastric contents remain leading anesthesia-related causes of maternal death. Table 3 describes the main recommendations to general anesthesia for cesarean delivery.

Brief algorithm of preparation to general anesthesia for cesarean delivery
1. Perform preanesthetic assessment and obtain informed consent; 2. Prepare necessary medications and check equipment and monitors; 3. Perform a "time-out" to verify patient identity, position, operative site, and procedure; 4. Place patient supine with left uterine displacement; 5. Consider the use of a nonparticulate antacid orally within 20 minutes before induction or metoclopramide 10 mg and/or ranitidine 30 mg intravenously more than 30 minutes before induction; 6. Administer antibiotic prophylaxis (preferentially before skin incision); 7. Initiate monitoring (electrocardiogram, non-invasive arterial pressure monitoring and pulse oximetry); 8. Provide 100% oxygen with a tight-fitting face mask for 3 minutes or longer. Alternatively, instruct the patient to take 4 to 8 vital-capacity breaths immediately before induction of anesthesia; 9. After the abdomen has been prepared and operative drapes are in place, verify that the surgeon and assistant are ready to begin surgery; 10. Initiate rapid-sequence induction (thiopental 4 to 6 mg/kg or propofol 1.5 to 2.5 mg/kg and succinylcholine 1 mg/kg; wait up to 45 seconds; The use of cricoid pressure is still recommended; 11. Perform endotracheal intubation. Confirm correct placement of endotracheal tube by using capnography; 12. Provide maintenance of anesthesia (usually by using volatile anesthetics); 13. Treat hypotension episodes by using phenylephrine or ephedrine; 14. Observe and support delivery of baby; 15. Begin a small bolus (up to 3 units) followed by a continuous infusion of oxytocin; consider other uterotonic agents (e.g., methylergometrine, misoprostol, prostaglandin F2α) if uterine tone is inadequate. Monitor cautiously the amount of blood loss; 16. Adjust maintenance anesthesia technique after delivery of the infant (reduced concentration of a volatile anesthetic to avoid a significant reduction in the uterine tonus); 17. Consider the high risk of awareness and recall in these patients. Cogitate administration of benzodiazepines (e.g., midazolam); 18. Provide adequate multimodal analgesia and prophylaxis for postoperative nausea and vomiting; 19. Perform extubation when neuromuscular blockade is fully reversed and the patient is awake and responds to commands; 20. Evaluate postoperative signs and symptoms (e.g., pain, nausea, vomiting, shivering, etc).

OBS: This algorithm may need to be modified accordingly case-by-case circumstances (e.g., emergency care for cesarean delivery).

Table 3. Main recommendations to general anesthesia for cesarean delivery

3.3 Hemodynamic monitoring: main techniques and recent advances

During cesarean delivery with neuraxial anesthesia, ECG changes have a reported incidence of 25% to 60% and are believed to be due to hyperdynamic circulation, circulating catecholamines, or altered hormone concentration ratios [60,61]. However, the significance of the ECG findings as an indicator of cardiac pathology remains controversial, but measurement of cardiac troponin indicates that rarely obstetric patients experience myocardial ischemia [62]. In a prospective study of 254 healthy women undergoing cesarean delivery with spinal anesthesia, Shen and colleagues have shown that the incidence of first- and second-degree atrioventricular block was 3.5% for each, severe bradycardia was 6.7%, and multiple premature ventricular contractions was 1.2%. The investigators speculated that a relative increase in parasympathetic activity occurred as a result of spinal blockade of cardiac sympathetic activity. Most of the dysrhythmias were transient and resolved spontaneously [63]. However, prompt management with vasoactive drugs should be performed if dysrhythmias persist.

An indwelling urinary catheter is used in almost all women undergoing cesarean delivery [64]. A urinary catheter helps avoid overdistention of the bladder during and after surgery. In cases of hypovolemia and/or oliguria, a collection system that allows precise measurement of urine volume should be used.

In regard to central invasive hemodynamic monitoring, there is insufficient literature to examine whether pulmonary artery catheterization or minimally invasive methods to evaluate cardiac output (pulse-wave analysis methods) are associated with improved maternal, fetal, or neonatal outcomes in women with pregnancy-related hypertensive disorders [65]. Additionally, there is an important lack of evidence regarding the management of obstetric patients with central venous catheterization. However, the routine use of pulmonary artery catheterization, pulse-wave analysis methods to evaluate cardiac output or central venous does not reduce maternal complications in severely preeclamptic women [6]. Therefore, the decision to perform invasive hemodynamic monitoring should be individualized and based on clinical indications that include the patient's medical history and cardiovascular risk factors.

3.4 Intravenous fluid replacement and preloading

Numerous techniques have been attempted to prevent hypotension following spinal anesthesia, with varying success. The most important preventive measure is to ensure left uterine displacement so as to avoid the supine hypotensive syndrome [66]. Prehydration or preloading is not necessarily an effective measure to prevent hypotension and several strategies of prehydration have been used elsewhere [67-69]. Some studies have found a smaller incidence of hypotension in the prehydrated patients as compared with the control (no prehydrated) patients. However, the total amount of fluid and vasoconstrictors, and the severity of the hypotension usually not differ between groups [67-69]. Nevertheless, neonatal outcomes, as measured by Apgar score and umbilical cord blood gas and pH measurements, are improved when the parturient is prehydrated [70]. Although there are some conflicting findings, the literature still supports the use of intravenous fluid preloading for spinal anesthesia since it seems to reduce the frequency of maternal hypotension when compared with no fluid preloading. Of note, though fluid preloading reduces the frequency of maternal hypotension, initiation of spinal anesthesia should not be delayed to administer a fixed volume of intravenous fluid.

Colloid prehydration may be promising, but still deserves further study. Ueyama and colleagues demonstrated that the incidence of hypotension was 75% in those who received lactated Ringer's, 58% in those who received 500 mL of hydroxyethylstarch, and only 17% in those who received 1000 mL of hydroxyethylstarch [69]. Future studies should address the use of colloids in the obstetric setting in order to demonstrate efficacy and safety.

3.5 Rationale for the use of vasoconstrictors

In regard to the use of vasoconstrictors in the obstetric setting especially for spinal anesthesia, the literature supports the administration of ephedrine, but suggests that phenylephrine is effective in reducing maternal hypotension during neuraxial anesthesia for cesarean delivery. The literature is equivocal regarding the relative frequency of patients with breakthrough hypotension when infusions of ephedrine are compared with phenylephrine; however, lower umbilical cord pH values are reported after ephedrine administration as compared to the $alpha_1$-agonist phenylephrine. Although recent data indicates that $alpha_1$-agonists are more effective to avoid hypotension following spinal anesthesia for cesarean delivery, ephedrine is acceptable for treating hypotension during neuraxial anesthesia. Therefore, intravenous ephedrine and phenylephrine are both acceptable drugs for treating hypotension during neuraxial (spinal or epidural) anesthesia. In the absence of maternal bradycardia, phenylephrine may be preferable because of improved fetal acid-base status in uncomplicated pregnancies. Of note, some countries routinely use metaraminol as an $alpha_1$-agonist instead of phenylephrine in the obstetric setting without significant adverse events. This drug seems to be similarly effective as phenylephrine. Of note, prophylactic intravenous ephedrine or phenylephrine before spinal anesthetic placement has been studied to prevent hypotension, and is generally not recommended because of the risk of reactive hypertension [71,72].

4. Recovery from anesthesia

4.1 Postoperative (post-cesarean) analgesia: the role of neuraxial opioids

For improved postoperative analgesia after cesarean delivery during epidural anesthesia, the literature supports the use of epidural opioids compared with intermittent injections of intravenous or intramuscular opioids. However, a higher frequency of pruritus was found with epidural opioids. The literature is insufficient to evaluate the impact of epidural opioids compared with intravenous PCA. In addition, the literature is insufficient to evaluate spinal opioids compared with parenteral opioids. However, there is sufficient evidence that neuraxial opioids improve postoperative analgesia and maternal satisfaction. Therefore, we can argue that, for postoperative analgesia after neuraxial anesthesia for cesarean delivery, neuraxial opioids are preferred over intermittent injections of parenteral opioids [6]. Studies are equivocal regarding doses regimen, especially for epidural opioids (morphine). In spinal anesthesia for cesarean delivery, morphine doses are usually between 60 and 100 μg. Epidural morphine is usually administered in doses between 2 and 3 mg. However, controversy exists and new studies regarding efficacy and adverse effects are warranted.

4.2 Oral intake, removal of urinary catheter and discharge

Mangesi and Hofmeyr performed a systematic review of six randomized clinical trials comparing early with delayed oral intake of fluids and foods after cesarean delivery [73]. The authors found that the early consumption (within 4 to 8 hours) was associated with a shorter time to return of bowel sounds and a shorter hospital stay. No differences were reported in nausea and vomiting, abdominal distention, time to bowel activity, paralytic ileus, or need for analgesia.

There are no differences in the incidence of urinary retention after general anesthesia and epidural anesthesia following cesarean delivery [74]. Risk factors for postpartum urinary retention after cesarean delivery include the use of postoperative opioid analgesia (particularly when given via an epidural catheter), multiple gestations, and a low body mass index [75]. Most urinary catheters are removed either immediately following cesarean delivery, before discharge from the postoperative care unit or within 24 hours, but there are no differences between these options in regard to postoperative urinary retention, infection, dysuria, urgency, fever, or length of hospital stay [76].

In regard to the postoperative discharge, the anesthesiologist should routinely assess for recovery of motor and sensory function if a neuraxial technique was administered. Patients should be reassured that breast-feeding is safe, even after general anesthesia, and that postoperative analgesics have a favorable safety profile. Early mobility and ambulation should be stimulated.

5. Cesarean delivery: Anesthetic complications

The main anesthetic complications in cesarean delivery include, but are not limited to: hypotension, failure of neuraxial blockade, high blockade levels, dyspnea, nausea and vomiting, postoperative pain, pruritus, and shivering.

Hypotension is a common consequence of neuraxial anesthetic techniques and, when severe and sustained, can lead to impairment of uteroplacental perfusion, resulting in fetal hypoxia, acidosis, and neonatal depression [77]. Severe maternal hypotension can also have adverse maternal outcomes, including unconsciousness, pulmonary aspiration, apnea, bradycardia, and even cardiac arrest. The definition of maternal hypotension is controversial, but many investigators accept the following definition: a decrease in systolic blood pressure of more than 20% from baseline measurements or a systolic blood pressure lower than 100 mmHg [78]. Neuraxial anesthetic techniques produce hypotension through blockade of sympathetic nerve fibers, which control vascular smooth muscle tone. Preganglionic sympathetic fiber blockade primarily causes an increase in venous capacitance, which shifts a major portion of blood volume into the splanchnic bed and the lower extremities, thereby reducing venous return to the heart. The rate and extent of the sympathetic involvement, and subsequently the severity of hypotension, are determined by the onset and spread of the neuraxial blockade [79]. Consequently, hypotension may be less common with epidural anesthesia than with spinal anesthesia because of the slower onset of blockade. The delayed onset of hypotension with epidural anesthesia may also allow earlier treatment before hypotension becomes more severe.

A failure of neuraxial blockade can be defined as blockade insufficient in extent, density, or duration to provide anesthesia for cesarean delivery. Approximately 4% to 13% of epidural and 0.5% to 4% of spinal anesthetics fail to provide sufficient anesthesia for the initiation or completion of cesarean delivery [33,80]. Epidural techniques are more often associated with failure, given the fact that the catheter is often placed during early labor, and over time the catheter may migrate out of the epidural space. Factors that may correlate with failed extension of labor epidural anesthesia for cesarean delivery include a higher number of bolus doses for the provision of labor analgesia, patient characteristics (e.g., obesity, catheter positioning), and the time elapsed between placement of the catheter and cesarean delivery [33,80].

It is not uncommon for the parturient to report mild dyspnea or reduced ability to cough, especially if the neuraxial blockade has achieved higher than a T_4 level. If impaired phonation, unconsciousness, respiratory depression, or significant impairment of ventilation occurs, administration of general anesthesia is recommended. High neuraxial blockade may also result in cardiovascular collapse, including severe bradycardia and hypotension. This complication may be caused by several mechanisms, including an exaggerated spread of spinal or epidural drugs and unintentional intrathecal or subdural administration of an "epidural dose" of local anesthetic.

Nausea and vomiting are regulated by the chemoreceptor trigger zone and the vomiting center, which are located in the area postrema and the medullary lateral reticular formation, respectively. The vomiting center receives impulses from the vagal sensory fibers in the gastrointestinal tract, the semicircular canals and ampullae (labyrinth) of the inner ear, higher cortical centers, the chemoreceptor trigger zone, and intracranial pressure receptors. Impulses from these structures are influenced by dopaminergic, muscarinic, tryptaminergic, histaminic, and opioid receptors, which are subsequently the targets for antiemetic agents. Efferent impulses from the vomiting center are transmitted through the vagus, phrenic, and spinal nerves to the abdominal muscles, which causes the physical act of vomiting [81].

Preventing maternal hypotension may be the best means of preventing nausea and vomiting. Additionally, several options exist for the pharmacologic prophylaxis of nausea and vomiting, and several different classes of drugs are available. Although various algorithms have been developed to prevent postoperative nausea and vomiting, primarily targeting the nonpregnant patient population, none has been universally successful [82]. However, the prophylactic use of these agents either before or after cord clamping during cesarean delivery with neuraxial anesthesia has been demonstrated to be highly effective. Notably, multimodal therapies combining different medications may eventually prove the most effective. Several drugs have been shown to be effective, but most frequently used include intravenous ondansetron 4 mg after cord clamping, metoclopramide 10 mg prior to surgery or after cord clamping, droperidol 0.625 - 1.25 mg at end of surgery, dimenhydrinate 25 - 50 mg, and/or dexamethasone 4 - 8 mg, both possibly after cord clamping or at end of surgery.

Postoperative pain may have at least two components, somatic and visceral. A multimodal approach seems to provide the most effective post-cesarean delivery analgesia. Such an approach often includes administration of a nonsteroidal anti-inflammatory drug (NSAID), acetaminophen and dipyrone. Concerns have been expressed regarding possible adverse effects (platelet dysfunction, uterine atony), but these agents are widely used and seem to be safe. Some investigators have expressed concern about the role of NSAIDs on breast-feeding, but the American Academy of Pediatrics has stated that ibuprofen and ketorolac are compatible with breast-feeding [83].

The administration of opioids can cause pruritus. The incidence is as high as 30% to 100%, and pruritus is more commonly observed when opioids are administered spinally than epidurally. Pruritus is typically self-limited and may be generalized or localized to regions of the nose, face, and chest. Opioid-induced pruritus appears to be influenced by the particular combination of local anesthetic and opioid; of interest, the addition of epinephrine to an opioid–local anesthetic solution appears to augment the pruritus [84]. Notably, this side effect does not represent an allergic reaction to the neuraxial opioid. If flushing, urticaria, rhinitis, bronchoconstriction, or cardiac symptoms also occur, allergic reaction to another drug should be considered as a differential diagnosis. The cause of neuraxial opioid–induced pruritus is not known, although multiple theories have been proposed. They include μ-opioid receptor stimulation at the medullary dorsal horn, antagonism of inhibitory transmitters, and activation of an "itch center" in the central nervous system [85]. Pharmacologic prophylaxis or treatment of pruritus may include an opioid antagonist, an opioid agonist/antagonist, droperidol, a serotonin antagonist (e.g., ondansetron), and/or a subhypnotic dose of propofol [85]. Yeh and colleagues observed that ondansetron significantly reduced the incidence of spinal morphine–induced pruritus [86]. Although opioid antagonists, such as naltrexone and naloxone, and partial agonist/antagonists, such as nalbuphine, are probably the most effective treatments for pruritus, the use of any of these agents, either as a single dose or in continuous intravenous infusion, may also reverse analgesia. Antihistamines are often prescribed but are largely ineffective because the mechanism of pruritus is not related to histamine release.

Intraoperative and postoperative shivering may also have several etiologies but is usually related to a decrease in central temperature related to peripheral vasodilation. Several treatments are effective, but most frequently used include intravenous meperidine 10 - 30 mg, clonidine 15 - 150 μg, and alfentanil up to 250 μg [87].

6. Anticoagulation, coagulopathies and regional anesthesia in obstetrics

Concern exists that an epidural/spinal hematoma may develop after the administration of neuraxial anesthesia in patients with coagulopathy or using anticoagulants. There are only a few published cases of epidural hematoma after the administration of neuraxial anesthesia in pregnant patients [88,89]. This fact suggests that epidural hematoma after neuraxial anesthesia either is very uncommon or is underreported. However, in view of the serious effects of an epidural hematoma, the risks and benefits of performing neuraxial anesthesia should be carefully considered in a patient with either clinical or laboratory evidence of coagulopathy or pregnant women using anticoagulants.

Clearly, severe coagulopathy represents a well-known contraindication to the administration of neuraxial anesthesia, even in obstetric patients. The anesthesiologist can use laboratory tests (e.g., prothrombin time/International Normalized Ratio, partial thromboplastin time, activated clotting time measurements or thromboelastography) to assess the extent of anticoagulation and the effectiveness of reversal in patients receiving standard unfractionated heparin or oral anticoagulation therapy. If use of a neuraxial anesthetic technique is considered in a patient with a congenital coagulopathy, results of the factor assays should be within the normal range before neuraxial anesthesia administration [90].

Thrombocytopenia is relatively common in pregnant women with severe preeclampsia. Asymptomatic thrombocytopenia also may occur in healthy obstetric patients. Previous studies have reported that administration of neuraxial anesthesia is safe in healthy pregnant women with thrombocytopenia (i.e., platelet count less than 100,000/mm^3). In this context, the anesthesiologist should always consider the following factors: clinical evidence of bleeding, recent platelet count, recent changes in the platelet count, quality of platelets, coagulation factors, and, most importantly, the risk/benefit ratio of performing neuraxial anesthesia [91].

Most pregnant women who require long-term anticoagulation receive low molecular weight heparin (LMWH) or standard unfractionated heparin throughout pregnancy. LMWH (e.g., enoxaparin) is considered to be more efficacious for thromboprophylaxis than standard unfractionated heparin and has been used safely in pregnant women [92]. However, several cases of epidural/spinal hematoma after neuraxial anesthesia in non-obstetric patients receiving LMWH have been reported [93,94]. This apparent increase in the risk for an epidural hematoma may be related to the use of higher doses of LMWH and its relatively greater bioavailability and longer half-life in comparison with standard unfractionated heparin. Guidelines recommend that in patients receiving LMWH for thromboprophylaxis, needle placement should occur at least 10 to 12 hours after the last LMWH dose. In patients receiving higher doses of LMWH (e.g., enoxaparin 1 mg/kg every 12 hours or enoxaparin 1.5 mg/kg daily), needle placement should not occur until at least 24 hours after the last dose of LMWH [92]. In patients receiving a single daily dose of LMWH thromboprophylaxis, the first postoperative LMWH dose should be administered only 6 to 8 hours after surgery. An indwelling epidural catheter may be safely maintained in these patients; however, it should be removed at least 12 hours after the last dose of LMWH, and the next dose of LMWH should be administered at least 2 hours after catheter removal. In patients receiving higher doses of LMWH, the first dose of LMWH should be delayed for 24 hours postoperatively, and an indwelling catheter should be removed at least 2 hours before initiation of LMWH therapy [92].

There is a large experience with the use of standard unfractionated heparin and a large number of patients have received neuraxial anesthesia while receiving subcutaneous thromboprophylaxis with standard unfractionated heparin, without significant neurologic complications. In this context, guidelines recommend that subcutaneous thromboprophylaxis with standard unfractionated heparin does not contraindicate the use of neuraxial anesthesia. However, the platelet count should be assessed before the administration of neuraxial anesthesia or catheter removal in patients who have received standard unfractionated heparin for more than 4 days [92].

If oral anticoagulants (e.g., warfarin) are administered during pregnancy, it is usually replaced by LMWH or standard unfractionated heparin before the onset of labor. If a pregnant woman begins labor while she is still taking oral anticoagulants, the effects can be reversed by intramuscular administration of vitamin K. Because reversal of anticoagulation requires time for the synthesis of new procoagulants, acute reversal can be accomplished by the administration of 10 to 20 mL/kg of fresh frozen plasma [91].

Low-dose aspirin does not significantly prolong the bleeding time in pregnant women [95]. Therefore, there is no recommendation to obtain a bleeding time measurement in patients who have received low-dose aspirin during pregnancy. Moreover, a large number of women receiving low-dose aspirin therapy for the prevention or treatment of preeclampsia have undergone epidural analgesia for labor and delivery without complications [96].

Notably, the contraindication of regional anesthesia in pregnant women displaying mild or isolated abnormalities in blood coagulation tests is somewhat controversial. However, it is clear that the prophylactic administration of low-molecular-weight heparin is a clinical risk factor that warrants caution in the administration of neuraxial anesthesia. The anesthesiologist should weigh the risks and benefits of neuraxial anesthesia and general anesthesia for the individual patient. It is preferable not to administer neuraxial anesthesia to a patient with a persistent laboratory coagulation abnormality. However, in selected circumstances, neuraxial anesthesia may be offered to a patient with an isolated laboratory abnormality and no clinical evidence of coagulopathy. In such patients, frequent neurologic examinations should be performed to facilitate the early detection of an epidural hematoma during the postpartum period.

7. Contraindications to regional (neuraxial) anesthesia in obstetrics

Regional (neuraxial) anesthesia is usually considered the first choice for most cesarean delivery procedures. However, similarly to other non-obstetric procedures, some contraindications can be pointed out. Contraindications for neuraxial anesthesia in the obstetrics setting usually include the following: patient refusal or inability to cooperate, severe coagulopathy, uncorrected maternal hypovolemia or significant hemodynamic instability, increased intracranial pressure, skin or soft tissue infection at the site of needle puncture. Severe anatomical abnormalities of the spine could also be related to significant difficulties to provide neuraxial anesthesia. The often-cited relative contraindication of preexisting neurologic disease is not usually based on medical criteria but rather on legal considerations [97]. The anesthesiologist should always weigh the risks and benefits of neuraxial anesthesia for each patient.

8. Summary of the main recommendations in anesthesia for cesarean delivery: the anesthetic procedure can change obstetric outcomes?

8.1 Perianesthetic evaluation

- Before providing anesthesia care, conduct history a focused on relevant obstetric history, maternal health and anesthetic history;
- Brief physical examination focused on airway and heart and lung examination and back examination when neuraxial anesthesia is planned;
- Baseline blood pressure measurement (at least two measures);
- Order a platelet count, blood type, and cross-match based on a patient's history, physical examination, clinical signs, and anticipated hemorrhagic complications. Of note, a routine platelet count and blood cross-match are not necessary in the healthy parturient and uncomplicated parturients;

- Oral intake of modest amounts of clear liquids may be allowed for uncomplicated patient undergoing elective cesarean delivery up to 2 h before induction of anesthesia. Pregnant women with additional risk factors for aspiration may have further restrictions of oral intake, determined on a case-by-case basis. Women undergoing elective cesarean delivery should undergo a fasting period for solids of 6–8 h depending on the type of food ingested;
- In selected patients, consider preanesthetic administration of nonparticulate antacids (sodium citrate), H_2 receptor antagonists (ranitidine), and/or metoclopramide for aspiration prophylaxis;

8.2 Anesthesia for cesarean delivery

- Equipment and support personnel available in the delivery operating room should be comparable to those available in the main operating rooms;
- Equipment and support for the treatment of potential complications (e.g., failed intubation, hypotension, etc) should be available in the delivery operating room;
- Appropriate equipment and support personnel should be available to postoperative care for obstetric patients recovering from major neuraxial or general anesthesia;
- Neuraxial techniques are preferred to general anesthesia for most cesarean deliveries. The decision to use a particular anesthetic technique should be individualized based on anesthetic, obstetric, or fetal risk factors, the preferences of the patient, and the judgment of the anesthesiologist;
- If spinal anesthesia is chosen, pencil-point spinal needles should be used instead of cutting-bevel spinal needles;
- An indwelling epidural catheter may provide equivalent onset of anesthesia compared with initiation of spinal anesthesia for urgent cesarean delivery
- General anesthesia may be the most appropriate choice in some circumstances (e.g., profound fetal bradycardia, ruptured uterus, severe hemorrhage, severe placental abruption);
- Intravenous fluid preloading may be used to reduce the frequency of maternal hypotension following spinal anesthesia for cesarean delivery. However, initiation of spinal anesthesia should not be delayed to administer a fixed volume of intravenous fluid;
- Uterine displacement (usually left displacement) should be maintained until delivery regardless of the anesthetic technique used;
- Intravenous ephedrine and alpha$_1$-agonists (phenylephrine or metaraminol) are both acceptable drugs for treating hypotension during neuraxial anesthesia. In the absence of maternal bradycardia, alpha$_1$-agonists, particularly phenylephrine, may be preferable because of improved fetal acid-base status in uncomplicated pregnancies;

8.3 Recovery from cesarean delivery

- For postoperative analgesia after neuraxial anesthesia for cesarean delivery, neuraxial opioids are preferred over intermittent injections of parenteral opioids

9. References

[1] Berghella V, Baxter JK, Chauhan SP. Evidence-based surgery for cesarean delivery. Am J Obstet Gynecol 2005; 193:1607-1617.

[2] Pallasmaa N, Ekblad U, Gissler M. Severe maternal morbidity and the mode of delivery. Acta Obstet Gynecol Scand 2008; 87:662-668.
[3] Ecker JL, Frigoletto Jr FD. Cesarean delivery and the risk-benefit calculus. N Engl J Med 2007; 356:885-888.
[4] Rollins M, Lucero J. Overview of anesthetic considerations for Cesarean delivery. Br Med Bull 2012; 101: 105-125.
[5] Toledo P. What's new in obstetric anesthesia? The 2011 Gerard W. Ostheimer Lecture. Anesth Analg 2011; 113:1450-1458.
[6] American Society of Anesthesiologists Task Force on Obstetric Anesthesia. Practice guidelines for obstetric anesthesia: an updated report by the American Society of Anesthesiologists Task Force on Obstetric Anesthesia. Anesthesiology 2007; 106:843-863.
[7] Practice advisory for preanesthesia evaluation: an updated report by the american society of anesthesiologists task force on preanesthesia evaluation. Anesthesiology 2012; 116:522-538.
[8] Rosaeg OP, Yarnell RW, Lindsay MP. The obstetrical anaesthesia assessment clinic: A review of six years experience. Can J Anaesth 1993; 40:346-356.
[9] Rai MR, Lua SH, Popat M, et al. Antenatal anaesthetic assessment of high-risk pregnancy: A survey of UK practice. Int J Obstet Anesth 2005; 14:219-222.
[10] Broaddus BM, Chandrasekhar S. Informed consent in obstetric anesthesia. Anesth Analg 2011; 112:912-915.
[11] Lanigan C, Reynolds F. Risk information supplied by obstetric anaesthetists in Britain and Ireland to mothers awaiting elective caesarean section. Int J Obstet Anesth 1995; 4:7-13.
[12] Wong CA, McCarthy RJ, Fitzgerald PC, et al. Gastric emptying of water in obese pregnant women at term. Anesth Analg 2007; 105:751-755.
[13] Wong CA, Loffredi M, Ganchiff JN, et al. Gastric emptying of water in term pregnancy. Anesthesiology 2002; 96:1395-1400.
[14] Dewan DM, Floyd HM, Thistlewood JM, et al. Sodium citrate pretreatment in elective cesarean section patients. Anesth Analg 1985; 64:34-37.
[15] Cohen SE, Jasson J, Talafre ML. Does metoclopramide decrease the volume of gastric contents in patients undergoing cesarean section? Anesthesiology 1984; 61:604-607.
[16] Ewart MC, Yau G, Gin T, et al. A comparison of the effects of omeprazole and ranitidine on gastric secretion in women undergoing elective caesarean section. Anaesthesia 1990; 45:527-530.
[17] Yau G, Kan AF, Gin T, et al. A comparison of omeprazole and ranitidine for prophylaxis against aspiration pneumonitis in emergency caesarean section. Anaesthesia 1992; 47:101-104.
[18] Tsai PS, Huang CJ, Hung YC, et al. Effects on the Bispectral Index during elective caesarean section: A comparison of propofol and isoflurane. Acta Anaesthesiol Sin 2001; 39:17-22.
[19] Shibli KU, Russell IF. A survey of anaesthetic techniques used for caesarean section in the UK in 1997. Int J Obstet Anesth 2000; 9:160-167.
[20] Afolabi BB, Lesi FE, Merah NA. Regional versus general anaesthesia for caesarean section. Cochrane Database Syst Rev 2006; CD004350.
[21] Chestnut DH. Anesthesia and maternal mortality. Anesthesiology 1997; 86:273-276.

[22] Tsen LC, Pitner R, Camann WR. General anesthesia for cesarean section at a tertiary care hospital 1990-1995: Indications and implications. Int J Obstet Anesth 1998; 7:147-152.
[23] Morgan BM, Aulakh JM, Barker JP, et al. Anaesthetic morbidity following caesarean section under epidural or general anaesthesia. Lancet 1984; 1(8372):328-330.
[24] Hawkins JL, Koonin LM, Palmer SK, et al. Anesthesia-related deaths during obstetric delivery in the United States, 1979-1990. Anesthesiology 1997; 86:277-284.
[25] Hawkins JL, Chang J, Palmer SK, et al. Anesthesia-related maternal mortality in the United States: 1979-2002. Obstet Gynecol 2011;117:69-74.
[26] Hawthorne L, Wilson R, Lyons G, et al. Failed intubation revisited: 17-yr experience in a teaching maternity unit. Br J Anaesth 1996; 76:680-684.
[27] Mhyre JM, Riesner MN, Polley LS, et al. A series of anesthesia-related maternal deaths in Michigan, 1985-2003. Anesthesiology 2007; 106:1082-1084.
[28] Reynolds F, Seed PT. Anaesthesia for Caesarean section and neonatal acid-base status: A meta-analysis. Anaesthesia 2005; 60:636-653.
[29] Hawkins JL, Gibbs CP, Orleans M, et al. Obstetric anesthesia work force survey, 1981 versus 1992. Anesthesiology 1997; 87:135-143.
[30] Riley ET, Cohen SE, Macario A, et al. Spinal versus epidural anesthesia for cesarean section: A comparison of time efficiency, costs, charges, and complications. Anesth Analg 1995; 80:709-712.
[31] Corke BC, Datta S, Ostheimer GW, et al. Spinal anaesthesia for caesarean section. The influence of hypotension on neonatal outcome. Anaesthesia 1982; 37:658-662.
[32] Garry M, Davies S. Failure of regional blockade for caesarean section. Int J Obstet Anesth 2002; 11:9-12.
[33] Pan PH, Bogard TD, Owen MD. Incidence and characteristics of failures in obstetric neuraxial analgesia and anesthesia: A retrospective analysis of 19,259 deliveries. Int J Obstet Anesth 2004; 13:227-233.
[34] Kuhnert BR, Philipson EH, Pimental R, et al. Lidocaine disposition in mother, fetus, and neonate after spinal anesthesia. Anesth Analg 1986; 65:139-144.
[35] Bucklin BA, Hawkins JL, Anderson JR, et al. Obstetric anesthesia workforce survey: Twenty-year update. Anesthesiology 2005; 103:645-653.
[36] Choi PT, Galinski SE, Takeuchi L, et al. PDPH is a common complication of neuraxial blockade in parturients: A meta-analysis of obstetric studies. Can J Anaesth 2003; 50:460-9.
[37] Russell IF. Problems with a continuous spinal anaesthesia technique for caesarean section. Int J Obstet Anesth 2010; 19:124-125.
[38] Alonso E, Gilsanz F, Gredilla E, et al. Observational study of continuous spinal anesthesia with the catheter-over-needle technique for cesarean delivery. Int J Obstet Anesth 2009; 18:137-141.
[39] Brownridge P. Epidural and subarachnoid analgesia for elective caesarean section. Anaesthesia 1981; 36:70.
[40] Carrie LE, O'Sullivan G. Subarachnoid bupivacaine 0.5% for caesarean section. Eur J Anaesthesiol 1984; 1:275-283.
[41] Davies SJ, Paech MJ, Welch H, et al. Maternal experience during epidural or combined spinal-epidural anesthesia for cesarean section: A prospective, randomized trial. Anesth Analg 1997; 85:607-613.

[42] Yun EM, Marx GF, Santos AC. The effects of maternal position during induction of combined spinal-epidural anesthesia for cesarean delivery. Anesth Analg 1998; 87:614-618.

[43] McNaught AF, Stocks GM. Epidural volume extension and low-dose sequential combined spinal-epidural blockade: Two ways to reduce spinal dose requirement for caesarean section. Int J Obstet Anesth 2007; 16:346-353.

[44] Thoren T, Holmstrom B, Rawal N, et al. Sequential combined spinal-epidural block versus spinal block for cesarean section: Effects on maternal hypotension and neurobehavioral function of the newborn. Anesth Analg 1994; 78:1087-1092.

[45] Kucukguclu S, Unlugenc H, Gunenc F, et al. The influence of epidural volume extension on spinal block with hyperbaric or plain bupivacaine for Caesarean delivery. Eur J Anaesthesiol 2008; 25:307-313.

[46] Russell IF. Levels of anaesthesia and intraoperative pain at caesarean section under regional block. Int J Obstet Anesth 1995; 4:71-77.

[47] Russell IF. A comparison of cold, pinprick and touch for assessing the level of spinal block at caesarean section. Int J Obstet Anesth 2004; 13:146-152.

[48] Bourne TM, de Melo AE, Bastianpillai BA, et al. A survey of how British obstetric anaesthetists test regional anaesthesia before caesarean section. Anaesthesia 1997; 52:901-903.

[49] Burns SM, Barclay PM. Regional anaesthesia for Caesarean section. Curr Anaesth Crit Care 2000; 11:73-79.

[50] Garry M, Davies S. Failure of regional blockade for caesarean section. Int J Obstet Anesth 2002; 11:9-12.

[51] Kestin IG. Spinal anaesthesia in obstetrics. Br J Anaesth 1991; 66:596-607.

[52] Greene NM. Distribution of local anesthetic solutions within the subarachnoid space. Anesth Analg 1985; 64:715-730.

[53] Carvalho B, Durbin M, Drover DR, et al. The ED50 and ED95 of intrathecal isobaric bupivacaine with opioids for cesarean delivery. Anesthesiology 2005; 103:606-612.

[54] Sarvela PJ, Halonen PM, Korttila KT. Comparison of 9 mg of intrathecal plain and hyperbaric bupivacaine both with fentanyl for cesarean delivery. Anesth Analg 1999; 89:1257-1262.

[55] Vercauteren MP, Coppejans HC, Hoffmann VH, et al. Small-dose hyperbaric versus plain bupivacaine during spinal anesthesia for cesarean section. Anesth Analg 1998; 86:989-993.

[56] Ben-David B, Miller G, Gavriel R, et al. Low-dose bupivacaine-fentanyl spinal anesthesia for cesarean delivery. Reg Anesth Pain Med 2000; 25:235-239.

[57] Bryson GL, Macneil R, Jeyaraj LM, et al. Small dose spinal bupivacaine for Cesarean delivery does not reduce hypotension but accelerates motor recovery. Can J Anaesth 2007; 54:531-537.

[58] Sakura S, Sumi M, Kushizaki H, et al:. Concentration of lidocaine affects intensity of sensory block during lumbar epidural anesthesia. Anesth Analg 1999; 88:123-127.

[59] Kodali BS, Chandrasekhar S, Bulich LN, et al. Airway changes during labor and delivery. Anesthesiology 2008; 108:357-362.

[60] Zakowski MI, Ramanathan S, Baratta JB, et al. Electrocardiographic changes during cesarean section: A cause for concern?. Anesth Analg 1993; 76:162-167.

[61] Palmer CM, Norris MC, Giudici MC, et al. Incidence of electrocardiographic changes during cesarean delivery under regional anesthesia. Anesth Analg 1990; 70:36-43.

[62] Moran C, Ni Bhuinneain M, Geary M, et al. Myocardial ischaemia in normal patients undergoing elective Caesarean section: A peripartum assessment. Anaesthesia 2001; 56:1051-1058.

[63] Shen CL, Ho YY, Hung YC, et al. Arrhythmias during spinal anesthesia for Cesarean section. Can J Anaesth 2000; 47:393-397.

[64] Tully L, Gates S, Brocklehurst P, et al. Surgical techniques used during caesarean section operations: Results of a national survey of practice in the UK. Eur J Obstet Gynecol Reprod Biol 2002; 102:120-126.

[65] Auler JO Jr, Torres ML, Cardoso MM, et al. Clinical evaluation of the flotrac/Vigileo system for continuous cardiac output monitoring in patients undergoing regional anesthesia for elective cesarean section: a pilot study. Clinics (Sao Paulo) 2010; 65:793-798.

[66] Scott DB. Inferior vena caval occlusion in late pregnancy and its importance in anaesthesia. Br J Anaesth 1968; 40:120-128.

[67] Rout CC, Rocke DA, Levin J, et al. A reevaluation of the role of crystalloid preload in the prevention of hypotension associated with spinal anesthesia for elective cesarean section. Anesthesiology 1993; 79:262-269.

[68] Park GE, Hauch MA, Curlin F, et al. The effects of varying volumes of crystalloid administration before cesarean delivery on maternal hemodynamics and colloid osmotic pressure. Anesth Analg 1996; 83:299-303.

[69] Ueyama H, He YL, Tanigami H, et al. Effects of crystalloid and colloid preload on blood volume in the parturient undergoing spinal anesthesia for elective cesarean section. Anesthesiology 1999; 91:1571-1576.

[70] Caritis SN, Abouleish E, Edelstone DI, et al. Fetal acid-base state following spinal or epidural anesthesia for cesarean section. Obstet Gynecol 1980; 56:610-615.

[71] Kee WD, Khaw KS, Lee BB, et al. A dose-response study of prophylactic intravenous ephedrine for the prevention of hypotension during spinal anesthesia for cesarean delivery. Anesth Analg 2000; 90:1390-1395.

[72] Kee WD, Khaw KS, Ng FF. Prevention of hypotension during spinal anesthesia for cesarean delivery: An effective technique using combination phenylephrine infusion and crystalloid cohydration. Anesthesiology 2005; 103:744-750.

[73] Mangesi L, Hofmeyr GJ. Early compared with delayed oral fluids and food after caesarean section. Cochrane Database Syst Rev 2002.CD003516.

[74] Sharma KK, Mahmood TA, Smith NC. The short term effect of obstetric anaesthesia on bladder function. J Obstet Gynaecol 1994; 14:254-264.

[75] Liang CC, Chang SD, Chang YL, et al. Postpartum urinary retention after cesarean delivery. Int J Gynaecol Obstet 2007; 99:229-232.

[76] Onile TG, Kuti O, Orji EO, et al. A prospective randomized clinical trial of urethral catheter removal following elective cesarean delivery. Int J Gynaecol Obstet 2008; 102:267-270.

[77] Corke BC, Datta S, Ostheimer GW, et al. Spinal anaesthesia for Caesarean section: The influence of hypotension on neonatal outcome. Anaesthesia 1982; 37:658-662.

[78] Cyna AM, Andrew M, Emmett RS, et al. Techniques for preventing hypotension during spinal anaesthesia for caesarean section. Cochrane Database Syst Rev 2006.CD002251.
[79] Mark JB, Steele SM. Cardiovascular effects of spinal anesthesia. Int Anesthesiol Clin 1989; 27:31-39.
[80] Eappen S, Blinn A, Segal S. Incidence of epidural catheter replacement in parturients: A retrospective chart review. Int J Obstet Anesth 1998; 7:220-225.
[81] Balki M, Carvalho JC. Intraoperative nausea and vomiting during cesarean section under regional anesthesia. Int J Obstet Anesth 2005; 14:230-241.
[82] Kranke P, Eberhart LH, Gan TJ, et al. Algorithms for the prevention of postoperative nausea and vomiting: An efficacy and efficiency simulation. Eur J Anaesthesiol 2007; 24:856-867.
[83] American Academy of Pediatrics Committee on Drugs. The transfer of drugs and other chemicals into human milk. Pediatrics 2001; 108:776-789.
[84] Douglas MJ, Kim JH, Ross PL, et al. The effect of epinephrine in local anaesthetic on epidural morphine-induced pruritus. Can Anaesth Soc J 1986; 33:737-740.
[85] Szarvas S, Harmon D, Murphy D. Neuraxial opioid-induced pruritus: A review. J Clin Anesth 2003; 15:234-239.
[86] Yeh HM, Chen LK, Lin CJ, et al. Prophylactic intravenous ondansetron reduces the incidence of intrathecal morphine-induced pruritus in patients undergoing cesarean delivery. Anesth Analg 2000; 91:172-175.
[87] Kranke P, Eberhart LH, Rower N, et al. Pharmacological treatment of postoperative shivering: A quantitative systematic review of randomized controlled trials. Anesth Analg 2002; 94:453-460.
[88] Vandermeulen EP, Van Aken H, Vermylen J. Anticoagulants and spinal-epidural anesthesia. Anesth Analg 1994; 79:1165-1177.
[89] Loo CC, Dahlgren G, Irestedt L. Neurological complications in obstetric regional anaesthesia. Int J Obstet Anesth 2000; 9:99-124.
[90] Roqué H, Funai E, Lockwood CJ. von Willebrand disease and pregnancy. J Matern Fetal Med 2000; 9:257-266.
[91] Sharma SK. (2009). Hematologic and Coagulation Disorders. In Chestnut DH, Polley LS, Tsen LC, Wong CA (Eds.), Obstetric Anesthesia: Principles and Practice (pp. 943-957).
[92] Horlocker TT, Wedel DJ, Rowlingson JC, et al. Regional anestesia in the patient receiving antithrombotic or thrombolytic therapy (ASRA evidence-based guidelines). Reg Anesth Pain Med 2010; 35:64-101.
[93] Horlocker TT, Wedel DJ, Benzon H, et al: Regional anesthesia in the anticoagulated patient: Defining the risks. (The second ASRA Consensus Conference on Neuraxial Anesthesia and Anticoagulation.). Reg Anesth Pain Med 2003; 28:172-197.
[94] Horlocker TT, Wedel DJ. Neuraxial block and low-molecular-weight heparin: Balancing perioperative analgesia and thromboprophylaxis. Reg Anesth Pain Med 1998; 23:164-177.
[95] Williams HD, Howard R, O'Donnell N, et al. The effect of low dose aspirin on bleeding times. Anaesthesia 1993; 48:331-333.

[96] CLASP (Collaborative Low-dose Aspirin Study in Pregnancy) Collaborative Group. A randomized trial of low-dose aspirin for the prevention and treatment of pre-eclampsia among 9364 pregnant women. Lancet 1994; 343:619-629.

[97] Wong CA, Naveen N, Brown DL. (2009). Hematologic and Coagulation Disorders. In Chestnut DH, Polley LS, Tsen LC, Wong CA (Eds.), Obstetric Anesthesia: Principles and Practice (pp. 223-242).

6

Neurological Complications of Regional Anesthesia

José Ricardo V. Navarro[1], Javier Eslava-Schmalbach[2], Daniel P. R. Estupiñán[3] and Luis A. Carlos Leal[4]
[1]*School of Medicine, Universidad Nacional de Colombia and Obstetric Anesthesia Rotation, Instituto Maternoinfantil-Hospital La Victoria, Bogotá*
[2]*Clinical Research Institute, School of Medicine, Universidad Nacional de Colombia*
[3]*Anesthesiology, Universidad Nacional de Colombia, Bogotá,*
[4]*Surgery, Universidad Nacional de Colombia, Bogotá, Colombia*

"The man with ideal education not necessarily is the wise man, but that who loves the correct things".
Lin Yutang: Importance of life

1. Introduction

The difference between a complication and an adverse event is that a complication can occur directly or indirectly as a result of the procedure; whereas an adverse event must have three conditions: it is an injury not related to the patient's illness, it occurs involuntarily, and happens during medical care of the patient.

According to Philip R. Bromage, neurological complications and its sequels can be divided into three classes (1, 2):

- Neurological complications produced by non-anesthetic causes
- Complications related to underlying pathology in which regional anesthesia can be a contributing factor
- Neurological complications related to regional anesthesia

Nonanesthetic causes: a pre-existing condition can coincide with the administration of regional anesthesia; like neurological injuries caused by abnormal medullary circulation like diabetes mellitus, atherosclerosis, and cervical injury which can lead to the infarction of the anterior two thirds of the spinal cord producing flaccid paralysis of the lower limbs (3). A case report of an intervertebral disc prolapse has been described after labor in obstetric patients that had received epidural analgesia with subsequent paresthesia in the legs (4). Arterial cerebrovascular events during labor or puerperium can also produce neurological injuries (5). Cerebral venous thrombosis secondary to pregnancy hypercoagulability and stasis have been described most commonly in the first week postpartum (6). Neoplasia, tumors or medullary metastasis of breast or lung cancer can produce medullary compressions with an incidence of 70% of thoracic, 20% of lumbar and 10% of cervical level (7).

The occurrence of spontaneous epidural abscess attributed to bacteremia or a neighboring infectious process, although very infrequent (1/50.000 patients) (8) can coincide with a regional anesthesia or analgesic procedure.

Rare cases like viral infections of the spinal cord like Guillain-Barré syndrome, multiple sclerosis, etc. can occur insidiously in these patients (8).

The recommendation of many authors when an unusual neurological deficit appears (motor deficit of only one limb, fever and severe pain of the spine, general well-being compromise, etc.), is to perform an exhaustive exploration emphasizing the central nervous system to exclude a pre-existing or co-existing neurological disease along with the anesthetic procedure (9,10).

Causes in which anesthesia can be a contributing factor: epidural hematomas can happen in obstetric patients with abnormal coagulation or low platelets (11). Two axioms should always be considered in medicine: always consider the risk-benefit analysis, as not all procedures are indicated for all patients; and second the anesthetist should titrate all medications and therapeutic options.

There are other case reports of epidural hematomas in chronic renal failure (12), hepatic cirrhosis (13), and liver failure (14).

Peltola et al (15) emphasize that bleeding in the epidural, subdural or subarachnoid space as a result of a vascular injury with the needle or the catheter can worsen to become a compressive hematoma even though the coagulation tests of the patient are within normal limits.

The American Society of regional anesthesia (ASRA) (16), have made these recommendations (available online at www.asra.com) in patients with antiplatelet or anticoagulant therapy that require neuraxial regional anesthesia:

- Aspirin and NSAIDs do not increase the risk of spinal hematoma in neuraxial blocks
- Cox-2 inhibitors do not alter platelet function and do not contraindicate neuraxial regional anesthesia
- The risk of spinal hematoma in patients receiving thienopyridines (clopidogrel and ticlopidine) and GP IIb/IIIa platelet receptor antagonists like (abciximab, eptifibatide and tirofiban) is unknown. It is recommended that clopidogrel be suspended 7 days, ticlopidine 14 days, abciximab 24-48 hours, and eptifibatide 4-8 hours before neuraxial puncture
- The insertion of epidural or spinal catheters who are receiving at the same time anticoagulants and antiplatelet agents is contraindicated
- The prophylactic doses of low molecular weight heparins (LMWH) (enoxaparin 40 mg SC/day or dalteparin 5000 units/day) should be administered at least 12 hours before spinal or epidural puncture
- When full anti-coagulation is required with low molecular weight heparins (enoxaparin 1 mg/kg bid or dalteparin 120 units/kg bid) the neuraxis should not be accessed until after 24 hours of its last administration

- Removal of the epidural catheter should be performed at least 12 hours after the last dose of prophylactic LMWH. The administration of the next dose of LMWH should be administered at least two hours after removing the catheter
- If a single dose of LMWH is administered the epidural catheter can be kept in the postoperative period
- Cancel the prophylactic administration of two doses of LMWH per day or anticoagulant doses is not recommended when an epidural catheter is in place
- When the spinal or epidural puncture has been traumatic the next dose of LMWH should be delayed 24 hours
- In patients receiving warfarin, neuraxial blocks should not be performed unless it has been suspended and the INR is below 1.5. This is the INR recommended to remove an epidural catheter
- And INR should always be obtained when a single dose of warfarin has been administered 24 hours before surgery or if the patient has received a second dose
- Herbal medications do not seem to increase the risk of spinal hematoma in neuraxial anesthesia
- The new thrombin inhibitors and fundaparinux currently exert an unknown risk and the insertion of epidural catheters should be avoided when the patient is receiving these medications.

Among the distinct factors associated with increased risk of spinal hematoma with neuraxial blocks are: female sex, older age, patient and anesthesia related factors, traumatic insertion of the needle or catheter, epidural versus subarachnoid puncture, LMWH dose, twice a day LMWH, use of epidural catheter with LMWH, immediate preoperative, intraoperative or immediate postoperative LMWH administration, concomitant use of anticoagulants or antiplatelet agents in patients whose neuraxis is accessed (16).

Neuraxial hematomas usually locate in the epidural space because of the dilated epidural venous plexus, the absence of vessels in the subarachnoid space, and the fact that if there is subarachnoid bleeding the blood is diluted with the CSF and drained in the segmental vessels along the exiting spinal nerves. (17)

Chronic adhesive arachnoiditis is another condition with poor prognosis and multifactorial in nature (18). It presents as a severe meningeal inflammatory response to different agents (trauma, surgery, infections, tumors, etc.). Its prognosis depends on the extent and formation of septums and adhesions that can trap and collapse the spinal blood vessels, which compromise the spinal cord circulation. Some researchers have associated the appearance of this complication with the use of chemicals substances present as preservatives of anesthetic agents like benzyl alcohol, methylparaben, and sodium bisulfite (19). This author established epidemiologically that the arachnoiditis that occurs after a subarachnoid anesthesia is an extremely rare complication, and no direct association between this pathology in the use of local anesthetic has been proved; and currently with the asepsis, antisepsis, disposable equipment use, absence of preservatives in subarachnoid medications, and worldwide standardized doses and concentration of anesthetics, this complication has virtually disappeared (20).

The incidence of back pain with regional anesthesia is not different from that in patients with general anesthesia (2 %). Obstetric patients with or without regional analgesia or anesthesia have an incidence of up to 40% of back pain that can last 24 hours, and which worsens with ambulation (2).

Obstetric nerve palsies can happen with the positions maintained during labor and delivery, specifically compromising the nerves crossing the pelvic rim; many others are associated with cephalopelvic disproportion, difficult or instrumented deliveries. Up to 25% can occur in normal deliveries with an incidence between 1: 2100 to 1: 2600 births (2).

Neurological complications related to regional anesthesia: these complications range from superficial, transient and minor injuries to serious and severe injuries that can be permanent or even compromise the patient's life. In general these type of complications are very infrequent and it is important to recognize them to prevent them and treat them promptly in an appropriate way to guarantee more safety and comfort to the patient. Highlighting Dr. Bromage's words: "no anesthetic is completely safe and many failed to provide the unique set of conditions that epidural analgesia can provide" (2).

2. Failure in blocks or analgesia

Failed blocks are the most frequent cause of immediate and minor complications in regional anesthesia, up to 15% in epidurals in teaching hospitals, or 2.35% of failure among all regional anesthesia techniques as reported in Fundación Santa Fe de Bogotá (21). In world literature, the incidence ranges from 2.8% overall for all regional anesthesia techniques, up to 5 to 25% with techniques other than subarachnoid puncture (22).

Generally, the approach and technique of these procedures is considered easy, but it must be considered that it not only consists of placing a catheter in a specific position and injecting the anesthetic; the anesthesiologist must also be capable of deciding the type, concentration an adequate dose of the anesthetic, individualizing each patient according to the time, anesthetic level and surgical procedure to be performed. Failure in the block or analgesia is an event that is immediately identified as the patient will refer pain and the surgical procedure cannot be performed. Failed blocks should not be dealt by repeating the technique, as the injection of more anesthetic in the subarachnoid space can lead to morbidity because of the high concentration in a subarachnoid space (22).

Failure of block has not been well defined as some describe it as the inability to locate the space, and obtain cerebrospinal fluid (CSF) after three punctures, which suggests incapability of the anesthesiologist to identify the space and impossibility to administer a dose of anesthetic. Others extend the concept, including every case that requires the use of general anesthesia at any point during the anesthetic or the surgery (23).

The causes can be divided in three groups (23):

1. **Technical factors**: related to the selection of the needle in terms of type and gauge, the position and localization of the space by the anesthesiologist. Among these factors in anesthesia or analgesia it is important to consider that identifying the epidural space with air can produce outcomes as serious as tetraplegia; because of high doses of air injected in the subarachnoid space. In adult patients, this can produce headache, multiradicular or compressive medullary syndrome. When fluid is used instead of air, the main complication is the increase in anesthetic level (24). Other key issue in this

technique is the final location of the catheter, as it determines the distribution of the injected medications in the desired site so that complications like total spinal anesthetic, epidural venous puncture or spinal myoclonias do not happen, which represent 6.2% of all inserted catheters (25). In the obstetric patient usually the spinal catheter is not left in place in cesarean section and does not represent greater risks

a. Total spinal anesthetic

It is produced by the administration of the epidural anesthesia medication (20 to 30 ml in volume) in the subarachnoid space because of poor positioning of the catheter or the epidural needle rupturing the dura, which can extend desired lumbar block to an inadvertent cervical, brachial plexus and sacral roots block which produce clinical symptoms depending of the level reached. As the level is more cephalad, motor and sensitive block increases until the patient develops unconsciousness, respiratory arrest, severe hypotension and pupillary dilation which can lead to cerebral ischemia in total amnesia of the event (26). These events happen within a period of one to 5 min.

The treatment for this type of complication is to secure the airway with an orotracheal tube or supraglottic device, in case of unconsciousness and loss of airway reflexes; to provide immediate thoracic compressions and intravenous hemodynamic support including intravenous fluids like crystalloids (at least 1000 ml); the use of vasoconstrictors like ephedrine initially with 10 to 30 mg and then with a continuous infusion to maintain a systolic blood pressure about 100 mmHg and incremental doses of 0.3 mg of atropine to treat bradycardia; while the patient recovers from the anesthetic overdose. One maneuver that can help is to use a head down position 10 to 20° with minimal lateralization to improve venous return (26).

b. Epidural venous puncture (27)

This represents 9% of the complications related to catheter positioning and produces a dramatic effect on obstetric patients. There are five technical factors which reduce the incidence of this complication: the introduction of the catheter in lateral position decreases the risk from 11.9% to 6.7%; distending the space with air reduces it from 12.9% to 6.7%; using single hole needles reduces it from 10% to 6.8%; avoiding introducing the needle more than 6 cm reduces it from 12.9% to 6.4%; and using catheters lined with polyurethane instead of polyamide. These catheters not only decrease the risk of venous cannulization but also have a decreased incidence of paresthesias. The position and previous distention of the space with air are the most effective measures. The median or paramedian techniques, or the needles gauge 16 or 18 G have not demonstrated any protection.

c. Spinal myoclonus

These are focalized involuntary movements muscle groups in a patient with a spinal catheter. With myelography it has been shown to be produced by the persistent stimuli of the catheter on a nerve root or in the medullary conus, and is corrected with the repositioning of the catheter away from these nerves (28).

To avoid this type of complication that catheter's position can be verified with fluoroscopy which allows the detection of the spread of the fluid with anterior posterior or lateral projections and thus reposition it in the correct space (29); this can also allow the detection of internal knots and posterior complications like rupture within the space that require surgical treatment.

2. **Patient factors**: basically related with anatomical abnormalities during pregnancy or obesity which make these procedures more difficult because of changes in the spinal canal's anatomical conformation, tissues, skin, internal CSF distribution, etc.
3. **Factors of the anesthetic solution**: there are multiple factors related to these agents ranging from the adequate choice by the anesthesiologist individualizing each patient and procedure, to the production technique of the solutions by the different manufacturing companies and the storage methods throughout the time for an optimal effect. It is important to verify expiration date, administration route, and contraindications of these medications before used in the different techniques. An example of such happened in the case of duritis after the erroneous infusion of potassium chloride through a subarachnoid catheter for postoperative analgesia with serious impact on the patient's health like hemodynamic abnormalities, motor activity changes and a dramatic increase in blood pressure (30).

As each anesthetic procedure is individualized for each patient, the management of block or analgesia failure should be personalized according to the situation or to painful stimuli control achieved.

3. Traumatic puncture

3.1 Post dural puncture headache (PDPH)

It is one of the most common neurological complications in patients subject to regional anesthesia with a median incidence of 3% between epidural and spinals (31,32). It is more common in patients under 40 years old, basically in children under 10, with a difference in gender more commonly in women, mainly in obstetric patients (33,34), in whom the complication is more common producing an increase in hospital stay up to 49% (34). This complication depends on factors like the gauge and design of the selected catheter. There is currently a debate regarding the design of the needles, and it is believed that atraumatic needles could produce less injury in the dura mater (33) which can decrease PDPH, however some studies using electronic microscopy found that pencil point needles produced more trauma in the dura with more irregular borders and more edema which accelerates the closure of the orifice and thus reduces its incidence (33).

The headache can also appear after the insertion of the epidural catheter when it accidentally ruptures or injures the dura. Different studies have been done to decrease its incidence, among them one reveals that the use of fluid to verify the loss of resistance compared to air decreases the incidence. The risk difference was 0.015. In addition and according to this metanalysis, among obstetric patients, there were no significant differences between mediums (35). Pathophysiologically this phenomenon is explained by the loss of CSF which drains faster than produced, generating a difference in pressures and traction of the intracranial contents in upright position (36). The imbalance is generated from the orifice of the dura after the puncture, and a depends on its shape and size (36). It occurs in the first 15 to 48 hours after the puncture (33).

The main characteristic as its name suggests is the severe headache observed mainly with positional changes, and other symptoms that can occur are vomiting, nausea as well as sixth cranial nerve palsy which produces diplopia. It is important to perform an appropriate diagnosis as prolonged and intense headache after spinal anesthetics has been related to intracranial hemorrhage, meningitis, and subdural hematoma (37), for which it is important to identify any change in symptoms or the appearance of alarming signs like meningeal stigmata, photophobia, fever, focalization and seizures (34,35).

The development of new needles with smaller gauges has decreased its incidence (37). Different studies have shown that the incidence of this complication decreases clearly and statistically significant with both the decrease in gauge of the needle as well as the selection of needles that produce lesser trauma to the dura during insertion (Table 1) (36).

Needle	Gauge	Incidence PDPH
Quincke	22G	40%
Quincke	25G	25%
Quincke	26G	2-12%
Quincke	27G	2.7%
Whitacre	27G	0.37%
Punta de lapiz	27G	0.01 - 1.7%
Quincke	29G	< 2%

Source: table made by authors from data of: Mordecai M, Bruell S. Spinal anesthesia. Current Opinion in Anaesthesiology. 2005; 18: 527-33.

Table 1. Incidence of PDPH with needle gauge

The initial treatment of PDPH is conservative based on adequate hydration, intravenous boluses of normal saline, rest, anti-inflammatory analgesics, methylergonovine and caffeine in doses of 300 to 500 mg IV or ingestion of caffeinated beverages (33,34). However, it has been described that this syndrome can correct spontaneously up to 50% of the cases in five days, and 90% at 10 days (33). If this conservative treatment fails and the headache either is steady or is severe, an epidural blood patch can be applied in the puncture site. The volume described is of 10 to 20 mL of autologous blood injected in the same intervertebral space where the traumatic puncture was performed (33). Jeskins determined in a retrospective study, that the blood patch has a short term benefit, as in longer terms it did not reduce the pain symptoms. He determined that the success rate of the first blood patch was 33%, and of the second blood patch required by 29% of the patients who did not improve was 50% in treating long-term pain (37). It is important to recognize that if this treatment is ineffective, or if the headache worsens and other alarming signs appear, it is important to extend the studies to exclude other type of complications or basal conditions of the patient (34).

3.2 Nerve and root injury

This important complication is produced when the anesthesiologist inserts the catheter for the administration of anesthetic solutions through the nervous fibers, or nerve bundles or performs a high puncture (above L1) injuring spinal cord. When advancing too much a catheter in children, complications like pneumothorax or serious vascular injury can result (24). The studies revealed that the estimate of the intervertebral level by the anesthesiologist compared to MRI is poor, as only 29% was in the desired space, whereas 68% were 1 to 4 spaces above the level desired (38). During the insertion of the catheter to provide regional anesthesia it is not uncommon that patients complain of paresthesias or severe radicular pain. Cheney et al (39) reviewed the complaint database of the American Society of Anesthesiologists finding that 92% of the injuries were related to the technique and that patients complained about paresthesias and pain during insertion. This is why it is recommended to perform this type of anesthetic in awake patients, capable of communicating any anomaly or complaint that occurs during the anesthetic procedure (40). It is important to be aware of these complaints and to do an appropriate follow-up, as these are the symptoms associated with nerve injuries that can lead to sequelae if not treated appropriately. Auroy et al (41) found that two thirds of the patients with neurological complications described these symptoms during different periods of the anesthetic, and even though many anesthesiologists stopped the procedure when the symptoms appeared, the complication still happened, which do not allow the identification of when to stop the procedure.

It is difficult to calculate its incidence as the report of these cases is not very frequent (1), however some estimate an incidence of this 0.3 among 2500 (42). Other study revealed that the incidence of paresthesias during epidural catheter insertion increases with each additional dose, and the postoperative neurological deficit increased from 0.13% with a single dose to 0.66% with a continuous catheter, explained by the evidence of demyelination and inflammatory process adjacent to the catheter (43,44).

To avoid this type of complications an appropriate puncture site should be selected avoiding spaces where intervertebral discs protrusions could happen which can produce a tight canal (44), and to never puncture above L1 to L2 (45). Giebler et al. (46) noticed an incidence of 0.2% of postoperative radicular pain in patients with thoracic catheters. In obstetric patients difficulties are common, and identification of the puncture site is commonly erroneous as they cannot flex their knees on the abdomen which generates cephalization of the Tuffier line; in addition their hips are wider than their shoulders which alters the horizontal spine line (47). A new anatomical reference point for the identification of the intervertebral space has been radiologically described showing that the 10th intercostal arch is aligned to L2's spinous process. Others have used other imaging tools during puncture and regional anesthesia including fluoroscopy, with the disadvantage of subjecting the patient to radiation, to ultrasound, both demonstrating a reduction in complications as there is less needle manipulation to reach the desired space and performance of the puncture avoiding injuring any vascular or neurological structure (36,47).

The incidence of back pain after epidural anesthesia has been observed to be between 18 and 19% in rich retrospective studies (48, 49, 51) and between 21 and 53% in prospective studies (50, 51)

3.3 Lumbar pain and sacral numbness

There are multiple studies in obstetric patients that demonstrate that there is no real association between back pain and regional anesthesia, and have probably the same incidence of the obstetric population without any neuraxial intervention with a 63% risk of developing back pain during the first year postpartum (48-51).

Many reports have described patients presenting non specific dull back pain after neuraxial procedures for C-section that improve spontaneously within eight weeks without associated abnormalities like dysesthesias or motor abnormalities. This type of pain is known as sacral numbness. The ethiology of this type of pain is unknown (40).

4. Chemically related injury related

The susceptibility of the different nervous fibers is determined by their location, myelination and blood supply, as when they are exposed to a foreign substance in more perfused and higher degree of myelination areas, it is easier for it to be cleared. The nerves of the subarachnoid space are more prone to pharmacological neurotoxicity than those of the of the epidural space as the latter are covered by the pia matter, to a degree that case reports have been made where substances as thiopental, potassium chloride or antibiotics injected into the epidural space have not produced any neurological injury or sequelae. Sacral roots are also at risk from local injury because of their poor myelination. That is why when instilling foreign substances into space so well protected against infections and other antigens, it can be presumed that local anesthetics, catheter debris, glove talcum, etc. can generate immune responses that can produce direct allergic reactions both locally or systemically, like in the cauda equina syndrome, transient neurological syndrome, adhesive arachnoiditis and epidural fibrosis.

4.1 Cauda equina syndrome

The incidence of cauda equina syndrome is in general terms very low, 0.73 per 10,000 subarachnoid anesthetics (40). This syndrome is described after the administration of intrathecal lidocaine, after repeat administrations of anesthetic in failed spinal blocks, after unique doses or infusions during combined spinal anesthesia, or even with a single dose during the administration of a regional anesthesia because of very high concentrations medication in a small area of the medulla. It has also been associated with the very slow injection of medications, like what happens with the administration through microcatheters (33). This syndrome is characterized by bladder atony, loss of micturition control, and injury of the lower motoneuron including paraplegia (41).

4.2 Transient neurological syndrome (TNS)

Reported for the first time in 1993 by Schneider et al., it is characterized by transient pain in the lumbar area related more to intrathecal lidocaine rather than bupivacaine, happening after 12 hours of the complete resolution of an uncomplicated spinal anesthetic. The patient has a normal neurological examination and the main characteristic is that there are no sequelae. The pain is typically described as neural localized in the gluteal area and can extend to both inferior limbs, worsening at nights, improves with ambulation and NSAIDs, with a complete resolution in 90 % of the cases between the second and fifth postoperative day. Its incidence is lower in obstetric patients comparing to the general surgical population, (0 to 7% versus 10 to 30% respectively (44)), with a 1 to 7 ratio in patients who are administered lidocaine for spinal anesthesia (41). Its cause is still unknown, and is usually related more to the position during surgery and lidocaine administration (11.9%) independent of its concentration, than to bupivacaine (1.3%), prilocaine, procaine, or tetracaine (1.3%) (33). A randomized prospective study reported an incidence of 16% of TNS both in patients who received 5% hyperbaric lidocaine with epinephrine, and received 2%

isobaric lidocaine (*Pollock J.E., 1999)* (33). A higher incidence of TNS has been reported in patients undergoing arthroscopy or genitourinary surgery with hip flexion (24.3%) than in those operated supine position (3.1%) (52) (Table 2)

Transient neurological symptoms (TNS)			
Agent	**Presentation**	**Position**	**Approximate TNS incidence**
Lidocaine	**Hyperbaric 2%-5%**	**Lithotomy**	**30%-40%**
	Hyperbaric 0.5%-5%	**Knee arthroscopy**	**20%-30%**
	Hyperbaric 5%	**Supine/not specified**	**5%-10%**
Bupivacaine	**Isorbaric/Hyperbaric**	**Lithotomy / others**	**Rare**
Tetracaine	**Hyperbaric**	**General use**	**Rare**
	Hyperbaric + Fenilefrina	**Lower limbs/ perineum**	**12%**
Procaine	**Hyperbaric 5%**	**Knee arthroscopy**	**6%**
	Isorbaric 5%	**Supine/not specified**	**1%**
Mepivacaine	**Hyperbaric 4%**	**Lithotomy / others**	**30%-40%**
	Isorbaric 1.5%	**Knee arthroscopy**	**Rare**
Ropivacaine	**Hyperbaric 0.25%**	**Supine volunteers**	**Rare***
*** 30% of the volunteers reported persistent back pain but denied extended symptoms**			

Taken from: Hodgson PS, Liu SS. New Developements in Spinal Anesthesia. Anesthesiology Clinics of North America. 2000;18(2):235-49. Reproduced with permission.

Table 2. Transient neurological symptoms

Some anesthesiologists believe TNS is the beginning of a cauda equina síndrome, but there is no literature supporting this. The management is individualized for each patient (44).

4.3 Epidural fibrosis

Is a common complication associated with the prolonged use of infusion of epidural medications. Epidurography has demonstrated that this fibrosis produces an encapsulation, stenosis and deviation of the epidural space. It can be suspected in patients resistant to the analgesic effect when referring lumbar pain. JA Aldrete suggested that the etiology instead of being a direct reaction to the medications, corresponded to direct meningeal injury from the catheter (53).

5. Infections

Epidural anesthesia or analgesia comprise 5.5% of the patients with epidural spinal abscesses (54). The incidence of meningitis and spinal abscesses occur more frequently in patients with interventions injuring the dura and less in obstetric patients than the general population *(Sweden 1990–1999).* In fact it happens more in women after delivery with spinal analgesia, than with C-section. The incidence of meningitis in obstetric patients is estimated at one every 39,000 after neuraxial procedures compared to the global epidural abscesses incidence standing at one every 302,757 patients (55).

Two access routes can explain the infections: endogenously from the normal flora of the patient, or exogenously by colonization of microorganisms through the breach of the blood brain barrier after dural puncture (33). Schneeberger et al reported four cases of iatrogenic meningitis by the same anesthetist with recurring pharyngitis and who did not use facemask during the procedures (33). Reynolds reported in 2008, 16 epidural abscess all related to the use of epidural catheters observing higher risk with prolonged duration, poor asepsis and traumatic insertions (56). Holt et al. reported an epidural catheter colonization rate of 6%, with the *Staphylococcus* being the most common microorganism, which was confirmed by Steffek et al. (26).

5.1 Spinal abscess

Spinal abscesses have a mortality of 18% and an incidence of 1/250,000 healthy patients, which increases to 1/2000 in patients with diabetes or immunodeficiency. Epidural abscess symptoms appear 4 to 10 days after the insertion of the catheter. The most common symptoms are severe back pain which increasing intensity and general weakness associated with fever, nuchal rigidity, headache or local symptoms like rash, erythema and pruritus, with increasing white blood cell count, and erythrocyte sedimentation rate in the initial phases of the disease, or associated with radicular pain, sacrum numbness, reflects loss, and bladder dysfunction as late symptoms of the disease (44). The symptoms can progress as rapidly as weakness becoming paralysis of the lower limbs in less than 24 hours (33). Fluid may ooze from the catheter insertion site. The most common microorganism is *Staphylococcus aureus* from direct contamination of the skin or blood borne from the vagina. Treatment success is based on early suspicion and identification of the symptoms. The gold standard for diagnosis is magnetic resonance imaging with gadolinium, although either a myelogram or CAT scan can confirm the diagnosis. Lumbar puncture is contraindicated when an epidural abscess is suspected. The American Society of Regional Anesthesia and Pain Medicine recommend the use of chlorexidine and alcohol as the best antiseptic technique for regional anesthesia, accompanied by hand wash, jewelry watches and pendants removal, use of sterile gloves, gown and sterile drapes (41,45). In 1991, Du Pen et al determined the relative risk of infection related to the catheter use in cancer patients with chronic pain at one every 1702 days of catheter use, which decreases in half with the use of external percutaneous catheters (De Jong, 1994) (41). The management is basically the immediate removal of the catheter and the initiation of an aggressive antibiotic scheme. The recovery of neurological function depends on the severity and progression of the symptoms like with epidural hematomas (33).

5.2 Meningitis

The mortality of this type of infection can be as high as 30%. Teele et al showed 15% of meningitis in children with bacteremia who underwent lumbar puncture against 1% in those without it (56). The most common microorganism is *Streptococcus viridans* type *salivarius, sanguis and uberis* which colonize the upper respiratory, the female genital and gastrointestinal tract, and which grow rapidly in aqueous media like cerebrospinal fluid but not in conventional laboratory culture media. The main mechanism of transmission is poor antiseptic technique and saliva particles when not using facemask. Common symptoms are: fever, headache, photophobia, nausea, vomiting and nuchal rigidity. Other symptoms are confusion, lethargy, and positive Kernig sign. Laboratory diagnoses is made with a lumbar puncture which reveals an increase in proteins and white blood cells in the cerebrospinal fluid and a decrease in the glucose levels compared with blood levels and with special cultures for *S. viridans.* The first-line treatment is the use of vancomycin with third-generation cephalosporin, begun immediately with clinical suspicion, not waiting for laboratory confirmation. Even though some authors have reported antibiotic treatment with infusion pumps or intrathecal catheters to limit the infection without their removal after suspicion of an epidural abscess *(Boviatsis, 2004),* this is not true in meningitis where the removal of infectious pockets is mandatory. Another cause of meningitis is chemical agents which is difficult to differentiate from bacterial infection (41).

Patients with confirmed bacteremia or septicemia benefit much more from an epidural than a spinal technique, only if an antibiotic scheme has begun before the block with an adequate clinical response. An example of such is the study of Bader et al. sin 1990 who used regional anesthesia in 293 women with chorioamnionitis without any infectious complication, even though only 43 had antibiotic treatment (33).

There is not contraindication for regional anesthesia among HIV- infected obstetric patients. There is no evidence of accelerated disease progression in the rate of infectious or neurologic complications in the neuraxial anesthesia. In HIV patients 40% of patients have neuropathic symptoms, the neurological symptoms as aseptic meningitis, headache, or polyneuropathy are indistinguishable and not related with the regional anesthetic technique used (33). Antibiotic prophylaxis is recommended against *Staphylococcus* in this type of patients, as well as patients with cancer, myelodysplastic diseases, low white blood cell count, diabetes and other immunodeficiency scenarios. The identification of infections in these patients can be delayed because they do not develop general symptoms like fever or leukocytosis (56). In patients infected with herpes virus no increase in infections has been demonstrated (55).

5.3 Discitis

It is a rarer complication reported after injection of steroids in L2 L3 level as well L4-L5. It is related to an infection with *Pseudomona aeruginosa.* Specific intravenous treatment with antibiotic is recommended with good results (57).

5.4 Arachnoiditis

This complication can happen days, weeks, or months after anesthesia. It produces a progressive weakness until paraplegia, caused by meningitis, spinal trauma or neurotoxic chemicals. Most are idiopathic and can occur by medication errors during administration (58).

5.5 Epidural collection of CSF

There are case reports of symptoms similar to epidural hematoma where the cause of compression has been the collection of cerebrospinal fluid in the epidural space, initially presenting as a post puncture headache from the loss of subdural CSF that is collected in the epidural space. It is difficult to diagnose because the imaging techniques cannot differentiate between CSF, blood or pus. It is mainly a clinical diagnosis and can be managed conservatively without any neurological sequelae with the same treatment as a post dural puncture headache (33).

5.6 Intrathecal granuloma

It consists basically in the formation of a mass of inflammatory characteristics around insertion point of the catheter, believed to form from the activation of the mitogen activated protein kinase cascade triggered from high concentrations of opioid infusions.

The prevalence is not well known and is estimated at 0.1 to 5%.

The symptoms are severe pain that can be accompanied by neurological symptoms depending on its size. The gold standard for diagnosis MRI, diagnosed usually .5 to 72 months after the opioid infusion. If symptoms of neurologic compression appear the clinical suspicion increases (33).

6. Miscellaneous

6.1 Palsy of cranial nerves VI and VII

This can happen before or after a post dural puncture headache, and has been related to the Tuohy needle (24), with similar etiology, as it is produced by the traction of the nerve that occurs from a deficit of CSF. The most common palsy is of the sixth and seventh cranial nerves showing diplopia or hearing loss. It usually resolves spontaneously. A blood patch may be useful if administered before symptoms, afterwards it does not show any efficacy (58).

7. Conclusion

All procedures demand maximum patient care, for which international organizations like the WHO and PAHO recommend the surgical checklist and safe anesthetic for a safe patient (59).

Complications and associated injuries will continue to occur as there are many factors to consider, some of them as previously reviewed, depend on conditions not related to medical care; however, it is essential that the anesthesiologist have a role in the postoperative care when any incident, complication or adverse event occurs, that he reports it and practices an effective follow-up to improve the patient's recovery.

The obstetric patients with diabetes and obesity are increasing every day (60), for which the anesthesiologists should be prepared to face these challenges with the availability of proper equipment and supplies, surgical tables, medications, infusion pumps, specialized care units, etc. in order to provide proper and professional care to these patients.

The interest and respect of care provided will determine the patient's evolution both physically and mentally with the implications for or against the people who cared for him.

Many neurological sequelae are the result of a delayed diagnosis and treatment (61), and in some cases there is poor follow-up and induced healthcare requirements.

It's worth adding that in spite of the several complications described, their incidence is relatively low and hence, regional anesthesia as compared to general anesthesia, still the preferable anesthetic option among pregnant women undergoing cesarean section

8. References

[1] Bromage PR. Neurological complications of subarachnoid and epidural anaesthesia. Acta Anaesthesiol Scand 1997; 41: 439-444

[2] Bromage PR. Complicaciones y contraindicaciones. En Analgesia epidural. Salvat Editores. Barcelona-España. 1984; 14: 493-535

[3] Wikinski JA, Bollini C. Complicaciones neurológicas de origen no anestésico. En Complicaciones neurológicas de la anestesia regional periférica y central. Editorial médica Panamericana. Buenos Aires Argentina 1999; 5: 69-84

[4] Forster MR, Nimmo GR, Brown AG y col. Prolapsed intervertebral disc after epidural analgesia in labor. Anaesthesia 1996; 51: 773-775

[5] Amias AG. Cerebral vascular diseases in pregnancy. II: Occlusion. J Obst Gynecol 1956; 74: 844-855

[6] Bousser MG, Chiras J, Bories J y col. Cerebral venous thrombosis. A review of 38 cases. Stroke 1985; 16: 199-213

[7] Byrne TN. Spinal cord compressions from epidural metastases. N Engl J Med 1992; 327: 614-619

[8] Renck H. Neurological complications of central nerve blocks. Acta Anaesthesiol Scand. 1995; 39: 859-868

[9] Dahlgren N, Törnebrandnt K. Neurological complications after anaesthesia. A follow-up of 18.000 spinal and epidural anaesthetics performed over three years. Acta Anaesthesiol Scand 1995; 39: 872-880

[10] Lee JA, Atkinson RS. Punción Lumbar y analgesia espinal. Editorial Salvat. Barcelona España 1981: 183

[11] Naulty JS, Becker RA. Bloqueo del neuroeje para el parto por cesárea. En Analgesia y anestesia epidural y raquídea temas contemporáneos. Clínicas de Anestesia de Norteamérica. Nueva editorial Interamericana, México DF. 1992: 122

[12] Grajda S, Ekllis K, Arino P. Paraplegia following spinal anesthesia in a patient with renal failure. Reg Anesth 1989; 14: 155-157

[13] Morisaki H, Doi J, Ochiai R y col. Epidural hematoma after epidural anesthesia in a patient with hepathic cirrhosis. Anesth Analg 1995; 80: 1033-1035

[14] Laglia A, Fisenberg R, Weinstein P y Col. Spinal epidural hematoma after lumbar puncture in liver disease. Ann Intern Med 1978; 88: 515-516

[15] Peltola J, Sumelahti ML, Kumpulainen T y col. Spinal Epidural hematoma complicating diagnostic lumbar puncture (Letter). Lancet 1996; 347: (8994) 131

[16] Horlocker TT, Wedel DJ, Benzon H, et al. Regional anesthesia in the anticoagulated patient: defining the risks (the second ASRA Consensus Conference on Neuraxial Anesthesia and Anticoagulation). Reg Anesth Pain Med 2003; 28: 172-197.

[17] Ptaszynski A, Huntoon M. Complications of spinal injections. Techniques in Regional Anesthesia and Pain Management. 2007; 11: 122-132

[18] Wikinski JA, Arlía R, Torrieri A. Aracnoiditis adhesiva crónica y anestesia. ¿Causalidad, riesgo o fatalidad?. Rev Arg Anest. 1992; 50: 159-167

[19] Kane RE. Neurologic deficits following epidural or spinal anesthesia. Anest Analg 1981; 60: 150-161

[20] Wikinski JA, Bollini C. Complicaciones neurológicas asociadas con procesos predisponentes y la anestesia regional como factor contribuyente. EnComplicaciones neurológicas de la anestesia regional periférica y central. Editorial médica Panamericana. Buenos Aires Argentina 1999; 9: 152

[21] Degiovanni JC, Chaves A, Moyano J, Raffán F. Incidencia de complicaciones en anestesia regional, análisis en un hospital universitario. Estudio de corte transversal. Rev Col Anest. 2006; 34: 155-162.
[22] Ballantyne JC, Kupelnick B, Mcpeek B, Lau J. Does the evidence support the use of spinal and epidural anesthesia for surgery? Journal of Clinical Anesthesia. [Review Article]. 2005;17:382-91.
[23] Bouchacourt V. Causas de falla del bloqueo subaracnoideo; formas de evitarlas. Anestesia Analgesia Reanimacion. 2005; 20(1): 31-37.
[24] Giaufré E. Risk and complications of regional anaesthesia in children. Baillière's Clinical Anaesthesiology. 2000;14(4):659-71.
[25] Mhyre JM, Greenfield ML, Tsen LC, Polley IS. A systematic review of randomized controlled trials that evaluate strategies to avoid epidural vein cannulations during obstetric epidural catheter placement. Anesthesia and Analgesia. 2009; 108(4): 1232-42.
[26] Steffek M, Owczuk R, Szlyk-Augustyn M, Lasinska-Kowara M, Wujtewicz M. Total spinal anaesthesia as a complication of local anaesthetic test-dose administration through a epidural catheter. Acta Anaesthesiologica Scandinavica. [Case Report]. 2004; 48: 1211-15.
[27] Mannion D, Walker R. Extradural vein puncture: an avoidable complication. Anaesthesia. 1991;46: 581-87.
[28] Ford B, Pullman SL, Khandji A. Spinal myoclonus induced by an intrathecal catheter. Move disorders 1997;12:1042-45.
[29] Mcintyre P, Deer T, Hayek S. Complications of spinal infusion therapies. Techniques in Regional Anesthesia and Pain Management. 2007;11:183-92.
[30] Litz RJ, Kreinecker I, Hübler M, Albrecht DM. Inadvertent infusion of a high dose of potassium chloridre via toracic epidural catheter. European Journal of Anaesthesiology. 2001;18(10):695-9.
[31] Steel AC, Harrop-Griffiths W. Lumbar puncture and spinal anaesthesia. Anaesthesia and Intensive Care Medicine. 2006; 7(11): 418-21.
[32] Lybecker H, Andersen T, Nielsen H. Incidence and prediction of postdural puncture headache: A prospective study of 1021 spinal anesthetics. Anesth Analg 1990; 70: 389-394
[33] Horlocker TT. Complications of spinal and epidural anesthesia. Anesthesiology Clinics of North America. 2000; 18(2): 461-85.
[34] Stamer UM, Wulf H. Complications of obstetric anaesthesia. Current Opinion in Anaesthesiology. 2001;14:317-22.
[35] Schier R, Guerra D, Aguilar J, Pratt G, Hernández M, Boddu K. Epidural space identification: a metaanalysis of complications after air versus liquid as the medium for loss of resistance. Anesthesia and Analgesia. 2009; 109(6): 2012-2022.
[36] Mordecai M, Bruell S. Spinal anesthesia. Current Opinion in Anaesthesiology. 2005; 18: 527-33.
[37] Jeskins GD, Moore AS, Lewis M. Long-term morbidity following dural puncture in an obstetric population. Int J Obstet Anesth 2001; 10: 17-24.
[38] Wong CA. Nerve injuries after neuroaxial anesthesia and their medicolegal implications. Best Practice and Research clinical Obstetrics and Gynaecology. 2009;4:367-81.
[39] Cheney FW, Domino KB, Caplan RA, Posner KL. Nerve injury associated with anesthesia, a closed claims analysis. Anesthesiology. 1999; 90: 1062-1069.
[40] Faccenda KA, Finucane BT. Epidural block: technical aspects and complications. Current Opinion in Anaesthesiology. 2002; 15: 519-523.
[41] Ptaszynski A, Huntoon M. Complications of spinal injections. Techniques in Regional Anesthesia and Pain Management. 2007;11:122-32.

[42] Auroy Y, Narchi P, Messiah JM, et al. Serious Complications related to regional anesthesia. Anesthesiology 1997; 87: 479-486
[43] Yoshi WY, Rottman RL, Rosemblatt RM et al. Epidural catheter-induced traumatic radiculopathy in obstetrics. One center experience. Reg anesth 1994; 19: 132
[44] Brooks H, May A. Neurological complications following regional anaesthesia in obstetrics. British Journal of Anaesthesia. 2003;3(4):111-14.
[45] Myers RR, Sommer C. Methodology for spinal neurotoxicity studies. Reg anesth. 1993; 18: 439-447
[46] Giebler RM, Scherer RU, Peters J. Incidence of neurologic complications related with toracic epidural catheterization Anesthesiology. 1997;86:55-63.
[47] Greensmith JE, Murray WB. Complications of regonal anesthesia. Current Opinion in Anaesthesiology. 2006; 19: 531-537.
[48] Russell R, Groves P, Taub N, O´Dowd J, Reynolds F. Assessing long term backache after childbirth. BMJ. 1993; 306:1299-1303
[49] MacArthur C, Lewis M, Knox EG, Crawford JS. Epidural anaesthesia and long term backache after childbirth. BMJ. 1990; 301: 9-12
[50] Mackathur A, Macarthur C, Weeks S. Epidural anaesthesia and low back pain after delivery: a prospective cohort study. BMJ. 1995; 311:1336-1339
[51] Macarthur AJ, Macarthur C, Weeks S. Is Epidural Anesthesia in labor Associated with Chronic Low Back Pain? A Prospective Cohort Study. Anesthesia and Analgesia. 1997;85:1066-1070.
[52] Hodgson PS, Liu SS. New Developements in Spinal Anesthesia. Anesthesiology Clinics of North America. 2000;18(2):235-49.
[53] Aldrete JA. Epidural Fibrosis after permanent catheter insertion and infussion. Pain Symptom Manage 1995;10:624-31.
[54] Reihsaus E, Waldbaur H, Seeling W. Spinal epidural abscess: a meta-analysis of 915 patients. Neurosurgery. 2000;23(4):175-204.
[55] Reynolds F. Neurological infections after neuraxial anesthesia. Anesthesiology Clinics. 2008;26:23-52.
[56] Teele D, Dashefsky B, Rakusan T. Meningitis after Lumbar Puncture in Children with Bacteremia. New England Journal of Medicine. 1981;305:1079-81.
[57] Broadman I. Non-Steroidal antiinflamatory drugs, antiplateled medications and spinal axis anesthesia. Best Practice and Research Clinical Anaesthesiology. 2005;19(1):47-58.
[58] Aronson PL, Zonfrillo MR. Epidural Cerebrospinal Fluid Collection After Lumbar Puncture. Pediatric Emergency Care. 2009;25(7):467-8.
[59] Navarro R, Eslava J. La seguridad y la anestesia. En Memorias Curso Anual SCA 2008. Seguridad del paciente y prevención del error médico. Charlie´s Impresores. Sociedad Cundinamarquesa de Anestesiología (SCA). Bogotá-Colombia 2008: 9-10
[60] Navarro JR, Aldana JL, Eslava JH. Gestacional obesity as a determinant of general technique for caesarean delivery: a case report. Rev Fac Med Univ Nac de Colomb 2009; 57 (3): 281-286
[61] Navarro JR, Luqueta JA, Tejada E. Lesión nerviosa periférica secundaria a anestesia regional subaracnoidea en paciente ginecobstétrica. Reporte de caso. Rev Col Anest 2009; 37: 71-78

7

Caesarean Section and Maternal Obesity

Vicky O'Dwyer and Michael J. Turner
UCD Centre for Human Reproduction,
Coombe Women and Infants University Hospital
Ireland

1. Introduction

In developed countries in women of reproductive age an increase in obesity levels has been widely reported with an associated increase in maternal obesity (Yu et al, 2006, Heslehurst et al, 2008, Huda et al, 2010). Obesity in pregnancy is associated with an increased incidence of medical complications including gestational diabetes mellitus, pre-eclampsia and venous thromboembolism (Huda et al, 2010). As a result, in part, obesity is associated with a higher incidence of obstetric interventions such as caesarean section, as well as an increase in pregnancy complications including haemorrhage, infection and congenital malformations (Yu et al, 2006, Heslehurst, 2008). The World Health Organization criteria define a Body Mass Index (BMI) <18.5kg/m^2 as underweight, 18.5-24.9 as normal weight, 25.0-29.9 as overweight and > 29.9 as obese. Obesity can be further subcategorised into class one obese which is 30.0-34.9, class two 35.0-39.9 and class three >40.0.

2. Rising caesarean section rates

In 1985, the World Health Organization (WHO) concluded that the caesarean section (CS) rate in every region should account for 5-15% of all births (Lancet, 1985). Yet by 2006, the CS rate in high-income countries ranged from 14% in the Netherlands to 40% in Italy and Mexico (OECD, 2009). In Ireland, the CS rate now exceeds 26% (O'Dwyer and Turner, 2011).

The caesarean section rate in the United States (US) has increased further in the last 13 years. The CS rate increased from 21% in 1994 to 32% in 2007. When the CS rate was analysed by the US Department for Health and Human Sciences, the CS rate was found to increase in all ages, racial groups and gestations. This may be due to more conservative clinical practice and legal pressures (MacDorman et al, 2008).

In a 2007 meta-analysis examining strategies to reduce the CS rate, audit and feedback and a multifaceted approach were found to reduce the CS rate without compromising maternal and fetal outcomes. Multifaceted strategies included the use of clinical guidelines, hospital payment policies, malpractice reform and identification of barriers to change. However, WHO has since finessed its position on CS rates by stating that the most important issue is that every woman who needs a CS should have one. It acknowledges that there is little scientific evidence to support a 15% CS rate (Chaillet and Dumont, 2007).

3. Rising obesity levels and rising caesarean section rates

With rising adult obesity levels there has been an associated increase in maternal obesity. A Scottish study found that the prevalence of obesity had increased from 9.4% to 18.9% over a 12 year period (Kanagalingam et al, 2005). In other studies in Britain and Ireland, nearly a fifth of women booking for antenatal care were obese (Fattah et al, 2010; CMACE 2010). The severity of obesity is also increasing. Based on the WHO sub-categorisation of obesity, a recent UK national audit of pregnant women found that 5.0% had Class 2 or moderate obesity and 2.0% had Class 3 or severe obesity (CMACE, 2010).

Rising levels of obesity in women of child-bearing age and gestational weight gain have been reported which has implications for the woman's lifelong health as well as for the pregnancy itself (Sherrard et al, 2007). In the US concerns are so great that the Institute of Medicine (IOM) has published new guidelines for weight gain during pregnancy (IOM, 2009). The new 2009 guidelines are based on the WHO BMI categories with a specific, relatively narrow range of recommended gain for obese mothers of 5.0 – 9.0 kgs.

Numerous studies have reported an association between maternal obesity and an increased CS rate (Weiss et al, 2004; Cedergren et al, 2004; Rode et al, 2005). It has been estimated that each 1% decrease in the number of obese mothers in the United States would translate into 16,000 fewer CS per annum.

There have been three recent meta-analyses which studied the issue of obesity and caesarean section. In the 2007 analysis, the risk of CS overall was increased by 2.05 (95% CI 1.86-2.27) in obese women, and 2.89 (95% CI 2.28-3.79) in morbidly obese women (Chu et al, 2007).The 2008 meta-analysis found that the overall CS was twice as high in the obese BMI category compared with the ideal BMI (MacDorman et al, 2008). The increase was significant for emergency sections (n=6 studies), but not for elective sections (n=3 studies). In the 2009 systematic review and meta-analysis of 11 cohort studies, the risk of CS was increased by 2.26 (95% CI 2.04-2.51) in obese women and by 3.38 (95% CI 2.49-4.57) in morbidly obese women compared with women with a normal BMI (Poobalan et al, 2009). This study was confined to primigravidas. There was an increase in both elective (OR 1.87) and emergency CS (OR 2.23) in the obese women.

A 2011 study found that maternal obesity, based on accurate calculation of BMI in the first trimester, was associated with an increase in emergency CS in primigravidas and an increase in elective CS in multigravidas (O'Dwyer et al, 2011). The increase in emergency CS in obese primigravidas was associated with induction of labour and a high rate of CS for fetal distress. The increase in elective CS in multigravidas was associated with a high rate of repeat elective CS.

4. Pre-conceptual counselling for obese women

Pre-pregnancy lifestyle changes including a healthy diet and exercise should be advised. If obese women lose weight prior to pregnancy this can prevent some of the pregnancy complications associated with obesity including neural tube defects and miscarriage. Obese women have a higher risk of neural tube defects (Rasmussen et al, 2008). Therefore it has been recommended that they start high dose folic acid supplementation pre-pregnancy (CMACE, 2010).

It has been reported that maternal obesity is associated with an increased risk of spontaneous miscarriage after spontaneous and assisted conception (Metwally et al, 2008). Increased rates of miscarriage also occur in obese women with polycystic ovarian syndrome (Lashen et al, 2004; Bellver et al, 2003). In a Finish study the miscarriage rate was found to be higher at the extremes of weight compared with normal weight women (Veleva et al, 2008). In a study examining the probability of pregnancy after assisted reproduction the odds ratio was 0.73 for obese Class 1 women and 0.5 for obese Class 2-3 women, compared with women in the normal BMI category (Wang et al, 2000; 2002).

Recurrent miscarriage is defined as three consecutive miscarriages. It affects 1% of couples. In a study of 491 women with a history of recurrent miscarriage the miscarriage rates in subsequent pregnancies were higher in obese women compared with normal weight women (Metwally et al, 2010). In another study the risk of recurrent miscarriage was four times higher in obese women compared with normal weight controls. Diabetes mellitus is a known cause of recurrent miscarriage but, in this study the prevalence was low in obese women and it did not explain their higher risk of miscarriage (Lashen et al, 2004).

5. Pregnancy after bariatric surgery

Pregnancy after bariatric surgery is safe once a woman's weight has stabilised, usually 1 -2 years after surgery. Antenatal care should include monitoring nutrition and appropriate gestational weight gain in these women (Karmon et al, 2008). The risk of maternal and neonatal adverse outcomes is lower in women post bariatric surgery than in obese women. In a systematic review of pregnancy after bariatric surgery there were lower rates of gestational diabetes mellitus, pre-eclampsia, low birth weight babies and macrosomia among women after bariatric surgery compared with obese women (Maggard et al, 2008).

A caesarean section is not required for delivery after bariatric surgery. The risk of caesarean section may be lower due to the lower risk of pregnancy complications in women after bariatric surgery compared with obese women. However, some studies have reported a higher risk of caesarean section in women after bariatric surgery. In a study period of 159,210 deliveries, of which 298 deliveries (0.2%) occurred in patients with previous bariatric surgery there were higher rates of CS among the bariatric operation group (25.2% vs 12.2%; odds ratios, 2.4; 95% confidence interval, 1.9-3.1; $p<0.001$) (Sheiner et al, 2004).

6. Antenatal care for the obese woman

Hypertension in pregnancy, including pre-eclampsia, occurs in almost 8% of pregnancies and is an important cause of pregnancy complications for both mother and baby. Pre-eclampsia is defined as hypertension (a systolic blood pressure of > 140 mmHg and/or a diastolic blood pressure of > 90 mmHg) measured on at least two separate occasions at least 6 hours apart with proteinuria (> 300 mg over 24 hours) after 20 weeks gestation. Epidemiological reviews have reported an association between pre-eclampsia and maternal obesity, based on a Body Mass Index (BMI) > 29.9kg/m^2 (Weiss et al, 2004; Abenheim et al, 2007).

To avoid misdiagnosing pregnancy-induced hypertension or pre-eclampsia women with a mid-arm circumference (MAC) >33cm should have their blood pressure measured with a large cuff. Previous studies have reported a MAC >33cm in 44% of class 1 (BMI < 35kg/m2) obese women and 100% of class 2-3 (BMI ≥ 35 kg/m2) obese women (Hogan et al, 2010). There is a higher rate of caesarean section in women with pre-eclampsia probably due to a higher rate of induction of labour (Kim et al, 2010). It is highly desirable that a CS for an unsuccessful labour induction is avoided in obese women especially if the induction may have been medically unnecessary. Therefore it is important that blood pressure is measured accurately in obese women.

Gestational Diabetes Mellitus (GDM) affects 1.1-14.3% of the pregnant population depending on the population studied and on the diagnostic criteria used (SOGC, 2002; Reece et al, 2009; Torloni et al, 2009). There is a higher rate of induction of labour and caesarean section in women with GDM. Previous studies have reported an association between increased rates of Gestational Diabetes Mellitus (GDM) and maternal obesity, based on a Body Mass Index (BMI) categorisation > 29.9kg/m^2. In a meta-analysis of 20 studies, the risk of developing GDM was about two, four and eight times higher among overweight, obese and severely obese women (Chu et al, 2007). Obese women should be offered a glucose tolerance test (GTT) at 24-28 weeks in countries where selective screening for GDM is performed (NICE, 2002). By identifying women with gestational diabetes the risk of neonatal mortality and morbidity such as congenital abnormalities, macrosomia, hypoglycaemia and jaundice may be reduced. There are, however, no studies that show that the diagnosis and treatment of GDM in obese women avoids the need for CS. Ideally, women should avoid prepregnancy obesity which may prevent the development of PET and GDM.

The HAPO study (2008) found an association between maternal hyperglycaemia and the rate of caesarean delivery and separately, gestational diabetes has been shown to be an independent risk factor for caesarean delivery (Rosenberg, 2005). However, others argue that obesity is an independent risk factor for caesarean section even when GDM is considered a confounder (Sebire et al, 2001; Ehrenberg et al, 2004; Rosenberg, 2005). Numerous studies have demonstrated pregestational diabetes to be independent risk factor for caesarean delivery (Sebire et al, 2001; Ray et al, 2001; Rosenberg, 2005). The complex interaction of obesity, diabetes, insulin resistance and the inflammatory milieu during pregnancy is the subject of ongoing research and these factors may have an effect on the progression of labour (Hauguel-de Mouzon, 2006; Chu, 2007; Schmatz, 2010). Ethnicity is also associated with the rate of caesarean delivery and studies have shown higher caesarean section rates in women of African descent (Rosenberg et al, 2005; Bragg et al, 2010).

There is an increased risk of congenital abnormalities, including neural tube defects, cardiac abnormalities and gastrointestinal anomalies in obese women compared to those with a normal BMI (Rasmussen et al, 2008; Waller et al, 2007). Detection of these anomalies is, however, more challenging in obese women (Paldini, 2009). This is due to poor visualisation of fetal anatomy because of the impaired acoustic window. The impaired acoustic window is due to the depth of insonation required and the absorption of energy by adipose tissue. Structures with low impedance such as the heart, kidneys, lips and cerebellum are difficult to visulaise. Despite technical advances such as lower emission frequencies, harmonic imaging and speckle reduction ultrasound imaging in obese women remains challenging.

7. Intrapartum care for the obese woman

In labour external abdominal fetal heart monitoring is hindered by the amount of subcutaneous tissue between the cardiotocograph and the uterus. Fetal scalp electrodes are often used instead of external monitoring when continuous fetal surveillance is required. In a recent review of intrapartum care for morbidly obese women there was a higher rate of invasive fetal monitoring and difficulty monitoring uterine contractions in the morbidly obese group compared with normal weight controls. Furthermore, fetal blood sampling can be challenging in obese women. Previous studies have described the technical difficulty and longer duration required to perform a fetal blood sampling (FBS) in obese women. There was also a higher rate of difficulty with vaginal examinations due to poor access to the perineum in the morbidly obese women (Ray et al, 2008).

Ideally morbidly obese women should be reviewed in an anaesthetic clinic as part of their antenatal care to access the possibility of peripheral venous access, regional and general anaesthesia. The anaesthetist on duty should also be informed when a morbidly obese woman presents in established labour. Peripheral venous access should be established early in labour. An epidural catheter should be placed early in labour in morbidly obese women so that there is no delay if an emergency caesarean section is required.

Induction of labour is known to be associated with a higher risk of caesarean section than spontaneous labour, especially in primigravidas (Seyb et al, 1990). Other studies have described a higher rate of failed induction and dystocia in labour for overweight and obese women compared with normal weight women (Yu et al, 2006; Vahration et al, 2003). In a Liverpool study of labour following induction for prolonged pregnancy the caesarean section rate was 38.7% in obese primigravidas compared with 23.8% in normal weight primigravidas (Arrowsmith et al, 2011).

8. Postpartum care

Obese women are less likely to intend, initiate and continue breastfeeding (Amir and Donath, 2007). Thus, obese women may need extra support after caesarean delivery with breastfeeding in the hospital and following discharge home (Mok et al, 2008).

Before discharging an obese woman home it is also a good opportunity for lifestyle advice and prepregnancy counselling for the future. A good diet and an exercise programme to lose weight postnatally are important.

Ideally obese women should optimise their weight before conceiving again. They should be advised that high dose folic acid is required to minimise the increased risk of neural tube defects associated with the low serum folate levels in obese women. Smoking cessation should also be advised.

It is important that obese women with gestational diabetes attend for their 6 week postnatal glucose tolerance test to identify those with type 2 diabetes mellitus. However, it is well described that attendance for postnatal glucose tolerance testing is poor (Russell et al, 2006; Persson et al, 2009). Obese women should be informed that even in the presence of a negative postnatal GTT they are at increased risk of type 2 diabetes later in life and that weight loss can reduce this risk.

9. Technical challenges of caesarean section in obese women

Ideally obese women should have an anaesthetic consultation before delivery as they are at high risk of complications due to obesity and medical co-morbidities. Obese women have higher rates of failure of epidural insertion, difficulty with inserting peripheral venous access, failed intubation and higher risk of aspiration (Yu et al, 2006). Regional anaesthesia in the obese can be technically challenging because of difficulties in identifying the usual bony landmarks. Ultrasound has been successfully used in the obese to help identify the epidural space and reduce the need for general anaesthesia (Adam & Murphy, 2000).

Special operating tables are required for morbidly obese women. It may be difficult to transfer an obese woman in a manner that is safe for both her and staff, and thus a hoist may be necessary. Surgery in the obese parturient can be challenging and requires a number of assistants with the increased use of retractors. The placement of the incision should be made at a site that will minimise the risk of wound infection. Vertical skin incisions should be avoided when possible. In a study of morbidly obese women undergoing primary caesarean section those who had a vertical skin incision had a higher rate of wound infection (OR 12.1, $p<0.001$) compared with a transverse skin incision (Wall et al, 2003).

10. Risks of caesarean section in obese women

One of the top ten recommendations from the Confidential Enquiries into Maternal and Child Health (CEMACH) report launched in 2007 refers to caesarean section. It states that whilst recognising that for some mothers and/or their babies' caesarean section (CS) may be the safest mode of delivery, however, mothers must be advised that caesarean section is not a risk-free procedure and can cause problems in current and future pregnancies. There are a number of complications associated with caesarean section and the risk of these complications is increased in obese women. Caesarean section is associated with haemorrhage, infection, damage to viscera, anaesthetic complications and long-term complications such as placenta accreta. In the 2008 meta-analysis of obstetric outcomes and obesity there was an increased risk of wound infection, endometritis and urinary tract infection for obese and morbidly obese women compared with those in the normal BMI category (Heslehurst et al, 2008). Another risk factor for postcaesarean section infectious morbidity is emergency caesarean sections, especially following a trial of labour or prolonged rupture of membranes. In a review of 81 clinical trials examining antibiotic prophylaxis for women undergoing caesarean section the reduction in endometritis and wound infection was significant enough to recommend routine antibiotic prophylaxis for these women (Smaill and Hofmeyr, 2002). In a review of 58 controlled trials, the use of routine antibiotic prophylaxis was not only found to decrease the risk of wound infection by 50-70% but also to decrease the cost of postnatal care by between £1300 and £3900/100 caesarean sections (Mugford et al, 1989). There is considerable variation in the timing of prophylactic antibiotic administration among surgical patients. In an American study there was a lower rate of infection among patients who received prophylactic antibiotics in the two hours prior to suregery (Classen et al, 1992). It is now recommended that antibiotic prophylaxis is given prior to skin incision. In an American study there was a decrease in infectious morbidity women who received cefazolin prior to skin incision compared to those who received cefazolin at cord clamping (relative risk [RR] = 0.4, 95% confidence interval

[CI] 0.18 to 0.87). In addition to this, studies recommend a higher dose of antibiotic prophylaxis for obese women undergoing caesarean section (ACOG, 2011).

The risk of complications increases with the number of repeat caesarean sections performed. (Silver et al, 2006). Bladder and bowel injury can occur at the time of caesarean section. Injury to the gastrointestinal tract occurs in 1 in 1300 caesarean deliveries. Increased pain medication requirement and longer hospital stay occur following caesarean section compared with vaginal delivery. Maternal obesity is also associated with a longer duration of hospital stay (Galtier-Dereure et al, 2000). Therefore, it is not surprising that maternal obesity has been associated with an increase in the use of healthcare resources (Heslehurst, 2008; Rowlands, 2010).

11. Thromboprophylaxis for obese women undergoing caesarean section

Pulmonary embolism (PE) is the leading cause of direct maternal death in the UK and the developed world (CMACE, 2001; Bourjeily et al, 2010). Maternal obesity has been associated with an increased risk of venous thromboembolism (VTE) (Bourjeily et al, 2010). A BMI > 29.9 kg/m^2 in early pregnancy is considered a moderate risk factor for VTE postpartum. An elective caesarean section is associated with twice the risk of the VTE risk postpartum when compared with a vaginal delivery, and an emergency caesarean section is associated with a four-fold increase in risk of VTE (RCOG, 2009).

There is scant evidence about the optimum administration of low molecular weight heparins (LMWH) to women during pregnancy and in the postpartum period (Tooher at al, 2010). Significant physiological changes occur during pregnancy and may last up to six weeks postnatally, thus the efficacy of LMWH doses which are based on studies of the non-pregnant population are unpredictable. Some evidence, for example, suggests that pregnancy affects the pharmacokinetics of tinzaparin (Norris et al, 2004). While the relative safety of LMWH use has been established, there is little evidence to guide the appropriate prophylactic dose in pregnancy and postpartum. Current guidelines by the Royal College of Obstetricians and Gynaecologists (RCOG) indicate suitable doses during pregnancy and the postpartum period. Suboptimal thromboprophylaxis in obese women has been described in a recent large scale study conducted by CMACE (CMACE, 2010).

12. Medication dosage in obese patients

Few studies have examined increased medication costs in obese populations. An Italian study detailing medication costs in 2622 patients showed that the obese group required more prescriptions annually with a 153% increase in annual medication cost over the normal weight group (Esposti et al, 2006). Another study found obesity resulted in a 47% increase in pharmacy claims by state employees in Arkansas (Hill et al, 2009).

There is an even greater dearth of information on obesity in pregnancy and the associated medication usage. A study investigating the influence of maternal obesity on healthcare costs for minor complications found an increase in the use of sodium alginate, insulin and anti-hypertensives (Denison et al (2009). However, the usage of these medications is most likely increased in obese patients whether they are pregnant or not. An increase in outpatient medication dispensed from community pharmacies has also been reported in obese women (Chu et al, 2008).

Antenatal medication usage is associated with increasing BMI. This appears to be related to the increase in complications during pregnancy with maternal obesity. A large population study involving 19,538 pregnancies in the USA describes an association between increased outpatient medication usage and increasing BMI (Chu et al, 2008). It also identified an increase in the total and postpartum length of hospital stay in women with an increased BMI. The effect of increased BMI on length of hospital stay was independent of the mode of delivery or the presence of a high-risk obstetric condition (diabetes mellitus, hypertension), but was not a significant factor when the authors adjusted for both.

13. Long-term consequences of caesarean section in obese women

Trial of labour after caesarean delivery (TOLAC) is a reasonable option for many women (Scott, 2011). In the US the increase in the caesarean section rate can be partly attributed to the fall in the vaginal birth after caesarean section (VBAC) rate (Mac Dorman et al, 2007). The success rate for a planned trial of labour for women with one prior caesarean is approximately 75%. It is positively influenced by a history of a vaginal delivery prior to caesarean section or a previous VBAC, spontaneous onset of labour, a baby weighing between 2.5 and 4kg and not requiring oxytocin augmentation in labour. A BMI ≥ 30 kg/m^2 has a negative influence on the success rate. In a retrospective cohort study of 8,246 singleton pregnancies in Dublin, the overall caesarean section (CS) rate was 45.3% in women with morbid obesity (BMI > 39.9 kg/m2) compared with 14.4% in women with a normal BMI ($p<0.001$). Morbid obesity was associated with an increase in both elective and emergency caesarean sections, and a decrease in vaginal birth after caesarean section (VBAC) compared with a normal BMI (25.0% vs. 63.5% $p<0.001$) (Farah et al, 2009).

There is higher maternal and neonatal morbidity associated with a failed trial of labour compared with an elective repeat caesarean section (Landon et al, 2004). The risk of uterine rupture is 0.5% for women with one prior lower transverse uterine incision. Certain practices can be used to minimise the risk of adverse outcomes in these women including uterine rupture. These include the use of colour coded partograms to highlight when a woman has a prior caesarean section, avoiding prostaglandin to induce labour and careful use of oxytocin to induce or augment labour (Turner, 2002).

With rising caesarean section rates the incidence of abnormal placentation is increasing. Abnormal placentation is a known risk factor for major obstetric haemorrhage and maternal morbidity and mortality (Turner et al, 2010). Thus, the CEMACH report also recommends that women who have had a previous caesarean section must have placental localisation in their current pregnancy to exclude placenta praevia and if present, further investigation to try to identify praevia accreta and enable the development of safe management strategies.

In a study of 97,799 women, in those who had a prior caesarean section the risk of placenta praevia was 0.26% with an unscarred uterus and increased almost linearly with the number of prior caesarean sections to 10% in patients with four or more. Patients presenting with a placenta praevia and an unscarred uterus had a 5% risk of clinical placenta accreta. With a placenta praevia and one previous caesarean section, the risk of placenta accreta was 24% (Clark et al, 1985). Another study of 41,206 women found that, in patients with placenta praevia the risk of accreta is 8 times greater with scarred uterus compared to unscarred uterus with placenta praevia. Furthermore, there was a higher risk of hysterectomy in 10% and 66% in women with placenta praevia and accreta and a prior CS (Chattopadhyay et al, 1993).

14. Conclusions

During the twentieth century there were remarkable advances in obstetric practices which led to great improvements in clinical outcomes for women and their offspring, particularly in well-resourced countries. However, overabundance of food and changes in physical activity levels in these countries have also led to rising levels of maternal obesity which risk reversing the improvements achieved in maternal and fetal outcomes. Caesarean delivery in the morbidly obese woman is both clinically and technically challenging. Ideally, morbid obesity is a modifiable risk factor that should be modified prepregnancy. If morbid obesity is present in early pregnancy, a comprehensive multidisciplinary plan is mandated to prevent complications and minimise interventions.

15. References

Abenheim HA, Kinch RA, Morin L, Benjamin A, Usher R. Effect of prepregnancy body mass index categories on obstetrical and neonatal outcomes Arch Gynecol Obstet 2007; 275: 39-43.

ACOG Practice Bulletin No. 120. Use of prophylactic antibiotics in labor and delivery. Obstet Gynecol. 2011; 117: 1472-83.

Adams JP, Murphy PG. Obesity in anaesthesia and intensive care. *Br J Anaesth* 2000; 85: 91–108.

Amir LH, Donath S. A systematic review of maternal obesity and breastfeeding intention, initiation and duration. BMC Preg Child 2007; 7:9.

Arrowsmith S, Wray S, Quenby S. Maternal obesity and labour complications following induction of labour in prolonged pregnancy. BJOG 2011; 118: 578-88.

Bellver J, Rossal LP, Bosch E, et al. Obesity and the risk of spontaneous abortion after oocyte donation. Fertil Steril 2003; 5: 1136–40.

Bourjeily G, Paidas M, Khail H, Rosene-Montella K, Rodger M. Pulmonary embolism in pregnancy. Lancet 2010; 375; 500-12.

Bragg F, Cromwell DA, Edozien LC, Guroi-Urganci I, Mahmood TA, Templeton A, et al. Variation in rates of caesarean section among English NHS trusts after accounting for maternal and clinical risk: cross sectional study. BMJ 2010; 341: c5065.

Cedergren MI. Maternal morbid obesity and the risk of adverse pregnancy outcome. Obstet Gynecol 2004; 103: 219–24.

Centre for Maternal and Child Enquiries (CMACE). Maternal obesity in the UK: Findings from a national project. London: CMACE, 2010

Centre for Maternal and Child Enquires and Royal College of Obstetricians and Gynaecologists Joint Guideline. Management of women with obesity in pregnancy. Centre for Maternal and Child Enquiries, March 2010

Chaillet N, Dumont A. Evidence-based strategies for reducing caesarean section rates: a meta-analysis. Birth 2007; 34: 53-64.

Chattopadhyay SK, Kharif H, Sherbeeni M. Placenta praevia and accrete after previous caesarean section. Eur J Obstet Gynecol 1993; 52: 141-6.

Chu SY, Schmid CH, Dietz PM, Callaghan WM, Lau J, Curtis KM. Maternal obesity and risk of cesarean delivery: a meta-analysis. Obes Rev 2007; 8: 385-94.

Clark SL, Koonings PP, Phelan JP. Placenta Previa/Accreta and Prior Cesarean Section. Obstet Gynecol 1985; 66: 89-92

Classen DC, Evans RS, Stanley L, Pestotnik R, Horn SD, Menlove RL et al. The timing of prophylactic administration of antibiotics and the risk of surgical-wound infection. N Eng J Med 1992; 326: 281-6.

Confidential Enquiries into Maternal Deaths in the United Kingdom. The fifth report: why mothers die 1997–1999. London, United Kingdom; RCOG Press: 2001.

Denison F, Norrie G, Graham B, et al. Increased maternal BMI is associated with an increased risk of minor complications during pregnancy with consequent cost implications. BJOG 2009; 116: 1467-72.

Ehrenberg HM, Durnwald CP, Catalano P, Mercer BM. The influence of obesity and diabetes on the risk of cesarean delivery. Am J Obstet Gynecol. 2004; 191: 969-74.

Esposti ED, Sturani A, Valpiani G, Di Martino M, Ziccardi F, Cassani AR et al. The relationship between body weight and drug costs: an Italian population-based study. Clin Ther 2006; 28: 1472–81.

Farah N, Maher N, Barry S, Kennelly M, Stuart B, Turner MJ. Maternal morbid obesity and obstetric outcomes. Obes Facts 2009; 2: 352-4.

Fattah C, Farah N, Barry S, O'Connor N, Stuart B, Turner MJ. Maternal weight and body composition in the first trimester of pregnancy. Acta Obstet Gynecol Scand 2010; 89: 952-5.

Galtier-Dereure F, Boegner C, Bringer J. Obesity and pregnancy: complications and cost. Am J Clin Nutr 2000; 71(5 Suppl):1242S–8S.

Hauguel-de Mouzon S, Guerre-Millo M The placenta cytokine network and inflammatory signals. Placenta. 2006; 27: 794-8.

Heslehurst N, Simpson H, Ells LJ, Rankin J, Wilkinson J, Lang R et al. The impact of maternal BMI status on pregnancy outcomes with immediate short-term obstetric resource implications: a meta-analysis. Obes Rev 2008; 9: 635-83.

Hill RK, Thompson JW, Shaw JL, Pinidiya SD, Card-Higginson P. Self-reported health risks linked to health plan cost and age group. Am J Prev Med 2009; 36: 468–474.

Hogan JL, Maguire P, Farah N, Kennelly MM, Stuart B, Turner MJ. Body Mass Index and Blood Pressure Measurement during Pregnancy. Hypertens Pregnancy. 2010 Aug 20. [Epub ahead of print]

Huda S, Brodie L, Sattar N. Obesity in pregnancy: prevalence and metabolic consequences. Sem Fet Neo Med 2010; 15: 70-76.

Kanagalingam MG, Forouhi NG, Greer IA, Sattar N. Changes in booking body mass index over a decade: retrospective analysis from a Glasgow Maternity Hospital BJOG 2005; 112: 1431-3.

Karmon A, Sheiner E. Pregnancy after bariatric surgery: a comprehensive review. Arch Gynecol Obstet. 2008; 277: 381-8.

Kim LH, Cheng YW, Delaney S, Jelin AC, Caughey AB. Is preeclampsia associated with an increased risk of cesarean delivery if labor is induced? J Matern Fetal Neonatal Med. 2010; 23: 383-8.

Landon MB, Hauth JC, Leveno KJ, Spong CY, Leindecker S, Varner MW et al. Maternal and perinatal outcomes associated with a trial of labor after prior cesarean delivery. N Engl J Med. 2004; 351; 2581-9.

MacDorman MF, Menacker F, Declercq E. Cesarean birth in the United States: Epidemiology, Trends, and Outcomes. Clin Perinatol 2008; 35: 293-307.

Maggard M, Yermilov I, Li Z, Maglione M, Newberry S, Suttorp M et al. Pregnancy and fertility following bariatric surgery. JAMA 2008; 300: 2286-96.

McGuire M, Cleary B, Sahm L, Murphy DJ. Prevalence and predictors of periconceptional folic acid uptake--prospective cohort study in an Irish urban obstetric population. Hum Reprod 25: 535-54

Metwally M, Ong KJ, Ledger WL, Li TC. Does high body mass index increase the risk of miscarriage after spontaneous and assisted conception? A meta-analysis of the evidence. Fertil Steril. 2008; 90: 714-26.

Mok E, Multon C, Piguel L, Barroso E, Goua V, Christin P, et al. Decreased full breastfeeding, altered practices, perceptions, and infant weight change of prepregnant obese women : a need for extra support. Pediatrics 2008;121:1319-24.

Mugford M, Kingston J, Chalmers I. Reducing the incidence of infection after caesarean section: implications of prophylaxis with antibiotics for hospital resources. BMJ 1989; 299: 103.

National Institute for Health and Clinical Excellence (Nice) guideline 63. Management of diabetes and its complications from pre-conception to postnatal period. 2002.

Norris LA, Bonnar J, Smith MP, Steer PJ, Savidge G. Low molecular weight heparin (tinzaparin) therapy for moderate risk thromboprophylaxis during pregnancy. A pharmacokinetic study. Thromb Haemost 2004; 92: 791–6.

Organization for Economic Co-Operation and Development (OECD). Health at a Glance. Health Statistics 2009; pp104-5.

O'Dwyer V, Turner MJ. Is the caesarean section rate in Ireland too high? Ir Med J. 2011; 104: 133-4

O'Dwyer V, Farah N, Fattah C, O'Connor N, Kennelly MM, Turner MJ. The risk of caesarean section in obese women analysed by parity. Eur J Obstet Gynecol Reprod Biol. 2011; 158: 28-32.

Paldini D. Sonography in obese and overweight pregnant women: clinical, medicolegal and technical issues. Ultrasound Obstet Gynecol 2009; 33: 720-9.

Persson M, Winkvist A, Mogren I. Surprisingly low compliance to local guidelines for risk factor based screening for gestational diabetes mellitus - A population-based study. BMC Pregnancy Childbirth. 2009; 16: 53.

Poobalan AS, Aucott LS, Gurung T, Smith WCS, Bhattacharya S. Obesity as an independent risk factor for elective and emergency caesarean delivery in nulliparous women-systematic review and meta-analysis of cohort studies. Obes Rev 2009; 10: 28-35.

Rasmussen SA, Chu SY, Kim SY, Schmid CH, Lau J. Maternal obesity and risk of neural tube defects: a metaanalysis. Am J Obstet Gynecol 2008; 198: 611-9.

Ray A, Hildreth A, Esen UI. Morbid obesity and intrapartum care. J Obstet Gynaecol 2008; 28: 301-4.

Reece EA, Leguizamon G, Wiznitzer A. Gestational Diabetes: the need for a common ground. Lancet 2009; 373: 1789-97.

Rode L, Nilas L, Wojdemann K, Tabor A. Obesity-related complications in Danish single cephalic term pregnancies. Obstet Gynecol 2005; 105: 537–42.

Rosenberg TJ, Garbers S, Lipkind H, Chiasson MA. Maternal obesity and diabetes as risk factors for adverse pregnancy outcomes: differences among 4 racial/ethnic groups. Am J Public Health. 2005; 95: 1545-51.

Rowlands I, Graves N, de Jersey S, McIntyre D, Callaway L Obesity in pregnancy: outcomes and economics. Sem Fetal Neonatal Med. 2010; 15: 94–9

Royal College of Obstetricians and Gynaecologists. Green-Top Guideline No. 37. Reducing the risk of thrombosis and embolism during pregnancy and puerperium. London: Royal College of Obstetricians and Gynaecologists, 2009.

Russell MA, Phipps MG, Olson CL, Welch GH, Carpenter MW. Rates of postpartum glucose testing after gestational diabetes mellitus. Obstet Gynecol 2006; 108: 1456-62.

Schmatz M, Madan J, Marino T, Davis J. Maternal obesity: the interplay between inflammation, mother and fetus. J Perinatol 2010; 30: 441-6.

Scott JR. Vaginal birth after caesarean delivery: a common-sense approach. Obstet Gynecol. 2011; 118: 342-50.

Sebire NJ, Jolly M, Harris JP, Wadsworth J, Joffe M, Beard RW et al. Maternal obesity and pregnancy outcome: a study of 287,213 pregnancies in London. Int J Obes Relat Metab Disord 2001; 25: 1175-82.

Seyb ST. Berka RJ, Socol ML. Dooley SL. Risk of Cesarean Delivery with Elective Induction of Labor at Term in Nulliparous Women. Obstet Gynecol 1990; 94: 600-7.

Sheiner E, Levy A, Silverberg D, Menes TS, Levy I, Katz M et al. Pregnancy after bariatric surgery is not associated with adverse perinatal outcome. Am J Obstet Gynecol 2004; 190: 1335e40.

Sherrard A, Platt RW, Vallerand D, Usher RH, Zhang X, Kramer MS. Maternal anthropometric risk factors for caesarean delivery before or after onset of labour BJOG 2007; 114: 1088-96.

Silver RM, Landon MB, Rouse DJ, Leveno KJ, Spong CY, Thom EA et al. Maternal Morbidity Associated With Multiple Repeat Cesarean Deliveries. Obstet Gynecol. 2006; 107: 1226-32.

Smaill F, Hofmeyr JG. Antibiotic prophylaxis for cesarean section (review). Cochrane Database of Systematic Reviews 2002, 3: Art. No.: CD000933.

Society for Obstetricians and Gynecologists of Canada (SOGC) clinical practice guidelines. Screening for gestational diabetes mellitus. J Obstet Gynecol Can 2002; 24: 894–903.

Sullivan SA, Smith T, Chang E, Hulsey T, Vandorsten JP, Soper D. Administration of cefazolin prior to skin incision is superior is superior to cefazolin at cord clamping in preventing postcesarean infectious morbidity: a randomized, controlled trial. Am J Obstet Gynecol 2007; 197: 455.e1-455.e5.

Tooher R, Gates S, Dowswell T, Davis LJ. prophylaxis for venous thromboembolic disease in pregnancy and the early postnatal period. Cochrane Database of Systematic Reviews 2010, Issue 5.

Torloni MR, Betran AP, Horta BL, Nakamura U, Atallah AN, Moron AF. Prepregnancy BMI and the risk of gestational diabetes: a systematic review of the literature with meta-analysis. Obesity Reviews 2009; 10: 194-203.

Turner MJ. Uterine rupture. Best Practice & Research Clin Obstet Gynecol 2002; 18: 69-72.

Turner MJ. Peripartum hysterectomy: an evolving picture. Int J Gynecol Obstet. 2010; 109: 9-11.

Vahration A, Zhang J, Troendle JF, Seiga-Riz AM, Savitz DA, Thorp J. Maternal obesity and labor progression in nulliparous women. Am J Obstet Gynecol 2003; 189: 202.

Veleva Z, Tiitinen A, Vilska S, Hyden-Granskog C, Tomas C, Martikainen H, Tapanainen JS. High and low BMI increase the risk of miscarriage after IVF/ICSI and FET. Human Reproduction 2008; 23: 878-84.

Wall PD, Deucy EE, Glantz JC, Pressman EK. Vertical skin incisions and wound complications in the obese parturient. Obstet Gynecol 2003; 102: 952-6.

Waller DK, Shaw GM, Rasmussen SA, Hobbs CA, Canfield MA, Siega-Riz AM et al. Prepregnancy obesity as a risk factor for structural birth defects. Arch Paediatr Adolesc Med 2007; 161: 1065-71.

Weight gain during pregnancy. http://iom.edu/Reports/2009/Weight-Gain-During-Pregnancy-Reexamining-the- Guidelines.aspx

Weiss JL, Malone FD, Emig D, Ball RH, Nyberg DA, Comstock CH et al. Obesity, obstetric complications and cesarean delivery rate - A population-based screening study. Am J Obstet Gynecol 2004; 190: 1091-7.

Yu CKH, Teoh TG, Robinson S. Obesity in Pregnancy. BJOG 2006; 113: 1117-25.

8

Breastfeeding After a Cesarean Delivery

Sema Kuguoglu[1], Hatice Yildiz[2],
Meltem Kurtuncu Tanir[3] and Birsel Canan Demirbag[4]
[1]*Gazikent University, College of Health Sciences, Division of Nursing, Pediatric Nursing Department,Gaziantep*
[2]*Marmara University Health Science Faculty, Division of Nursing, Obstetric and Gynecological Nursing Department*
[3]*Zonguldak Kara Elmas University Health School, Division of Nursing, Head of Pediatric Nursing Department*
[4]*Karadeniz Technical University, School of Nursing, Division of Nursing, Public Health Nursing Department*
Turkey

1. Introduction

A cesarean delivery (also known as a cesarean section) is the birth of the baby through surgical incision made in both the wall of the mother's abdomen and her uterus. Anesthesia (*general or regional*) is required for the procedure (Alexander et al., 2010). A cesarean birth can be scheduled (*may be on maternal request*) or unscheduled event; it may be an emergency procedure to save the mother and/or fetus such as fetal distress, abruption placentea, a prolapsed cord, cephalopelvic disproportion, total placenta previa, multiple pregnancies, cervical failure, herpes, etc. A cesarean delivery is sometimes necessary for the safety of the mother or the baby, but sometimes it may be on maternal request. However, there is considerable debate about this type of cesarean that performed depending on the mother's request. Whatever the reason, the cesarean rate is dramatically increasing in recent years (Alexander et al., 2010; Mayberry, 2006; Pasupathy & Smith, 2008; Mayberry, 2006; Towle, 2009).

Cesarean delivery also carries a risk to the mother and infant as compared with normal vaginal deliveries (Mayberry, 2006; Towle, 2009). Because of the extend of the abdominal incision, there is a increased loss of blood with a cesarean delivery. When the incision is made, there is an increased risk of damage to other internal organs especially the urinary bladder and uterine blood vessels. If the fetus is large, there is a risk of tearing the uterine incision causing more trauma to uterine tissue (Towle, 2009). Women who have a cesarean birth have a significantly increased risk of rehospitalization for uterine infection, complications from surgical wound (infection, and so on), anesthesia complications, and cardiopulmonary and thromboembolic complications (Mayberry, 2006; Simpson, 2008). Risk of maternal mortality after cesarean birth from anesthesia complications, puerperal infections, and venous thromboembolism is 3.6 times higher for women who have vaginal birth (Smith, 2010). Babies born via cesarean are at significantly increased risk for respiratory complications and admission to the neonatal intensive care unit (NICU) (Simpson, 2008). In addition, other maternal outcomes are significantly in favor of vaginal birth over cesarean birth in the postpartum period. These risks include postpartum hemorrhage, increased maternal hospital length of stay, and delayed or impaired breast feeding (Mayberry, 2006; Simpson, 2008).

The woman who has had a cesarean birth will require the same care as the woman who delivered vaginally, plus routine postoperative care (Towle, 2009). But, mothers who have cesarean delivery are had major abdominal surgery. Therefore, their hospital, postpartum, and breasfeeding experience will be different from the vaginal delivery mothers. Cesarean mothers usually stay in the hospital longer than vaginal delivery mothers, they have more discomfort, they may not be able to have rooming-in privileges (depending on hospital policies), and they may be more dependent on hospital staff (Rosenthal, 2000). The mothers and infant's experiences during labor and delivery may influence lactation in several ways. But, cesarean surgery is strongly associated with delayed lactogenesis, poorer infant suck, delayed in early breastfeeding, decrease in success of breastfeeding, more supplementation, and shorter duration of breastfeeding (Dewey et.al, 2002; Smith, 2010). So, mothers who delivery by cesarean section and their babies will need extended, intense, skilled, and knowledge able to help from maternity care team to establish and maintain exclusive breastfeeding (Smith, 2010).

2. How a cesarean can affect with breastfeeding

There are many factors that are thought to have influence on the breast-feeding after birth. When we look according to delivery types, breastfeeding after the cesarean birth is affected by these reasons:

2.1 Maternal pain, fear and stress, fatigue, and prolonged recovery

Mothers having cesarean section more experience complication, pain, prolonged recovery, readmitted to a hospital, fatigue, discomfort, stress and anxiety, and etc. then the mothers with vaginal birth (Lauwers & Swisher, 2011, B.M. Newman & P.R. Newman, 2009; Smith, 2010). Karlström et al.(2007) study found that women with cesarean section reported high levels of experienced pain during the first 24 hours. There was no difference between elective and emergency cesarean births in the levels of pain. Postoperative pain negatively affected breastfeeding and infant care. Therefore, mothers who had cesarean delivery need more post surgery pain relief drugs. The pain medication is also important for mother's comfort. However, the pain medication that is received during and after surgery is passed in to mother's milk. And, some post surgery pain relief drugs suppress breastfeeding, improve the amount of breastfeeding, and infant weight gain. Also, stress or fatigue can also lead to a decreased milk supply. Mothers who delivered by cesarean section often find it difficult to achieve a comfortable position for breastfeeding (Francis, 2007; Smith, 2010). Even though a mother experiences pain and discomfort after a cesarean section, breastfeeding should be started as soon as possible and should be help the mother put the baby to breast (Janke, 2008).

Stress clearly can affect people strongly. Mothers who had cesarean section have higher scores in somatic anxiety, muscular tension, and suspicion (Smith, 2010). Especially unscheduled cesarean sections (*due to mother or baby*) are often the result of fetal stress or serious maternal complications. Maternal and infant stress during labor and delivery can adversely affect the onset of milk production (lactogenesis). There is several possible mechanisms for this relationship. Maternal stress is known to affect the release of oxytocin and thus may inhibit the milk-ejection reflex. Infant stress may affect lactogenesis via weak or inadequate sucking ability or reduced infant demand (Dewey et al., 2002). If woman have had an unexpected cesarean, she may be worse feelings (robbed/separated from baby etc.) associated with her childbirth experience and this situation can affect her ability to breastfeed. If the cesarean was planned (elective) or if it's experienced more than one time, woman probably have not experience this kind of emotional upheavals (Rosenthal, 2000). Carlander et al.(2010) study reported that mothers with a vaginal delivery experienced breastfeeding less stressful than the mothers with a caesarean delivery. Three and nine months after delivery the mothers with a caesarean delivery on request reported more breastfeeding problems than mothers in the other groups.

2.2 Complications and separation of mother and baby

Some complications after cesarean delivery may interfere milk supply significantly in the postpartum period. Infant born by cesarean section have higher of respiratory distress, more likely to be taken to a newborn intensive care unit, more likely physically separate from the mother, and mother-infant attachment behaviors may more disrupt. Because of all these reasons, the stress hormones (cortisol and adrenaline) increase in mother and infant, establish breastfeeding more difficult, and more likely to have altered sucking patterns. Transfers less milk at breast on days 2-5, which increases the risk of early and unnecessary supplementation and leave excess milk in the mother's breast, suppressing lactogenesis (Smith, 2010). Women having a cesarean section have excessive blood loss as about twice amount than the women having a vaginal birth. If a woman experiences excessive blood loss during surgery, she may be experience anemia, and may be more sluggish and exhausted (Dewey et al., 2002). A report based on case studies has suggested that maternal postpartum hemorrhage may be risk factor for insufficient milk production. In this study, for all mothers are recommended as soon as possible early breastfeeding after birth (Willis & Livingstone, 1995). In multicentre cohort study reported that women with greater blood loss are less likely to initiate and sustain full breastfeeding and this may be related to delays in initial contact with their baby. These findings have implications for postnatal care as these women may require greater support, education and assistance in initiating and sustaining breastfeeding. In particular, enabling the opportunity for the newborn to suckle as soon as is practical should be encouraged (Thompson et al., 2010). In addition, mothers who are rehospitalized for infection stroke, or wound dehiscence after cesarean surgery are likely to experience suppressed or delayed onset of lactation (Smith, 2010). Therefore, management of factors that cause separation mothers and infants are important in the postpartum unit. In a pilot study has been tested the standardized intraoperative and postoperative nursing intervention protocol for maternal-infant separation after cesarean. And, in this study found that the standardized intervention protocol showed positively affecting maternal-infant outcomes after cesarean delivery (Nolan & Lawrence, 2009).

2.3 Delayed access to baby and supplementary feedings

Initial contact between mother and infant should be during the first hour postpartum. Because early contact is important to establish successful breastfeeding. But, mothers who delivered through cesarean section experienced a longer delay in making their first contact with their infant (B.M. Newman & P.R. Newman, 2009). Sometimes hospital practices in the immediate postpartum period that is associated with operative intervention in delivery can affect first mother-infant contact and initiation of breastfeeding the findings of a study confirmed that cesarean section and hospital practices was significant barrier to implementation of Baby-Friendly Hospital Initiative (Rowe-Murray & Fisher, 2002). Chalmers, et al.(2010) study found that more interventions in labor, women who had a cesarean birth after attempting a vaginal birth had less mother-infant contact after birth and less best breastfeeding practices (B.M. Newman & P.R. Newman, 2009). If mothers who had a general anesthetic cesarean may experience a bit more of delay to breastfeeding, since they'll need some time to come out of the anesthetic (*In this case, holding the baby close and cuddling can begin right after coming to and breastfeeding can begin shortly thereafter*) (Devroe, 2007; Rosenthal, 2000). Some mothers are able to nurse their babies' right on the table during surgery; most are told to wait until they are in the recovery room. This means a delay of almost a hour, and sometimes more. Although not ideal, this is not insurmountable. Some hospitals do also not permit women who have had a cesarean to have their babies' room in with them. All these situations can cause often delays the timing of the first breastfeeding, and the production of milk after cesarean birth, and also frequency of breastfeeding can reduce in the mothers who had cesarean (B.M. Newman & P.R. Newman, 2009). In a study that examined the factors associated with early breastfeeding, the breastfeeding within the first hour of life found that higher in mothers with vaginal birth than mothers with cesarean section. In the study, mothers with cesarean section and preterm birth were reported as vulnerable situations (Vieira et al., 2010). The study which made by Perez-Escamilla et al. (1996) examined the relationship between cesarean birth and breastfeeding, and they found that the cesarean section a risk factor for the initiation of breastfeeding. Leung et al. (2002) study found that the cesarean delivery was a risk factor for not initiating breastfeeding, for breastfeeding less than one month, and remained a significant hazard against breastfeeding duration. In another study was examined the effect of method of delivery and timing of breastfeeding initiation on the prevalence of breastfeeding at one and three months after delivery. And, odds of breastfeeding at one and three months after delivery found that a lower in the women with cesarean delivery. Also according to the findings emphasized that the importance of conservative use of operative obstetrical intervention due to its negative impact on breastfeeding (Chien & Tai, 2007).

The timing of the first breastfeeding is often delayed after cesarean birth. Delayed onset of milk production is a vexing problem by breastfeeding mothers. But, given a supportive hospital and home environment this need not adversely effect breastfeeding success. Because breastfeeding is very much a function of supply and demand, early and frequent breastfeeding is extremely important for establishing breastfeeding (Dewey et al., 2002). The more feedings of colostrum (the early milk) that the baby receives, the more immunological protection the baby gets. In addition, early and frequent breastfeeding can help lessen or treat a baby's tendency towards hypoglycemia, infants weight loss, and jaundice, problems common after birth scenarios that lead to cesarean (Dewey et al., 2002; B.M. Newman & P.R. Newman, 2009). Caglar et al.(2006) study found that the infants' weight loss and hypernatremia found associated with delay at initiation of first breastfeeding and cesarean section. And, the study reported that the mothers should have been helped and supported for breastfeeding their infants as soon as possible after delivery (Caglar et al., 2006).

Some mothers who have had cesarean birth are less often tending to start breastfeed according to mothers who have vaginal delivery. Most women plan to at least try to breastfeed, but sometimes theirs efforts may not be effective due to some physical or emotional reasons after cesarean. They may be groggy from drugs, woozy with pain, and exhausted from labor, surgery, and significant blood loss. Suddenly breastfeeding may seem overwhelming and too much trouble or they may be too out of it to try very effectively. In this situation, bottle feeding may be often seems easier and more convenient (Dewey, 2002; Towle, 2009; Smith, 2010). Babies who are born by cesarean section and separated from their mothers are also frequently given formula as a first feeding. But, many cesarean babies give routinely the bottles of formula in some hospitals. Sometimes, supplementary feedings are necessary to prevent hypoglycemia, or when the baby looses a great deal of weight after birth and does not regain it quickly, or for the test of baby's ability to suck. These and similar factors that delayed breastfeeding after cesarean could effect woman's confidence and desire to breastfeed (Lauwers & Swisher, 2011). In a study, the delayed onset of lactation and early lactation success found associated with primiparity, cesarean section, labor medications, use of non breast milk (fluids and/or pacifiers), etc. (Dewey et al. (2003).

Therefore, supplementary feedings should be avoided as much as possible. The labor and delivery staff can preserve and protect breastfeeding by avoiding these types of practices, which can hinder subsequent breastfeeding (Lauwers & Swisher, 2011).

All cesarean mothers should be encourage for rooming-in and her baby's care if there is not a complication that causes to baby to be separated from the mother. If the mother had a cesarean birth having a support person stay with her facilitates earlier rooming-in. Since frequent feedings are an important part of establishing milk supply in a timely manner, rooming in is an important part of helping cesarean mothers breastfeed more easily, and sleeping with the baby in your arms can help even more (Lauwers & Swisher, 2011). Breastfeeding, with skin-to-skin contact, should be initiated within an hour of birth. Because the baby's sucking movements reach a peak 45 minutes after birth and decline until at 2 hours. Early feedings are associated with mothers who breastfeed for a longer duration. Successful latch-on and sucking greatly reduce sucking disorganization or dysfunction later and contribute to increased breastfeeding duration. If the baby has not been feed within 2 hours, this situation may cause sucking disorganization or disfunction on baby's sucking movements. (Janke, 2008). If mothers with cesarean are start as soon as possible breast-feeding and are supported, they can be as successful as the mothers who have vaginally delivery (B.M. Newman & P.R. Newman, 2009).

2.4 Anesthesia and analgesia (delayed lactogenesis and poorer infant suck)

There is inadequate information on weather anesthesia or analgesia used during labor and delivery have any influence on lactation (Dewey et al., 2002). But on the other hand, clearly that the some anesthesia or analgesics given during delivery have the potential to interfere with the early development of breastfeeding behaviors and negatively influencing breastfeeding long term (Janke, 2008). But yet there is no consensus about what unintended affects obstetric anesthesia cause on breastfeeding (Devroe, 2007). Because, effect on breastfeeding of some anesthetic/analgesic drugs that used during birth related to type and amount, and timing of medication. Some drugs may delay effective feeding for hours to several days, some drugs may depress sucking behavior of infant, so pulsatile oxytocin may decrease, etc. The route of administration local, IV, or injected pain relief drugs cross very quickly enter the infant bloodstream via placental perfusion, in a matter of seconds to a few minutes. The drugs tend to sequester in infant brain tissue and effect central nervous system function. Also, the drugs are designed to numb sensory nerves in the mother. Therefore, they also affect sensory and mother nerves in the infant that affect rooting, sucking, and breathing. All these behaviors must be intact for the infant to begin breastfeeding. Administration of epidural anesthesia causes the level of beta-endorphins to fall dramatically. Beta-endorphins produced in labor and present in colostrums and milk protects the baby from pain. Epidurals may delay the onset of lacto genesis. Vaginally delivered mothers had significantly more oxytocin pulses than the cesarean section mothers. In addition, vaginally delivered mothers had significant rises in prolactine levels at 20-30 minutes after onset of breastfeeding, with the number of pulses correlated to duration of exclusive breastfeeding (Smith, 2010).

After delivery, levels of estrogen and progesterone in the body rapidly decrease, triggering the production of milk. Two hormones (prolactin and oxitocin) are released in response to a baby suckling (Alexander, 2010). Prolactin levels are high during about first ten days of postpartum and slowly decline over the next 6 months. Prolactin levels are also highest at night. It is thought that the frequent sucking acts as a stimulus to increase the binding capacity of prolactin receptor sites in the breast. This enhances tissue responsiveness, accounting for continued full milk production as prolactin concentrations decline over time. Nipple stimulation prompts oxitocin to be released from the pituitary gland in a pulsatile manner numerous times during each feeding. The sensation that accompanies the effect of oxytocin on breast tissue is called the letdown reflex or the milk-ejection reflex Oxytocin causes the network of myoepithelial cells surrounding the alveoli to contract and expel milk into the larger ductules, making it available to the newborn. Touch, massage, and skin-to-skin contact stimulate oxytocin release. Separating mothers and newborns should be discouraged unless there is a medical indication (Janke, 2008).

A caesarean section can be carried out under either regional or general anaesthesia. The type of anesthesia used for the cesarean can also influence breastfeeding rates. This may reflect the type of anesthesia, the amount of medications the baby received, the amount of separation of mother and baby after the operation, or many other factors, In addition, whether the cesarean was scheduled or unplanned also may make a difference in delayed onset of lacto genesis (Francis, 2007; Lauwers & Swisher, 2011; Rosenthal, 2000). Zanardo et al.(2010) study found that emergency and elective cesarean deliveries are similarly associated with a decreased rate of exclusive breastfeeding compared with vaginal delivery. General anesthesia tends to reach the baby strongly, and may depress baby's responses after birth for some time. Drugs may also result in the baby being less effective at suckling. Regional anesthesia results in lower doses of the various drugs crossing the placenta to the baby, so although baby may still be affected, he may not be affected as strongly as after general anesthesia. Also, breastfeeding frequency and longer breastfeeding periods after epidural anaesthesia are higher than after general anesthesia (Devroe, 2007; Lauwers & Swisher, 2011; Rosenthal, 2000). In a prospective, randomized, and double-blind study found that high-dose labor epidural Fentanyl were more likely to have stopped breastfeeding (Beilin et al., 2005). It has been reported that the women with cesarean sections given epidural anesthesia may be more likely to continue breastfeeding to 3 or 6 months postpartum than general anesthesia (Dewey et al., 2002). Because, if the mother receive general anesthesia during the cesarean section, the breastfeeding may be possible when mother awake and able to respond (Lauwers & Swisher, 2011). Baumgarder et al. (2003) study explored that the association between labor epidural anesthesia and early breast-feeding success in both epidural and nonepidural anesthesia groups. In this study it has been reported that labor epidural anesthesia had a negative impact on breast-feeding in the first 24 hours of life, even though it did not inhibit the percentage of breast-feeding attempts in the first hour. According to these studies' results, cesarean with general or epidural anesthesia effects sucking and breastfeeding success and lactogenesis negatively in different levels. However, if there is no complication in mother and her baby, these negative factors may be reduce with starting breastfeeding as early as possible, supporting and encouraging mothers about breastfeeding. At the same time, mothers should be willing and endeavour for breastfeeding their baby

Infant characteristics can also influence the timing of onset of milk production, the milk ejection reflex, and ultimately the volume of milk produced. Also babies born via cesarean section are often problematic babies. Such as, low birth weight infants and/or smaller size at birth infants has been associated with delayed lactogenesis. This may be due to reduced sucking strength, frequency or duration of feeds among smaller infants (Dewey et al., 2002). In a study found that the volume of milk transferred to infants born by caesarean section was significantly less than that transferred to infants born by normal vaginal delivery on days 2 to 5 (Evans et al., 2003). Cakmak & Kuguoglu (2007) study found that LATCH (*LATCH is a breastfeeding charting and scoring system that provides a systematic method for gathering information about individual breastfeeding sessions. Each letter of the acronym LATCH denotes an area of assessment. "L" is for how well the infant latches onto the breast. "A" is for the amount of audible swallowing noted. "T" is for the mother's nipple type. "C" is for the mother's level of comfort. "H" is for the amount of help the mother needs to hold her infant to the breast.*)scores for mothers who underwent cesarean sections averaged 6.27 for the first breastfeeding and 8.81 for the third breastfeeding, out of maximum possible score of 10 scores averaged 7.46 for the first breastfeeding and 9.70 for the third feeding in mothers who delivered vaginally. Riordan et al. (2000) used a scoring system to evaluate the effect of medications on neonatal suckling in 129 vaginally-delivered babies. Babies of medicated mothers scored lower in suckling effectiveness than babies of unmedicated mothers, and the scores were lowest in the group that received both epidurals and IV drugs. In summary, clearly that some anesthesia/analgesia drugs given during labor and birth may affect the baby's suckling response and feeding behaviors, and it's also clear that medication given to the mother can also affect her milk supply. The perinatal nurse maybe able to offset some of the side affect of labor medications by helping start breastfeeding early, keeping the mother and newborn together, and teaching the mother to recognize hunger cues and putting the newborn to breast (Janke, 2008).

3. Benefits of breastfeeding after a cesarean

The World Health Organization (WHO) recommends exclusive breastfeeding (EBF) the infant for the first six months of life, consistent with a previous recommendation by Unicef, to achieve optimal growth, development and health. Thereafter, appropriate complementary foods should be introduced, while breastfeeding continued up to two years of age or beyond. However, the prevalence of EBF is low globally in many of the developing and developed countries around the world. There is much interest in the effectiveness of breastfeeding promotion interventions on breastfeeding rates, in early infancy (Imdad et al., 2011)

Observational studies in low income populations, even in developing countries, have shown that fluids in addition to breast milk are unnecessary to maintain hydration.Furthermore, the addition of water, tea, or other liquids has adverse effects on the output of breast milk, growth, and morbidity and mortality due to infectious diseases (Black,2002)

The duration of breastfeeding is longer in mothers who start to breastfeed immediately after birth. Initiating breastfeeding as early as possible provides many health advantages, in addition to assuring longer breastfeeding duration. Therefore, mothers who had cesarean delivery, breastfeeding should have been start as soon as mother recovers, even if the mothers experience pain and discomfort after a cesarean birth. But, the mothers need help to put the baby to breast for the first day or two. Therefore, the mothers should be support in first few days. Breastfeeding offers many benefits such as faster uterine involution and controls bleeding immediately after delivery, and quicker weight loss after birth to the cesarean mother in particular. Cesarean babies who have been breastfeed also receive significant benefits such as immunological protections, and prevention/minimization of hypoglycemia and jaundice problems (Alexander, 2010; Francis, 2007; Janke, 2008; Lauwers & Swisher, 2011).

3.1 Uterine involution, postpardum bleeding and weight loss

After the baby's born, the uterus needs to start shrinking down in order to return to its normal size and state. Breast stimulation causes endogenous oxytocin to be released by the pituitary gland, stimulating uterine contractions, and helps the uterus to start shrinking more quickly and efficiently, and promote uterus involution (Janke, 2008; Towle, 2009). The increased oxytocin secretion because of suckling, contacts with the uterus more quickly and controls bleeding immediately after delivery (Janke, 2008; Lauwers & Swisher, 2011). Eventually, due to the increased levels of oxytocin from breastfeeding, the uterus returns to its normal size more quickly and the women experiences less postpardum bleeding, and speeds up mother's well-being. But, cesarean mothers may have more trouble with uterine involution (Rosenthal, 2000; Alexander, 2010). Negishi (1999) found that cesarean mothers tended to have larger uterine at one month postpartum than mothers who had had a vaginal birth, so uterine involution may be of special concern to women who have had cesarean. So, especially breastfeeding may be helpful in cesarean mothers.

Many mothers find it difficult to return to the pre-pregnancy weight after birth, and anecdotally, this may be particularly true after a cesarean. Restrictions on mobility, pain from the incision, anemia from blood loss, adhesions from the surgery, etc. may all combine to make a cesarean mother less active than one who has given birth vaginally, sometimes significant lengths of time may affect postpartum weight loss. Therefore, breastfeeding may also helps a woman to return to her pre-pregnancy wight more quickly, if a woman have difficulties to resume her activity level after a cesarean (Alexander et al., 2010).

3.2 Immunological protections, hypoglisemia, jaundice, bonding

Breastfeeding provides optimal nutrition for infants and improves maternal postpartum health (Devroe, 2007). Cesarean babies may be more at risk for infection for several reasons. Cesarean mothers also have higher rates of infection than mothers who have had vaginal births, thus potentially exposing their babies to this infection as well. Invasive procedures and equipment for the breathing problems common to cesarean babies may also further the risk for infection (Alexander et al., 2010; Simpson, 2008; Towle, 2009). And since cesarean babies stay in the hospital longer as their mothers recover, they are exposed to more germs and risk for infections (Rosenthal, 2000; Simpson, 2008; Towle, 2009). Breastfeeding decreases significantly incidence in many of the infant's complications after birth such as diarrhea, gastrointestinal difficulties, respiratory infections, ear infections, urinary tract infections, etc. (Alexander et al., 2010; Simpson, 2008; Towle, 2009). Also, breastfeeding known as a natural first vaccine. Because, colostrum (the first milk) is extremely high in protective antibodies that help for coat the baby's gastrointestinal system and protect it from harmful bacteria, and it also contains substances that help 'kick-start' the baby's own immune system (Alexander et al., 2010). İntestinal bacteria play an important role in the development of the infant immune system. If these infants who born via cesarean delivery are not support for early breastfeeding, colonization and physiological development of their intestinal flora is delayed (Walker, 2011). Chen et al.(2007) study found that primary intestinal bifidobacteria in neonates who born with caesarean may be disturbed more significantly than lactobacilli. If intestinal flora develop on an alternate trajectory as coused by a cesarean delivery and/or feeding with infant formula, the development of the immune system might also be different, leaving it vulnerable to a number of diseases. For example atopic diseases appear more often in infants who have experienced a cesarean delivery compared with those delivered vaginally (Walker, 2011). Therefore, considering the possible infection risk in many cesarean's babies, breastfeeding's immunological protections become especially important (Alexander, 2010).

Jaundice is common in premature babies, sick babies, babies of diabetic mothers, and when labor was induced or augmented artificially with pitocin. Many of these babies end up with cesareans. Thus jaundice is not an unusual finding in cesarean babies, not because of the cesarean itself but because of the conditions and drugs that tend to cause a higher cesarean rate. Much of the bilirubin in the first days is eliminated through the baby's meconium (stool). If the baby does not stool enough, the bilirubin is reabsorbed through the intestines. Thus breastfeeding frequently is one of the best ways to minimize jaundice. Because, colostrum begins the establishment of normal bacterial flora in the newborn's gastrointestinal tract and exerts a laxative effect that begins elimination of meconium, decreasing the potential reabsorption of bilirubin (Janke, 2008).

Breastfeeding is important to prevent hypoglycemia in infants immediately after delivery. Because of the possibility of low blood sugar after a difficult birth, many hospitals routinely give a bottle of glucose water to cesarean babies. Unfortunately, this tends to cause a quick spike in blood sugar followed by a crash, and this unstable blood sugar can be a problem for the baby, causing a vicious cycle of treatment and re-treatment. The colostrum has plenty of lactose to help raise the baby's blood sugar (Janke, 2008).

Bonding is often an issue after a cesarean. Many mothers report feeling distant and detached from their cesarean babies. Breastfeeding is important for cesarean mothers and babies not only for physiological reasons, for emotional ones too. Unfortunately, many hospitals do not place a priority on breastfeeding, or have routine protocols that actively interfere with breastfeeding. Breastfeeding can help restore the bond between mother and baby, healing the separation that has occurred. For many women, breastfeeding was the most healing thing in their lives after going through the cesarean (Alexander, 2010).

4. Breastfeeding positioning after cesarean

Successful breastfeeding is possible for mothers if they have had a c section. Epidural or spinal anesthesia is ideal because of it allows the mother to be awake and relatively pain free in the postoperative period, thus improving the chances for early initiation of breast feeding. Appropriate pain medication may aid during this period. But all pain relieving drugs should be passing to baby with breastfeeding.

Many mothers who deliver by cesarean appreciate the extra teaching opportunities they receive while they were staying in the hospital. They usually need more help to find a comfortable position because of the abdominal incision and pain related the movement. The women may need to void before beginning to breastfeed, and she should be instructed to wash her hands each time nurses her infant. (Lauwers, J.; Swisher A)

There are three common breastfeeding positions that can be used by most mothers. These positions are the *cradle hold, the football hold, and the side-lying* position. (Littleton & Engebretso, 2002). For some mothers, the best position for breastfeeding after surgery is the *"football position"* as the babies will not lie on the mothers' abdomen. Others put a cushion over the incision to reduce the pain (Filidel Rimon & Shinwell , 2005).

In the *football* (side sitting or Clutch) *hold* ; the mother holds the infant's back and shoulders in her palm and tucks the infant under her arm. Remind the mother to keep the infant's ear, shoulder, and hip in straight line. The mother supports the breast with her hand and brings it to the infant's lips to latch on. She continues to support the breast until the infant begins to breastfeeding. This position allows the mother to see the infant's mouth as she guides her infant (Ricci &Kyle,2008). Holding the baby's head in her right hand, she supports the child's body with her right forearm and raises his or her head to breast level.

The *Cross Cradle Hold* is a different take on the traditional cradle hold. In the *Cross Cradle, the* baby's head is at the mother's right breast but the baby's body is supported by the mother's left arm. Her left hand is at the base of the baby's neck. Supporting it and helping to direct the baby gentle. The mother's right hand is then free to help with breastfeeding or she would like (Weiss, 2010).

In the *side lying position*, the mother lies on her side with a pillow supporting her back and another pillow supporting the newborn in the front. To start, the mother props herself up on an elbow and support the newborn with that arm, while holding her breast with the opposite hard. Once breast feeding is started, the mother lies down in a comfortable position (Ricci & Kyle, 2008).

4.1 Breast feeding multiples after cesarean section

The three commonly used positions for bar simultaneous breastfeeding are as follows (Filidel Rimon & Shinwell, 2005)

1. *"Double football"*. An infant's head is supported in each of the mothers hand or on a pillow, with an infant's body lying under each of the mother's arms. Many mothers use these positions initially until they gather more experience.
2. *"Double crade"*.In this position each infant is held, in the cradle position. The two infants cross on the mother's abdomen. This position is ofen used when the mother is more experienced and the infants have better head control.
3. *"Combination of cradle with double football"*, one infant is held in the cradle position and the second in the football position.

5. Strategies for increasing breastfeeding success

The possible direct effect of cesarean delivery on the infant has been investigated with attention to the level of circulating catecholamine in umbilical plasma samples (Kroeger and Smith, 2004). Some researchers have found that neuro-behavioral depression caused by labor analgesia, particularly in cases where dosage intervals are short, may result in a delay in positive breast feeding behavior (Dennis, 2002). This has an adverse effect on breastfeeding. Another study showed that mothers who had cesarean encounter difficulties, feelings of fatigue, sleeplessness and breastfeeding problems in the process of both their own recuperation and in caring for their babies (Gungor et al., 2004).

5.1 The effect of cesarean section on breastfeeding

Cesarean delivery has negative effects on breastfeeding. After a surgical delivery, unassisted mothers are almost certainly unable to hold their newborns in the delivery room or for the frequent breastfeeding periods that follow (Mohrbacher, Stock, 2003), and bottle-feeding has become a common clinical practice in these cases (Perez et al., 1996; Chapman, 1999). In addition, feeding milk-based formulas will reduce the newborn's sucking capacity and consequently the mother's lactation stimulus. If the newborn becomes accustomed to bottle (formula) feedings, he or she may have difficulty adjusting to breastfeeding, which may cause the mother to become discouraged and to consider giving up breastfeeding (Welan et al., 1998).

Cesarean sections with local and general anesthesia are the factors that affect breastfeeding. Especially under general anesthesia, it takes mothers longer to recover from the effects of the anesthesia, being delayed in becoming sufficiently awake to hold and breastfeed their babies. It is obvious that the mode of delivery affects breastfeeding after birth and general anesthesia mothers are more likely to need support and help in breastfeeding compared with local anesthesia mothers. If you must have a Cesarean, prefer regional anesthesia (epidural, spinal, or combined spinal epidural) instead of general anesthesia (Vincenzo, 2010).

A prospective study by Janke likewise found no difference in breastfeeding outcomes by delivery method (Janke, 1998). This finding is important, because support and encouragement have been recognized as key indicators of breastfeeding success even after surgical births.

5.2 Lactogenesis after cesarean section

Lactogenesis is a function of a finely tuned feedback mechanism, which is potentially susceptible to pharmacological, physical, and psychological manipulations on the part of the mother, her infant, or both (Evans et al., 2003; Dewey, 2001). Whichever birth method is used, early breastfeeding is effective in the active secretion of breast milk. A study was carried out with two groups of mothers who delivered with Cesarean section. The first group started to breastfeed one hour after the delivery and the second group 20 hours after the delivery. The study concluded that early sucking after CD promotes significantly earlier colostrum or breast milk secretion (Kroeger and Smith, 2004). Nursing within the first hour after birth and frequently thereafter help bring the mature milk in sooner and increases supply. If possible, nurse the baby before the effects of the regional anesthesia wear off. You will be relatively alert and free of pain, which will help the first nursing go better than if you are worn out, in pain, or in need of sleep (Vireday, 2002).

5.3 Mother baby bond

Literature shows that Cesarean delivery may adversely affect the mother's bonding with her child, acting as an obstacle in the way of a positive mother and child relationship and making it difficult for the mother to accept the infant (Heck et al., 2003; Ince, 1998). In a

Cesarean section delivery, the mother is a surgical patient carrying the risks and problems that this entails (Kroeger and Smith, 2004). Thus, it is important in Cesarean section births that support is given to bring about the early initiation of a mother-and-child bonding.

If a bonding cannot be achieved soon after the birth for reasons related to the mother and child, the relation between the two is seen to adversely affect the physical care the mother gives to the child and also it affects the baby's relations with other people (Riorden, 1998).

5.4 Baby breastfeeding positions after cesarean section

Mothers delivering by cesarean are unable to offer their babies a satisfactory breastfeeding position because of their discomfort. In addition, they tend to initiate breastfeeding at a later time due to the effect of anesthetics (Heck et al., 2003; Ince, 1998). Mothers need more professional support in the early period after birth, particularly in holding the baby in breastfeeding position. It has been seen that this need is more pronounced in mothers who have delivered by cesarean section under general anesthesia (Cakmak and Kuguoglu, 2006)

The position of baby on the breast is very important to help establish breastfeeding and prevent nipple soreness. A mother should make sure her baby's body is close to her, chest to chest, chin to breast and nose away from the breast. The 'football' or 'clutch' hold is often more comfortable after a C-section. Women whose babies are born by cesarean delivery under general anesthesia can use cross-cradle position and side-lying position to be useful. The side-lying position is relaxing and gets mother much more needed sleep. This position is also beneficial for the mother who had a cesarean birth. Mothers need more professional support in the early period after birth, particularly in holding the baby in breastfeeding position. Utilize the support of a professional lactation consultant to help with positioning and latch-on concerns (Vireday, 2002).

5.5 The effects of early breastfeeding

The immediately after baby is born is a great time to start breastfeeding. The results demonstrate a dose—response relationship between early skin-to-skin contact and breastfeeding exclusivity (Mannel, 2011). As it is known, the hormones of labor will help breastfeeding get started sooner and more easily (Sozmen, 1992).

After a cesarean, breastfeeding should start as soon as possible. Try positioning the baby lying face down across the mother's breast (similar to cradle hold, but the baby is higher up and away from the mother's incision, and the mom is lying flat). When nursing in this position with a newborn, have someone nearby to make sure the baby's nose doesn't get blocked, since you both may be groggy from the meds. A partner or a nurse help position the baby, and use lots of pillows around the mother to help with support. In order to facilitate the secretion of milk soon after the Cesarean section, baby-mother communication must be established by supporting the general condition of the mother.

Breastfeeding carries certain benefits for a mother delivering by Cesarean section. The suckling action, it is known, stimulates the production of oxytocin which assists the process of healing in the postoperative uterus. Another useful aspect of it is the psychological satisfaction that a mother who has been unable to deliver naturally derives out of finally being able to participate actively in a maternal capacity (Dennis, 2002; Kroeger and Smith, 2004).

Whatever the mother's situation, it is generally reasonable to expect the acceptance of breastfeeding as a goal. In case where it is possible to introduce breastfeeding early on or even when time pass before the medical problems stabilize, the supporting role that the nursing staff will play is imperative to successful and satisfying lactation. The mother pursues regular and frequent feedings (at least 8-12 times in the first days and at least every 2-3 hours for the first several days to a week). Some babies nurse more efficiently than others, while some are sleepy at first and may take a long time to finish a feed. Babies don't need to nurse constantly, but neither should they be artificially limited to small amounts of time. Let your baby set its own feeding cues as long as it seems like they seem like they are getting enough. If there any doubt about baby's weight gain or whether there is sufficient intake, nurse frequently and don't limit time on the breast (Vireday, 2002).

5.6 The importance of education in effective breastfeeding

To encourage, support and achieve the continuation of breastfeeding, educational programs should be organized during the antenatal, natal and postnatal periods.

5.7 Family support in breastfeeding

Many studies have shown that family support to the mother is important in effective breastfeeding. Research has also shown that the prenatal education of fathers on the importance of breastfeeding encourages mothers in successful breastfeeding That the nursing staff who looks after the mother at home after the Cesarean section has enough information on the uses of breastfeeding is of great importance in that it encourages the mother to breastfeed (Lynn et al., 2011).

Partners have been encouraged to be present in the operating theatre, to share the birth of their babies. The father or relatives can be an important source of moral and physical support and be involved with their baby from birth. Have a family member (father or other relative) in the room too. Sleep with the baby, which can greatly ease regular feedings. Vincenzo et al (20) showed that the role of fatigue, stress, pain, and health complications in scheduled Cesarean deliveries is important in lactation. Lacking assistance, the mother may be unable to breastfeed initially, which can affect lactation and cause breastfeeding to fail (Vincenzo, 2010).

5.8 The importance of the relaxation of mother in effective breastfeeding

Before breastfeeding, the mother must be relaxed that she can succeed this. Those who will ensure this must be the medical team who are there. There is an association between the help of nursing staff and successful breastfeeding.

After cesarean, mother who has pain. So that nurse has to support to mother for breastfeeding. Nurse must to give relaxation of mother in effective breastfeeding. Don't limit time on the breastfeeding. Pursue regular, frequent feedings. Be sure that mother's nutrition is excellent and that the mother is getting plenty of extra fluids. If the mother has pains, she should take medicine as needed in order to be comfortable. A mother without pain will be breastfeed her baby more comfortably (Vireday, 2002).

If the mother is having trouble with milk supply, relaxation exercise and music can be effective. Use relaxation tapes and guided imagery to help decrease mother's stress and increase milk output. In order for the mother to feel relaxed, support from lactation consultants can be obtained. It should be born in mind that early breastfeeding help lactation by activating hormones.

The emotional condition of the mother also affects breastfeeding. Each mother experiences the postnatal period differently and therefore they should be given psychological support. If they experience problems, get expert help from a professional lactation consultant as soon as possible.

5.9 The effect of mother baby bond created by their coexistence in the same room on the effective breastfeeding

The coexistence of mother and baby in the same room after the birth is important for an effective breastfeeding. As soon as the baby starts to cry, the mother-baby contact starts. Have a family member in the room. Sleep with the baby, which can greatly ease regular feedings. Research shows that rooming in also increases breastfeeding rates. This is probably because the baby nurses more often (stimulating milk supply) and gets less supplementation. Because some hospitals do not permit women who have had Cesarean to have their babies room in with them, this can negatively affect breastfeeding rates.

5.10 Avoid supplements

Hospital staff shouldn't give any supplemental bottles or pacifiers, as these artificial nipples can cause problems (Righard, 1998). If supplements are medically required, hospital staff should use alternative method rather than by bottle (supplements should be given via cup or feeding syringe rather than a bottle to avoid the risk of nipple confusion)

5.11 Yeast infection

A yeast infection of the baby's mouth and/or the mother's nipples is a special concern after c-section. Any pain, redness, burning/itching of the mother's nipples, or white patches seen in baby's mouth may indicate that thrush has developed and needs to be treated. In such a case, the baby rejects breastfeeding.

6. Dealing with special situations

6.1 Hypoglycemia

A frequent concern regarding the newborn infant is hypoglycemia. Part of the challenge of health professionals in dealing with newborns is to discover whether the infant has hypoglycemia. Although no widely accepted standards for serum glucose levels have been set down as accurate criteria for determining whether an infant has the condition, there are various indications that are generally used in assessing hypoglycemia incidence across infant populations (Page-Goertz, 2010).

More recent views on defining hypoglycemia in infants accept the following blood sugar levels as normal in term neonates: 0-3 hours < 36 mg/dl (2.0 mmol/L), 3-6 hours < 25 mg/dl (.4 mmol/L), 6-24 hours < 30 mg/dl (.7 mmol/L), 24-48 hours < 40 mg/dl (2.2 mmol/L), and > 48 hours < 45 mg/dl (2.5 mmol/L) (Çetinkaya et al., 2006; Page-Goertz, 2010).

Hypoglycemia is a common and generally temporary condition in the early days of the infant. Whereas routine follow-ups of blood glucose levels in healthy term newborns are not necessarily a prescribed procedure, certain conditions are recognized as risk factors for hypoglycemia. Babies small or large for gestational age, a smaller twin, infants with a low birth weight or with diabetic mothers, or those with asphyxia, polycythemia, erythroblastosis fetalis, respiratory distress, or with any other similar condition before birth are considered to be at relatively more risk (Janke, 2008; Kliegman, 2002).

In some cases, cesarean birth can lead to the development of hypoglycemia in infants. Hypoglycemia in breastfed babies may be reduced or prevented with the use of methods that support breastfeeding. In this context, breastfeeding within an hour of birth, skin-to-skin contact between mother and newborn to prevent cold stress, increasing the infant's store of glucose, breastfeeding 8 to 12 times per day, not leaving the newborn to cry, and feeding the newborn every 1-2 hours with a spoon or cup if the baby is unwilling to suckle are methods that can be considered (Janke, 2008).

All high-risk babies should be evaluated for signs of hypoglycemia and treated, regardless of whether or not symptoms are present.

6.2 Jaundice

Jaundice is another potential complication that can arise as a result of difficult labor and cesarean birth.

6.2.1 Cause and types of jaundice

Newborn jaundice is a condition that is encountered in more than 60% of healthy babies and one that is more likely to appear as physiological jaundice. The condition reaches pathological levels that require treatment in only about 10% of cases. Jaundice is diagnosed when the total serum bilirubin (TSB) level exceeds 2 mg/dl in the adult and more than 5-7 mg/dl in newborns (Indriyani et al., 2009; Wong et al., 2006). Hyperbilirubinemia, seen in 60%-70% of term infants and in almost all preterms, is the most frequent reason for neonate presentation at the hospital and re-admittance after initial discharge (Maisels, 2006; Maisels et al., 2007; Maisels & McDonagh, 2008; Vatansever & Çelik, 2005).

Because of the potential toxicity of bilirubin, infants with severe hyperbilirubinemia must be promptly treated and closely monitored to avoid the development of acute bilirubin encephalopathy and/or kernicterus (American Academy of Pediatrics, 2004). The risk of developing kernicterus is higher in the premature infant compared to term babies due to the immaturity of the liver. The condition develops when indirect bilirubin levels in the blood rise because of extreme erythrocyte breakdown. When indirect bilirubin levels rise, the bilirubin penetrates the fetal blood-brain barrier, being released into the brain and causing damage to brain cells. The risk of developing hyperbilirubinemia is higher if the baby has acidosis, hypoxia or hypoglycemia, all of which prevent indirect bilirubin levels from bonding with albumin (Çavuşoğlu, 2011). Establishing standardized approaches and monitoring in the treatment of this physiological or pathological process has become a need recognized all over the world and countries such as the United States, Canada and Israel have prepared guidelines for this (American Academy of Pediatrics, 2004; Kaplan & Merlob, 2008; Sgro & Campbell, 2006).

Jaundice develops as one of several types. Abnormal jaundice appears in the first day or two following the birth of the infant and is usually associated with blood incompatibility or other similar problems. This type of jaundice requires a course of treatments, sometimes even blood transfusions (Kliegman, 2002).

6.2.2 Causes in relation to time from birth

6.2.2.1 Onset in less than 24 hours

This emergence of the condition is always pathological, likely to be a result of hemolysis (Rhesus disease, ABO incompatibility), and may be caused by an underlying serious disease such as sepsis and more rarely, other blood group incompatibilities, red cell enzyme defects (glucose-6-phosphate dehydrogenase deficiency (G6PD), and red cell membrane defects (hereditary spherocytosis) (Statewide Maternity and Neonatal Clinical Guidelines Program, 2009).

Early-onset jaundice appears in the first 24 hours of the infant's life, reaching its highest point on the third or fourth day and then beginning to decline until normal levels are attained after the first month. If processing is slow, concentrations of unconjugated bilirubin can increase. Since large amounts of unconjugated bilirubin are stored in the meconium, a delay in elimination for any reason may result in reabsorption of the bilirubin into the blood. Under normal conditions, the laxative effect of colostrum promotes the elimination of meconium, diminishing the level of unconjugated bilirubin and thus preventing resorption. In some hospitals, newborns are routinely given sugar-water. Infants given sugar-water have higher bilirubin levels; levels are lower in those given colostrum. This is because Dextrose (5%) water has 6 calories per ounce, and colostrum has 18 calories per ounce. By consuming sugar-water, the newborn fails to ingest two-thirds of the calories needed to ward off reabsorption of bilirubin. Effective breastfeeding management that relies on 8-12 feedings every 24 hours can reduce or prevent early-onset **pathological** jaundice (Janke, 2008).

6.2.2.2 Onset at 24 hours-10 days

The most frequently encountered reason for jaundice in newborns is increased levels of bilirubin. Jaundice that appears after the first 24 hours of life (after the first 48 hours in preterm infants) and does not exhibit a daily bilirubin increase of more than 5 mg/dl, and does not exceed a level of 12 mg/dl in healthy and term infants or 15 mg/dl in preterms, with a duration of not more than one week in term infants and no more than two weeks in preterms, is referred to as physiological jaundice (Törüner & Büyükgönenç, 2012).

"Breast milk jaundice" is jaundice that emerges most frequently at the end of the first week of life in breastfed babies. Although the reason for this type of jaundice is not fully known, it is believed that in some cases, mother's milk contains a substance that inhibits the activity of the liver enzyme glucuronyl transferase. It is thought that this maternal factor increases the reabsorption of indirect bilirubin in the intestinal tract. It is also asserted that genetic factors may also play a role. The type of jaundice seen in breastfed infants who do not get enough mother's milk in the first four days of life is considered early-onset breast milk jaundice whereas the type of jaundice that starts after the fourth day and steadily increases is referred to as late breast milk jaundice. When breastfeeding is stopped for 2-3 days, the level of indirect bilirubin falls within 24-48 hours. Breastfeeding does not need to be interrupted continuously. When breastfeeding is resumed, the jaundice may increase slightly and last for weeks but it will not reach the levels it had before breastfeeding was interrupted. Mothers should be informed about continuing to express milk during the period that breastfeeding is interrupted (Sivaslı, 2009; Törüner & Büyükgönenç, 2012).

6.2.2.3 Onset after 10 days (prolonged for more than 2 weeks

Causes include conjugated hyperbilirubinemia due to idiopathic neonatal hepatitis, infections (Hepatitis B, TORCH, sepsis), congenital malformations (biliary atresia, choledochal cyst, bile duct stenosis), and metabolic disorders (galactosaemia, hereditary fructose intolerance, Alpha-1 antitrypsin deficiency, tyrosinaemia, glycogen storage disease type IV, hypothyroidism), also, sepsis, hypothyroidism, and hemolysis. Late onset breast milk jaundice develops 4 to 7 days after birth, peaking at 7-15 days. This condition is less common (Statewide Maternity and Neonatal Clinical Guidelines Program, 2009).

6.2.3 Treatment

Treatment for hyperbilirubinemia (American Academy of Paediatrics, 2004; Janke, 2008; Maisels & Watchko, 2003)) includes the use of phototherapy, exchange transfusion, or pharmacological agents.

Because the level of bilirubin causing kernicterus cannot be determined and varies according to the individual infant, deciding upon the time to begin phototherapy is difficult. Newborns are generally introduced to phototherapy when bilirubin concentrations rise higher than 18-20 mg/dL after the first 48 hours after birth. The recommendation for bilirubin levels of over 18-20 mg/dL is more frequent breastfeeding and phototherapy (Agarwal et al., 2011).

Assessment of late-onset jaundice in a newborn is firstly based on an analysis of bilirubin levels, after which the baby is formula-fed for 24 hours followed by another bilirubin level analysis. Late-onset jaundice requires no treatment (Agarwal et al., 2011).

Treatment with an immediate exchange transfusion is indicated if the infant has jaundice and shows signs of intermediate to advanced stages of acute bilirubin encephalopathy, with possible symptoms of lethargy, hypotonia, poor feeding and a high pitched cry, hyper-alertness or irritability, hypertonia, arching, or retrocollis-opisthotonos, where the baby is obtunded or comatose, displays apnoea or seizures. The infant's condition must be reviewed by neonatology specialists before the start of pharmacological treatment (Statewide Maternity and Neonatal Clinical Guidelines Program, 2009).

6.3 Sleepy baby

One of the problems many mothers who have cesarean deliveries experience is a sleepy baby who has been affected by the medications administered during the birth and through the surgery. In general, babies show more interest in feeding when they are alert or awake, although they might be drowsy. In the first few hours after birth, babies are usually awake and eager to be fed but they may later become sleepy and then remain sleepy until they are a day old. The nurse will advise that the mother wake and feed the baby every three hours even if the baby does not demand the feeding on its own. Some babies may sleep for longer periods. Loosening the baby's covers, light massage, keeping the baby perpendicular, encouraging movement, changing the diaper, maintaining skin-to-skin contact or talking to the baby may be useful in waking the infant (The Childbirth Centre Queensway Carleton Hospital, 2005).

Mothers may think it unkind to wake a sleeping baby but they must be encouraged to do so in the first few days after birth. Particularly if there are medical concerns such as jaundice, it is important for the health of the baby that mother -led two-hour feeding schedules are set up.

6.4 Prematurity

A major difficulty for cesarean mothers is the birth of a premature baby. Many premature babies are born by cesarean and this situation is twice as hard on the mother, since she must cope with both the stress of recovering from surgery and with the problems of a premature infant. The powerful emotional and physical implications of these situations can prove to be overwhelming for some women. Because preterm babies are born without having completed their intrauterine growth, all of their systems are immature and thus prone to many problems. One of the issues that come up in the clinical environment is the feeding of preterm infants. There are three principal factors that complicate preterm feeding: the relative immaturity of the preterm's gastrointestinal systems; their being born in the 24th-36th gestational weeks, the period in which fetal growth is greatest; and the fact that their nutrient stores are still relatively poor. Other difficulties include the risk of aspiration and the need for maximum patience on the part of the mother because of the baby's need for a prolonged feeding time (Savaşer, 2002).

Preterms begin to be fed by mouth when their sucking, **cheek** and tongue movements have developed, there is enough coordination so that the uvula moves up and back to close the nasopharyx and the epiglottis closes the glottis, esophageal action is able to bring the milk down into the stomach, and hiccup reflexes are present (Çavuşoğlu, 2011; Murray & Mckinney, 2006; Neyzi ve Ertuğrul, 2002). In one study, compared to a control group in which feeding regulation was doctor-designed, premature infants encouraged to feed with oral nutritional pathways were 6 days earlier in making the transition to completely oral feeding (Kirk et al., 2007). Healthy infants weighing more than 1500 grams may feed orally in the first few hours after birth (Tengir & Çetinkaya, 2008).

Preterm feeding depends on the baby's gestational age, whether or not there is a pathological condition, and on the infant's individual tolerance. Babies at a gestational age of more than 32-34 weeks with normal sucking and swallowing reflexes can feed on a bottle/breast in the absence of a severe pathological condition. At the same time, the transition to bottle-feeding may prove to be too stressful for a preterm infant (Savaşer, 2002).

Preterms should not be forced to feed orally if they are not ready. Oral feeding should be discontinued at the first sign of discomfort; the baby should not be allowed to get worse. In the case of babies that are unable to suckle, the use of a spoon may be tried in place of bottlefeeding to encourage babies to get used to the breast. However, sucking-swallowing and breathing coordination must be developed before bottlefeeding is initiated (Savaşer, 2002).

While the goals of enteral feeding are to reduce the incidence of hypoglycemia and hyperbilirubinemia and to enhance cerebral and somatic development, the objectives of making the transition into bottlefeeding are to ensure sucking, swallowing and breathing coordination and to create an adequate tolerance for nutrient intake so that healthy growth and development can be encouraged (Satar, 2001; Savaşer, 2002).

To conclude, nurses should be able to observe symptoms of nutritional deficiency in premature babies, manage an appropriate feeding schedule, watch for complications related to nutrition, observe the effectiveness of caregiving in terms of feeding, as well as be able to determine and implement effective nursing interventions. Nurses should also never forget their role as nutritional educator and consultant to mothers and fathers before, during, and after feedings.

6.5 Breastfeeding in twins/triplets

Twin/triplet births are considered high risk. These infants are at risk of being premature or smaller relative to their gestational age. An ultrasound taken during pregnancy may be useful in determining the major issues in the infant's development (Çavuşoğlu, 2011; Kliegman, 2002, Murray & Mckinney, 2006). Multiple births have climbed significantly in the last 25 years, achieving unprecedented numbers in twins, triplets and other higher order multiples. Contributing to these rising rates have been the trend to delay childbearing and the increased interest in infertility therapy and assisted reproductive technologies (Bowers et al. 2008, Murray & Mckinney, 2006).

In multiple pregnancies, it is important to ensure that each of the babies get adequate care after birth. Any one of the infants may have problems that need immediate intervention (Çavuşoğlu, 2011; Kliegman, 2002). About 2% of twins are born with major structural deformities, a condition that is higher in prevalence in same-sex twins. The most frequently encountered abnormalities are cardiac malformations, neural tube defects, facial clefts, and gastrointestinal anomalies. The rate of cardiac defects and gastrointestinal anomalies in multiples is twice the rate for singletons. The striking incidence of congenital anomalies in all twins is almost exclusively related to the higher rate of anomalies in monozygotic twins (Bowers et al. 2008).

There are some abnormalities that are seen only in multiple gestations. Conjoined twins occur at a rate of 1/50,000 to 1/100,000 births, being three times more common in female fetuses than in male fetuses. Survival of conjoined twins is seen to be generally dependent on the extent of shared organs (Bowers et al. 2008). If twin infants have twin-to-twin transfusion syndrome (or feto-fetal transfusion syndrome), the donor twin of the transfusion suffers retarded growth, anemia, pallidity, hypovolemia and malnutrition. For this reason, these babies may have to be transferred to the intensive care unit. Parents' first encounter with the newborn is an important step in their relationship. Parents need guidance in this process (Çavuşoğlu 2011, Kliegman, 2002, Bowers et al. 2008).

Twins and triplets may be nourished like other babies according to their gestational age, their special needs, and the mother's preferences. Breastfeeding has various advantages for twin/triplet births. Firstly, breastfeeding is less time-consuming and more economic. In formula feeding, feeding bottles and specially prepared formulas are needed. It is important for the mother that she is nourished during the lactation period with a diet enriched with protein and calories, adequate fluids and plenty of rest. If care is taken to meet these requirements, the mother will generally have adequate milk for her babies because twins and triplets actually stimulate milk production. Breastfeeding two babies simultaneously will give the mother time to rest and engage in other activities. The mother must be guided in placing herself in an optimum position for breastfeeding. If the infants are being artificially fed, she should enlist the help of other members of the household at feeding times (Çavuşoğlu, 2011).

6.6 Failure to thrive syndrome

The most important characteristic that differentiates children from adults is the fact that children are in a consistent state of growth and development. The term "growth" refers to increases in body dimension and "development" to the changes and maturing of biological functions. Growth and development processes are slower or more rapid at various ages but they occur with continuity and follow a defined pattern (Kurul, 2011).

Children's growth after birth is divided into three main periods—infancy, childhood and adolescence. In the first six months of infancy, growth is a continuation of rapid development, independent of the growth hormones of the intrauterine stage. The most significant factor affecting growth in the child's first 2 years is nutrition (Neyzi ve Ertuğrul, 2002; Günöz et al., 2003). This is particularly important in the fetal stage. Postanatally, long-term protein and energy deficiency leads to malnutrition and growth retardation. This is also an important issue in infancy, which is a period of rapid growth (Günöz et al., 2003).

Because of the unique characteristics of the period of pregnancy, making sure that conditions are appropriate for the healthy birth of a baby of normal weight and length is relatively more important in this period compared to other periods in life (Neyzi ve Ertuğrul, 2002). Babies will generally lose weight shortly after birth but then start to gain steadily and predictably. If the infant does not gain the weight it is expected to gain or instead loses weight, this is referred to as "failure to thrive." This state may be caused by various different factors (Şahin, 2002). In the general population, failure to thrive affects 3-5% of infants. There is an organic explanation for a small minority. Non-organic failure to thrive brings with it an increased risk of physical illness, continued growth retardation as well as cognitive and emotional disturbances (Jaffe, 2011; Jolley, 2003).

In Organic Failure to Thrive (OFTT), organs involved in digestion and food absorption are either incomplete or malformed, meaning that the infant is unable to digest food. Non-organic Failure to Thrive (NOFTT) is the most common cause of FTT and refers to situations where the infant is unable to receive enough food because of economic reasons, parental neglect or psychosocial problems (Jaffe, 2011; Krugman & Dubowitz, 2003; Şahin, 2002).

6.6.1 Causes and symptoms

Sometimes babies are unable to take in, digest, or process food because of an underlying and inhibitive physical condition. Such conditions may involve the esophagus, stomach, small or large intestine, rectum or anus and are usually brought about by an incomplete development of the organ. Surgical correction is likely to be needed. Physical defects can usually be detected in the days immediately after birth. Failure to thrive may also be caused by an absence or poor quality of available food. Underlying this may be economic factors in the family, parental beliefs and concepts of nutrition, or child neglect. Additionally, in breast-fed infants, the problem may lie in the quality or quantity of the mother's milk. Psychosocial issues arising from poor parent-child relations can also bring about failure to thrive. The child's appetite may be less than desired because of depression caused by a lack of adequate attention from the parents. Failure to thrive is accepted as a diagnosis when infants and toddlers exhibit significantly less growth than expected (Krugman & Dubowitz, 2003; Şahin, 2002).

Conditions that disrupt the child's health cause deviations in the growth process. For this reason, each child needs to be monitored and evaluated periodically from birth. In the first two weeks of the neonate, weight increase should be assessed at frequent intervals (once a week or more). Subsequently, a follow-up should be made at the end of the first month. The growth and development of the child should from then on continue to be monitored once a month until the 6th month, every three months from 6th months of age to a year, every six months from age 2 to age 6, and annually from age 6 up until adulthood (Neyzi & Ertuğrul, 2002).

6.6.2 Diagnosis

It is known that children who are at risk of growth retardation have improvements in their prognosis when they have been diagnosed early and started on appropriate rehabilitation (Kurul, 2011). Babies are usually weighed at birth and that weight reading is used as a reference for future well-baby check-ups. When the baby shows signs of poor weight gain, this requires a more comprehensive examination by the health professional. If no physical deformities can be diagnosed in the digestive tract, the health professional will then review the circumstances of the child's environment. This will involve looking into the family history of height and weight as well asking questions about feedings, illnesses, and family routines. In the case of breastfeeding, an evaluation will also be made of the mother's diet, general health, and well being since it is known that this has an effect on the quantity and quality of mother's milk. The diagnosis of failure to thrive is confirmed where there is a positive growth and a behavioral response to enhanced nutrition (Jolley, 2003; Krugman & Dubowitz, 2003).

6.6.3 Treatment

Failure to thrive stems from many underlying factors and therefore the treatment of the syndrome should be based on a multidisciplinary or team approach. The team should make an assessment of feeding disorders and ideally comprise a pediatric dietician, a social worker, and a speech/occupational therapist. A team approach can provide a more comprehensive assessment of the family situation, which will ultimately be more effective in dealing with symptoms such as growth retardation. A focus on only the child may conceal other factors that may be largely contributing to the growth failure (Jolley, 2003).

In the event that there is a physical cause of failure to thrive, such as a disorder of the swallowing mechanism or intestinal problems, a corrective intervention might reverse the condition. If there are environmental factors involved, the physician will advise as to how the parents can obtain sufficient food for the infant. The physician's recommendation may also include maternal education and parental counseling. Hospitalization or the need for a more nurturing home may be indicated in extreme situations (Bergman & Graham, 2005).

6.6.4 Prevention

Physical defects that bring about failure to thrive cannot be prevented but corrective measures can be taken so that the infant is not under risk. When there is no physical defect, maternal education and emotional/ economic support systems are all effective in helping to prevent the syndrome (Şahin, 2002).

6.7 Polycystic Ovarian Syndrome (PCOS) and breastfeeding

The endocrine disorder PCOS affects 5%-10% of women of reproductive age and is characterized by high levels of androgens (male hormones such as testosterone) from the ovary. It is associated with insulin resistance (Grassi, 2008; Kelley, 2003).

6.7.1 Causes PCOS

There is no definitive and known cause of PCOS but there is wide research being carried out to understand the syndrome. It is thought that PCOS develops as a result of genetic factors. Polycystic ovaries have been found in young girls before puberty, indicating that this might be a congenital condition. There are other theories that set forth the hypothesis that PCOS may develop through exposure to high androgen levels in the womb (Grassi, 2008).

6.7.2 Diagnosis of PCOS

Currently, PCOS is diagnosed on the basis of two of the following three conditions: oligomenorrhea (period intervals of > 40 days) or amenorrhea; clinical and/or biochemical signs of hyperandrogenism; and polycystic ovaries on an ultrasound, with exclusion of other causes. A few questions asked of a patient may reveal undiagnosed PCOS (Grassi, 2008; Trent et al., 2002).

Milk supply problems may stem from PCOS and therefore, clinical evaluation and management are important in maintaining the breastfeeding relationship (Grassi, 2008).

6.7.3 Treatment of PCOS

Relief of PCOS symptoms can be attained with diet, exercise and insulin-lowering medications such as Metformin and Byetta or Rosiglitazone. The use of oral contraceptives may help to restore and regulate menstrual function and hormone levels, as well as decrease acne and hirsutism (Grassi, 2008). The main objectives in treatment are menstrual function regulation, reduction of androgen and insulin levels, and improvement of dermatological symptoms (Grassi, 2008).

Supplementing progesterone and metformin are methods used in maintaining healthy pregnancies in women with PCOS. This has the added advantage of enhancing the milk supply. A study reports that progesterone treatment administered before conception and through the first trimester of pregnancy improved breast morphology and achieved successful lactation in an infertile (but non-PCOS) patient (Kelley, 2003).

Low volumes of glandular tissue may indicate a lack of ductile support for breastmilk production. Lactation may be adversely affected as a result of hormonal imbalances such as elevated androgens, low prolactin levels and insulin resistance, all seen in PCOS. It is common for women with PCOS to produce milk normally and breastfeed without difficulty but whenever milk supply is a problem, an assessment should be made for the diagnosis of PCOS. In the study by Vanky et al (2008) 75% of the women with PCOS were breastfeeding exclusively at one-month postpartum and 14% did not breastfeed at all. In the control group, 89% were breastfeeding exclusively and 2% did not breastfeed. It was found that at three- and six-months postpartum, breastfeeding was equal in the two groups. Another study came to the conclusion that maternal androgen levels in mid-pregnancy are negatively associated with breastfeeding (Carlsen et al., 2010).

Breastfeeding rates in women with PCOS seem to be lower in the early postpartum period. It is possible that gestational dehydroepiandrosterone-sulphate might have a negative effect on the breastfeeding rate of women with PCOS. For this reason, breastfeeding women with the syndrome need additional emotional and clinical support. They should be strongly encouraged to breastfeed since they are usually able to carry this out successfully and it is highly beneficial for their infants (Vanky et al., 2008).

It is suggested that women with PCOS pump their milk from each breast for at least 10-15 minutes in order to maintain an adequate milk supply in the first 2 weeks of nursing. Milk production can be maximized with frequent feedings with full drainage along with an adequate diet and drinking fluids. Setting up strategies for breastfeeding early on during pregnancy, accessing resources from local support groups, and working with a certified lactation consultant soon after delivery are beneficial.

7. Breastfeeding and bonding after cesarean

7.1 Effect of cesarean birth on breastfeeding

In recent years, cesarean births occur more frequently than vaginal deliveries, all over the world and in Turkey. According to Turkish Population and Health Research (TNSA) data for 2008, 36.7% of all births are by cesarean section (Ergöçmen et al., 2009). This percentage is above the target set (15%) by the World Health Organization (World Health Statistics, 2011).

It is known that a cesarean delivery can affect the bonding between mother and baby and make it more difficult for the mother to accept her child (Yiğit et al., 2009). It is believed that the rise in cesarean birth rates stems from such factors as the rise in the ages of pregnant women, the increase in the percentage of first deliveries, the anxieties of mothers and doctors about the delivery, the preference shown to giving birth at private hospitals, and the desire to choose the time of birth (Olds et al., 2004; Usha Kiran & Jayawickrama, 2002; Yılmaz et al., 2009).

There are disadvantages involved in cesarean birth. These include the necessity for surgery, the risk of infection and hemorrhage, the relatively more painful process compared to normal delivery, the prolonged recovery time, problems with digestion and elimination, and the delayed return of the mother back to her normal life (Büyükkayacı Duman & Karataş, 2011; Murray & Mckinney, 2006). Because of these factors, the mother sometimes has difficulty taking the baby into her arms to breastfeed. Cesarean, however, is not an obstacle in the way of breastfeeding. Mothers who have given birth by cesarean section are as capable of breastfeeding their infants as mothers who have had normal deliveries (Yılmaz et al., 2009).

There is often a delay in the initiation of breastfeeding with cesarean mothers due to the fact that these mothers need extra time to recuperate and to feel well enough to nurse their babies. Breastfeeding can begin as soon as they can hold the baby when they are fully conscious and alert. Epidural anesthesia generally is generally effective in helping mothers to breastfeed their babies sooner and for longer periods than mothers who have had general anesthesia (Jonkers, 2005).

Cesarean babies are likely to be drowsy and lethargic, particularly if the mother was kept under anesthesia for a prolonged period during labor. Breastfeeding in these circumstances will still be successful but the milk supply may take longer to come in compared to what would occur after a vaginal birth. The lethargic baby may need encouragement and stimulation to be alert during feedings, but this period of lethargy is usually quick to pass (Ahmed & Najib, 2010).

After the birth, the nurse should make sure that the mother is provided the support needed from the husband and family to establish the mother-baby bond, initiate and maintain breastfeeding as early as possible, ensure that the infant is fed only mother's milk and that the baby rooms in with the mother. Moreover, during the mother's stay at the hospital, the nurse should provide her with information about lactation and the mechanism involved, breastfeeding methods, baby care, problems that may be encountered and their solutions, breast care, personal care, nutrition and exercise. The method used in breastfeeding should be observed and improvements made to help the mother take the optimum position for successful breastfeeding. It should be ensured that the mother will be able to breastfeed her child using the correct method on her own (Ilgaz, 2000; İnce, 2001; Savaşer, 2001; Yıldız, 2001).

The effects of educating mothers on mother-and-baby and family health have been clearly demonstrated. Information and consultation made available to the mother to eliminate deficiencies of knowledge about baby care has proved to increase competence, boost parents' self-confidence, reduce mothers' anxieties, and contribute to the growth and development of the baby. Social support has been found to have a positive effect on the psychological and social adjustment of the parents as well as on the bond between mother and baby (Gagnon & Bryanton, 2009).

7.2 The Importance of the mother-baby bond after a cesarean

The term "bonding" refers to the emotionally positive and mutually satisfying relationship established between the baby and the baby's care-givers. Bonding is the process in which the baby has the tendency to feel closer to certain people and safer in their presence (Görak, 2002; Murray & Mckinney, 2006; Sabuncuoğlu & Berkem, 2006).

Because of the biological immaturity of the baby's life systems, the baby is dependent upon his mother or caretaker for vital needs such as food, warmth, and protection. It is inevitable and natural that the baby should develop a bond with the person fulfilling its needs, the one who loves, protects and cares for him/her--the mother (Soysal et al., 2005; Tüzün & Sayar, 2006). Babies trust the person they bond to and they want to spend their time with her, feeling safe and happy, seeking that person out whenever there is a situation that provokes fear or discomfort. It is for this reason that the bonding concept in infancy includes all of the patterns of these emotions and behaviors (Soysal et al., 2005).

The togetherness of the family and the baby is a high quality and effective relationship that starts in the prenatal period, increases as the fetus becomes more active, coming to a peak with the actual birth. The process of connection between the family and the baby is different for the mother and the father. While bonding with their babies is a phenomenon that noticeably increases from around the fifth month of pregnancy for women, emotional development in this context is slower in the father and reaches the mother's level after the birth with the start of baby care (Driscol, 2008; Görak, 2002; Lowdermilk & Perry, 2007; Murray & Mckinney, 2006).

The period right after the birth is an emotional time in terms of mother-baby bonding. The time that the mother is most ready to bond with her baby and respond to the baby's needs is in the first 60-90 minutes after awakening. This is why the mother's contact with the baby is especially important in this time frame (Görak, 2002). Mothers who have difficulty developing bonding behavior are observed to be indifferent and inhibited toward the idea of touching their babies. The mother's ability to cope in this period is not only dependent upon the baby's medical risk status, the age of pregnancy and developmental factors, but also on the quality of the mother's social support, her skills in coping with stress, the marital relations of the mother and father, and is also said to be associated with the relationship of the mother with her own mother (Özbek & Miral, 2003).

Bonding frequently becomes problematic after a caesarean. There are mothers who indicate that they feel distant and detached from their caesarean babies. Part of these feelings may have to do with the fact that the mother cannot be a part of the actual birthing process and therefore is the last person to hold and cuddle the baby. Some women may feel suspicious about whether the baby is really their own. Others are so bothered by physical pain, grogginess and exhaustion that they are disappointed in not being able to feel particularly joyful and caring about the baby (Korte, 1998).

It is important for the cesarean baby to be nursed at an early stage after birth. This is because being nurtured with mother's milk helps to foster the mother-baby bond, facilitates and strengthens the development of a loving relationship. The mother who willingly and lovingly nurses her child instills a feeling of trust in the baby. A healthy biological and psychological closeness is created. Mothers that breastfeed are more compassionate with their babies and complain less about the baby's care and feeding (Brandt et al., 1998).

Goodfriend (1993) has shown that babies taken from their mothers into special care for one reason or another immediately after birth often experience slower development or a halt in development altogether, exhibiting a sad facial expression while not feeding and retreating from social contact (Soysal et al., 2000).

Lastly, starting off on a positive mother-baby relationship after a cesarean helps to instill a feeling of trust in the child and forms the foundation for the development of a healthy personality in later life. Nurses and other health professionals working with newborns have important responsibilities in helping to initiate this relationship.

7.3 Factors that affect the mother-baby bond (e.g. depression, hormonal factors, emotional factors, pain)

Although cesarean birth may appear to be a safe procedure, the fact that it is after all a surgical intervention causes it to be a traumatic experience with related adverse factors (McFarlin, 2004). The physical and psychological effects of cesarean birth have more of an impact on the mother compared to normal delivery. Besides the physical problems that may arise because of the surgical nature of the procedure, not being able to actively participate in the birth, being unable to see the baby immediately and the inability to take an interest in the infant are all factors that may riddle the entire experience of birth with negative feelings (Sayıner et al., 2009).

In terms of the attitudes families have toward their babies, it is reported that some of the factors that can influence the relationship are individual genetic backgrounds, the baby's reaction, the baby's being a planned and wanted child, the mother's feelings of trust, the family's socioeconomic and cultural situation, marital relations and marital support, relations with the mother's family and social circle, the length of labor and birth, the type of birth, the anxiety experienced in the first days after birth, the health of both mother and child, any anomaly that the baby may have, the baby's extended stay at the hospital, the nature of the bonding of the mother with her own mother when she was a baby (Görak, 2002; Steele et al., 2002; Tilokskulchai et al., 2002).

In one study, when mothers were asked when they felt love toward their baby, 41% responded "during the pregnancy", 24% said "at the delivery", 27% remarked "in the first week after the birth", and 8% commented "after the first week". Forty percent of first-time mothers noted that they felt nothing when they first held their babies in their arms. For this reason, evaluating the early reactions and emotions of mothers is important in terms of fostering a bond between mother and infant (Moehler et al., 2006). Another reason mothers may be ambivalent after a cesarean birth is that their pain may be so great that they forget about breastfeeding altogether or feel too uncomfortable to hold the baby in their arms (Ilgaz, 2000).

There are many factors that exacerbate mothers' emotional instability after the birth. Hormonal changes, psychological problems, unwanted or risky pregnancy, difficult birth, conflicts in the family, a lack of social support, not being able to get support from the health team during the birth, a stressful lifestyle, obstetrical complications, the stress created by baby care, and difficult babies can all be cited as potential troublemakers (Beck, 2001; Tammentie et al., 2002; Tezel 2006). In a study where the correlation of the level of social support with pregnancy and postpartum depression was explored, it was found that women whose social support system was lacking were at significantly higher risk both in pregnancy and for postpartum depression (Xie et al., 2009).

The mother's emotional status is a factor that affects the baby's adaptation period and its speed. About 50%-80% of mothers will experience "baby blues" or "postpartum blues" after the birth. Most women in this situation are unable to provide a logical explanation for their feelings, which are in generally affected by hormonal changes. Some women feel depressed because they feel that their bodies have become deformed after the birth, some are disappointed that the delivery did not go as planned, while others are sad because they haven't received the support that they were expecting from their families (Beji, 2010). In a study of mothers in depression, only 29% were identified as having problems with bonding (Brockington et al., 2001). It has been reported that the mother's emotional tie or bond with her baby and the behavioral relationship between mother and baby are often affected by psychological factors. In fact, the babies of mothers experiencing postpartum depression have been found to be lacking a trustful bond with their mothers even in their second year (Martins & Gaffan, 2000).

It is therefore important when there is a new arrival and the mother is trying to cope with adjusting to the baby, with postpartum discomfort, the new order in the family and the changes in her body, that there should be support and information available to the mother on baby care and the baby's needs (Murray & Mckinney, 2006).

7.4 The effect of rooming in on the mother-baby bond

A relationship of bonding and care is important for the healthy physical, mental and emotional development of the newborn. The role of the neonatal nurse is pivotal in the development of mother-baby bonding. The most important task of the nurse is to determine the needs of the mother as regards the child and to support the mother until she is able to take on the baby's care on her own. Elements that foster the development of the mother-baby relationship are the baby's being allowed to share the mother's room (rooming-in), skin-to-skin contact between the mother and the baby (kangaroo care), eye-to-eye contact, holding the baby, nursing, and participating in caring for the baby (Görak, 2002; İşler, 2007; Neyzi & Ertugrul, 2002).

7.5 The effect of rooming in on breastfeeding

The American Academy of Pediatrics (AAP) recommends that mothers feed their babies exclusively with mother's milk and continue to breastfeed for at least one year. To facilitate breastfeeding, the further recommendation is for mothers to sleep in close contact with their babies. It is emphasized that sleeping together makes breastfeeding easier over the course of the night. Some of the reasons mothers should sleep in contact with their babies include making the baby comfortable, increasing the time spent with the baby, strengthening the mother-baby bond, compensating for a situation where the baby has nowhere else to sleep. The most important reason cited in many studies for sleeping in close contact with the baby is being able to breastfeed (American Academy of Pediatrics 2005; Buswell & Spatz, 2006; Galler et al., 2006).

Feeding the baby breast milk strengthens the psychological bond between mother and child. In particular, breastfeeding in the first half-hour after birth and sharing the mother's room is known to create a bond between mother and baby (Çınar et al., 2010). It is for this reason that mothers and babies should be accommodated in the same room. The mother can then breastfeed for however long and at whatever frequency the baby demands. It is a fact that adequate milk production is dependent upon regular breastfeeding. The mother's being together with her baby in the same room will relax the mother and makes the baby feel safer. The baby's place is with the mother and a system whereby the baby can be in a bassinet but in the same room with the mother will have a positive effect on the baby's health. Putting babies to the breast at frequent intervals is the most important factor in achieving breastfeeding success. The mother should take the baby in her arms and breastfeed whenever the baby cries (Buswell & Spatz, 2006; Jansen et al., 2008).

The close contact of mother and baby after the birth and frequent breastfeeding is the best method of speeding up milk production. The mother should pick the baby up in her arms and breastfeed whenever she wants or whenever the baby cries. Rooming in provides healthy babies with the opportunity to suckle at frequent intervals. The rooming-in arrangement makes both mother and baby happier. Because problems such as crying and feeling hungry are solved on the spot, the baby can rest more peacefully. It has been observed that mothers in rooming-in situations are more successful at breastfeeding (Neyzi & Ertugrul, 2002).

In a study in which the relationship between breastfeeding and where the baby was kept was explored, Çınar et al (2010) reported that babies sleeping in the same room with their mothers were breastfed more than babies kept apart from their mothers and that the statistical difference between the two groups was highly significant. Other studies as well have shown that babies sleeping in the same room with their mothers are breastfed during the night three times more frequently than babies in separate rooms and that overall, this is twice the frequency experienced by babies in separate rooms (Blair & Ball, 2004). AAP recommends that, to make breastfeeding easier, the baby should be in the same room but sleeping in a separate bed (American Academy of Pediatrics, 2005).

Despite the existence of some studies that report that a baby's remaining in the same room with its mother has no effect on breastfeeding (Brenner et al., 2003; Flick et al., 2001), there are a great many studies that conclude that breastfeeding is positively affected when mother and child are in the same room together (Blair ve Ball, 2004; Galler et al., 2006).

Breastfeeding as early as possible after the birth starts mother and baby off on their bond together. When they are accommodated in the same room, mothers tend to more quickly adapt to their own roles and develop increasing interaction with their babies (Görak, 2002; Hofer, 2005). For this reason, in the first days after birth, together with the start of breastfeeding, nurses need to promote an adequate, successful, and sustained interaction between the mother and her baby (Soysal et al., 2005).

7.6 The effect of Kangaroo care on the mother-baby bond

Kangaroo care is a method that has many benefits for both mother and baby, the least of which is that by initiating an interaction between mother and baby, the method helps mothers feel closer to their babies. The method is also known to help to develop mothers' caregiving skills and also regulate babies' periods of sleep. Listening to the mother's heartbeat soothes a baby and promotes feelings of security and a deep sleep (Olds et al., 2004).

Kangaroo care is a cost-free, easy-to-implement method that gives the mother an active role in the baby's care and brings both parents and the baby numerous benefits. It is also regarded as a safe and non-pharmacological model of baby care (Derebent & Yiğit, 2006).

In various studies, it has been found that skin-to-skin contact between mother and child in the first 15-60 minutes after birth has a positive effect on the behavior of both mother and baby throughout the feeding period. Studies conducted since 1980 have found that babies exposed to skin-to-skin contact with their mothers after birth successfully seek the breast, grasping it and suckling without any help from mother (Bystrova et al., 2009; Renfrew et al., 2010).

The skin contact between mother and child not only helps in breastfeeding but also offers benefits for the process of bonding as well. This can be explained by the fact that prolactin and oxytocin secretion is stimulated in this way and the mother's milk supply increases (Matthiesen et al., 2001; Soysal et al., 2005). Early skin contact between the baby and mother has been shown to increase the time and the quality of time at the breast, strengthening the bond between the mother and child and encouraging the mother to be more caring for her baby. It has been observed that mothers who spend more time with their babies, who have more skin contact and practice massaging the baby are more successful at breastfeeding and are able to breastfeed for longer periods of time. In a study by Glover et al (2002), it was noted that mothers in postnatal depression who attended a massage course experienced an increase in the secretion of the hormone oxytocin.

Ali et al (2009), in their comparison of babies receiving and not receiving kangaroo care, reported that the group of infants receiving kangaroo care had good weight gain, shorter stays at the hospital, a lower incidence of hospital infection, reduced risk of hypothermia, and that they received high and exclusive quantities of mother's milk. In short, it can be suggested that parents of newborns be informed about kangaroo care and the advantages it provides so that the method can be practiced with more awareness and consequently with more benefits.

8. Conclusion

In conclusion, cesarean birth is not a hindrance to breastfeeding. Mothers who deliver by cesarean section can breastfeed their babies just like women who have had normal childbirth. Cesarean mothers may however encounter problems, some of them having to do with the mother, and some related to the baby. It is inevitable that nurses at hospitals and health clinics have major responsibilities in this context, as they are the health professionals that spend the most time with mothers giving childbirth. Since nurses/midwives are key figures in helping mothers to decide on and continue with breastfeeding, their duties and responsibilities in supporting breastfeeding starts from before the birth and should continue until the time the baby is weaned from the breast. Besides making sure that the baby is provided with good care and nutrition, the nurse should also have knowledge about breastfeeding mechanisms and methods and also the skills to assist mothers in coping with and solving the problems that they may encounter in breastfeeding. For this reason, breastfeeding methods should be observed and improvements suggested so that the mother can be in an optimum position to nurse her baby and to ensure that she will later be able to correctly breastfeed the infant on her own.

Health professionals should realize that breastfeeding and mother-baby bonding following a cesarean birth are multi-faceted processes. In this awareness, health personnel need to work to strengthen the coping strategies adopted by the baby's family at each contact with the baby. Their efforts should also go into increasing the parents' self-confidence about baby care and helping mothers and fathers to develop their respective parental roles.

9. Vignettes about the breastfeeding after a cesarean

9.1 Vignette 1

Mrs. Merih experienced her first delivery via elective cesarean section under general anasthesia. Her baby was female, healthy, and baby's weight was 3.300 g. She said that about her experiences and feelings after the caesarean section: "*When I met with my daughter, my consciousness was not totally open. The first thing I could remember, breastfeeding was tried to be done with my breasts by nurses instead of me. My first breastfeeding couldn't be in appropriate position. This problem continue until I felt myself well. And I had nipple cracks at the evening of first day. Then the breastfeed become both exciting and painful experience for me. Things that I most wanted after delivery were sitting comfortable, hugging my baby easily, breastfeed her troubleless and comfortable and dressing her up. I could make this my wishes after 7-8 hours from ceserean section. I had more trouble than the mothers who had a vaginal delivery. Because of these reasons I said "I wish, I had a normal delivery" and I felt guilty for being elective cesarean.*"

1. What kind of experiences this mother has about breastfeeding and which problems might be later on?
2. By thinking about how cesarean affect breastfeeding, what kind of a care plan should apply for this mother's needs and problems?

9.2 Vignette 2

Mrs Karabacak has 3 children. They are all girls. When Mrs Karabacak was 41 weeks pregnant, she was admitted to the hospital for Cesarean section. Mrs Karabacak's husband was not with her. The Karabacaks had not attented preparatory classes for childbirth. Mrs Karabacak's section progressed, and she had a baby girl. Mrs Karabacak was transferred to the postpartum unit, and the baby girl Karabacak was transferred to the nursery. Because Mrs Karabacak stated that she was tired and that she was not able to look after the baby at the time. Mrs Karabacak will breast-feed her baby. Until now, her husband has not come to the hospital yet. Mrs Karabacak is unhappy. During a conversation with the nurse, Mrs Karabacak said that if the baby had been a boy, her husband would have been very happy.

1. The nurse does an assesment of the baby girl Karabacak with her mother. Which further assesment will be more effective for breastfeeding?
2. The nurse and Mrs. Karabacak have discussed breast-feeding. What kind of strategies should the nurse follow for effective breastfeeding?

9.3 Vignette 3

9.3.1 Jaundice

Esra, 30 years old, has given birth for the first time to a live baby boy from her second pregnancy, delivered at term with C/S , birth weight 3180 grams. There is Rh incompatibility with her husband and as a result, Baby Ege has developed jaundice. Initial treatment was carried out immediately after the birth. The first jaundice reading was 15 and Ege was started on phototherapy. Baby Ege would start to cry each time he was laid down in the incubator. Each time they saw the baby cry, Esra and her husband couldn't help themselves and cried along with him. After two days of treatment, the reading came down to 11 and they were discharged. Within a month Ege's jaundice reappeared, the value this time going up to 16. The cause of the jaundice was not exactly known. Mother's milk was stopped for a 2-day interval; the baby was fed frequently but the reading failed to drop. Ultimately, inadequate liver enzymes were suspected and the baby was started on oral treatment. The medication regulated the enzymes. Following treatment, the value dropped down to 7 this time. The parents, however, were very anxious that the jaundice would return. Esra in particular was very despondent and exhausted. She said that her milk had dried up because she had been so upset. At the time they came in for a check-up after the dose of medicine was completed, the jaundice reading had fallen to 5. The mother began to cry from happiness. *"I'm so happy," she said.* "My baby doesn't have to suffer any more. They've been constantly drawing blood from his heels, his hands and his arms. His pain was piercing me to the core. Now he's saved from going through all that suffering."

9.4 Vignette 4

9.4.1 Postpartum depression

Ayşe and Ahmet have been married for two years. Ayşe had always wanted to have a baby but because her husband was in a different city due to his job, the husband felt that Ayşe would have trouble with a baby on her own so the couple decided to postpone pregnancy. Ayşe finally did get pregnant. Her mother-in-law stayed with her during the pregnancy. There were constant arguments at home. The pregnancy gave Ayşe a craving for certain foods but no one paid her any attention. Her husband was always away. She was very upset by all of this and she would cry herself to sleep almost every night. Finally, the day came for her to take her baby in her arms. Her husband Ahmet was by her side that day. Baby Arda came into the world a healthy baby; everything was going well. But when two hours later, the baby was brought to Ayşe's room, she didn't want to hold him at first and only threw furtive glances at him from the corner of her eye. When the baby started to cry, she almost threw him into her mother-in-law's arms. The nurse came into the room and said, "Let's see if we can breastfeed the baby, I'll help you get into position, there's nothing to worry about." Ayşe told the nurse that she didn't want to breastfeed the baby, that she "had pain and that she couldn't hold the baby in her arms." The nurse assisted her in picking the baby up but she burst out angrily, "Take him away from me, I don't have any milk anyway, why do you keep insisting?" And Ayşe started to cry... A consultation was requested from the psychiatric department and she was started on therapy...

10. Acknowledgment

We wish to acknowledge our families for their patience and support throughout the writing process especially summer time. We thank Sema's husband Irfan; Sons Okan Eren and Ismail Hakki; We thank Canan's husband Zihni; daughter Belemir Huda; Sons Alperen Taha and Atahan Gufran; We thank Hatice's daughter Ekin; and We thank Meltem's husband Murat and daughter Ipek. You nurtured our passion for babies, mothers, and family members.

11. References

Agarwal, R.; Aggarwal, R.; Deorari, A. & Paul, VK. (2011). Jaundice in the Newborn, 26.07.2011, Available from http://www.newbornwhocc.org/pdf/jaundice.pdf

Ahmed, HM. & Najib BM. (2010). Effect of Implementing Nursing Process on Women's Health after Cesarean Birth at the Maternity Teaching Hospital/Erbil City, *Proceedings of the World Medical Conference,* ISBN 978-960-474-224-0, Malta, September 15-17, 2010, 02.08.2011, Available from http://www.wseas.us/elibrary/conferences/2010/Malta/MEDICAL/MEDICAL-00.pdf

Alexander, L.L., LaRosa, J.H., Bader, H., Garfield, S., Alexander, W.J. (2010). *New Dimensions in Women's Health,*(Fifth edition), Jones and Barlett Publishers, ISBN: 978-0-7637-6592-7, Sudbury, USA.

Ali, SM.; Sharma, J.; Sharma, R. & Alam, S. (2009). Kangaroo Mother Care as Compared to Conventional Care for Low Birth Weight Babies. *Dicle Medical Journal,* Vol.36, No.3, pp.155-160, ISSN 1300-2945

American Academy of Pediatrics (February 2005). Breastfeeding and the Use of Human Milk. In: *Pediatrics,* Vol.115, No.2, ISSN 0031-4005, 22.07.2011, Available from http://aappolicy.aappublications.org/cgi/reprint/pediatrics;115/2/496.pdf

American Academy of Pediatrics, Provisional Committee for Quality Improvement and Subcommittee on Hyperbilirubinemia (2004). Management of Hyperbilirubinemia in the Newborn Infant 35 or More Weeks of Gestation, In: *Pediatrics,*Vol.114, No.1, 01.08.2011, Available from http://aappolicy.aappublications.org/cgi/reprint/pediatrics;114/1/297.pdf

Baumgarder, D.J., Muehl,P., Fischer,M., Pribbeno,B. (2003). Effect of labor epidural anesthesia on breast-feeding of healthy full-term newborns delivered vaginally. *J Am Board Fam Pract,* Vol.16, No.1, pp.(7-13), ISSN:1544-8770

Beck, CT. (2001). Predictors of Postpartum Depression: An Update. *Nursing Research,* Vol.50, No.5, pp.275-285, ISSN 00296562

Beilin, Y., Bodian,C.A.,Weiser,J., Hossain, S. Arnold, I., Feierman,D.E., Martin,G., Holzman, I. *(2005).* Effect of labor epidural analgesia with And without fentanyl on ınfant breast-feeding a prospective, randomized double-blind study. *Anesthesiology,* Vol.103, No.6, pp. (1211-7), ISSN: 0003-3022

Beji, NK. (2010). Pregnancy in Postpartum Period and Psychosocial Adaptation of the Family, In: *Perinatal Nursing,* 1. Baskı, Kömürcü N. (Ed.), pp.386-391, İstanbul Sağlık Müdürlüğü, ISBN 978-605-378-138-7, İstanbul

Bergman, P. & Graham, J. (September 2005). An approach to 'failure to thrive', In: *Reprinted from Australian Family Physician,* Vol.34, No.9, pp.725-729, 01.08.2011, Available from http://www.racgp.org.au/Content/NavigationMenu/Publications/AustralianFamilyPhys/2005Issues/SeptemberGrowth/200509bergman.pdf

Black, RE. (2002). Optimal duration of exclusive breast feeding in low income countries: Six months recommended by WHO applies to populations, not necessarily to individuals, in: *BMJ*. November 30; 325(7375): 1252–1253.

Blair, PS. & Ball, HL. (2004). The Prevalence and Characteristics Associated with Parent-Infant Bed-Sharing in ENGLAND. *Archives of Disease in Childhood,* Vol.89, No.12, pp.1106-1110, ISSN 0003-9888, 1468-2044 (online)

Bowers, NA.; Curran, CA; Comerford Freda M.; Krening, CF.; Poole, JH.; Slocum, J.; Burke Sosa ME. (2008). High-Risk Pregnancy, In: *Perinatal Nursing*, Simpson KR., Creehan PA. (Eds.), pp.240-276, Lippincott Williams & Wilkins, ISBN 13: 978-0-7817-6759-0, ISBN 10: 0-7817-6759-8, Phidelphia

Brandt, KA., Andrews, CM. & Kvale J. (1998). Mother-Infant Interaction and Breastfeeding Outcome 6 Weeks After Birth. *Journal of Obstetric, Gynecologic and Neonatal Nursing,* Vol.27, No.2, pp.169-174, ISSN 0884-2175, 1552-6909 (online)

Brenner, R.; Morton, BGS.; Bhaskar, B.; Revenis, M.; Das, A.; Clemens, JD. (2003). Infant-Parent Bed Sharing in an Inner-City Population.(reprinted). *Arch Pediatr Adolesc Med,* 157: 33-39, ISSN 1538-3628

Brockington, IF.; Oates, J.; George, S.; Turner, D.; Vostanis, P.; Sullivan, M.; Loh, C. & Murdoch, C. (2001). A Screening Questionnaire for Mother-Infant Bonding Disorders. *Archives of Women's Mental Health,* Vol.3, pp.133–140, ISSN 1435-1102

Buswell, SD. & Spatz, DL. (2006). Parent-Infant Co-Sleeping and Its Relationship to Breastfeeding. *Journal of Pediatric Health Care,* Vol.21, No.1, pp.22-28, ISSN 0891-5245

Büyükkayacı Duman N. & Karataş, N. (2011). The Effect of Home Care Service Gıven to Postpartum Early Dıscharged Women who Had a Cesarean Section on the Maternal Health and Power of Self-Care. *Journal of Health Sciences,* Vol.20, No.1, pp.54-67, ISSN 1018-3655

Bystrova, K.; Ivanova, V.; Edhborg, M.; Matthiesen, AS.; Ransjö-Arvidson, AB.; Mukhamedrakhimov, R.; Uvnäs-Moberg, K. & Widström, AM. (2009). Early Contact Versus Separation: Effects on Mother-Infant Interaction One Year Later. *Birth,* Vol.36, No.2, pp.97-109, ISSN 0730-7659, 1523-536X (online)

Caglar, M.K., Ozer, I., Altugan, F.S. (2006). Risk factors for excess weight loss and hypernatremia in exclusively breast-fed infants. *Braz J Med Biol Res,* Vol.39, No.4, pp. (539-544), ISSN: 0100-879X

Cakmak, H.,Kuguoglu,S. (2007). Comparison of the breastfeeding patterns of mothers who delivered their babies per vagina and via cesarean section: An observational study using the LATCH breastfeeding charting system. *International Journal of Nursing Studies,* Vol.44, pp. (1128-1137), ISSN: 0020-7489

Carlander, AK..K.,Edman,G., Christensson,K., Andolf,E.,Wiklund,I. (2010). Contact between mother, child and partner and attitudes towards breastfeeding in relation to mode of delivery. *Sexual & Reproductive Healthcare,* Vol.1, No.1, pp. (27-34), ISSN: 1877-5756

Carlsen, SM.; Jacobsen, G. & Vanky, E. (2010). Mid-pregnancy Androgen Levels are Negatively associated with Breastfeeding. *Acta Obstetricia Et Gynecologica Scandinavica,* Vol.89, No.1, pp.87-94, ISSN 0001-6349, 1600-0412 (online)

Cavuşoğlu, H. (2011). *Child Health Nursing,* 10th ed., System Offset, ISBN 975-94996-3-0, 975-94996-4-9, Ankara

Cetinkaya, M.; Köksal, N.; Sağlam, H. & Tarım, Ö. (2006). Evaluation of Our Cases With Neonatal Hypoglycemia. *Journal of Uludağ University Medical Faculty,* Vol.32, No.3, pp.87-91, ISSN 1300-414X

Chalmers, B., Kaczorowski,J., Darling,E., Heaman,M., Fell,D.B. O'Brien,B., Lee,L., for the Maternity Experiences Study Group of the Canadian Perinatal Surveillance System. (2010). Cesarean and vaginal birth in Canadianwomen: A comparison of experiences. *Birth,* Vol.37, No.1, pp.(44-49), ISSN: 1523-536X

Chapman, D.J., & Pertez, E. (1999). Identification of risk factors for delayed onset of lactation. *J Am Diet Assoc.* Vol.99, pp: 450-454. ISSN: 0002-8223

Chen,J.,Cai, W., Feng, Y.(2007). Development of intestinal bifidobacteria and lactobacilli in breast-fed neonates. *Clinical Nutrition,* Vol. 26, pp. (559–566), ISSN: 0261-5614

Chien, LY. Tai, CJ.(2007). Effect of delivery method and timing of breastfeeding ınitiation on breastfeeding outcomes in Taiwan. *Birth,* Vol.34, No.2, pp. (123-130), ISSN: 1523-536X

Cınar, N.; Sözeri, C.; Dede, C. & Cevahir, R. (2010). Effects of Breast Feeding of Mother and Baby Sleeping in the Same Room. *Maltepe University Nursing Science and Art E-Journal,* Special Edition, pp.235-241, ISSN 1308-4429

Dennis, C.L. (2002). Breastfeeding initiation and duration; a 1990-2000 literature review. *JOGNN.* Vol. 31(1), pp: 12-27. ISSN: 1552-6909

Derebent, E. & Yiğit, R. (2006). Pain in Newborn: Assesment And Management. *Journal of Cumhuriyet Universıty School of Nursing,* Vol.10, No.2, ISSN 1301-6865

Dewey, K.G. (2001). Maternal and fetal stress are associated with impaired lactogenesis in humans. *Journal of Nutrition.* 131, pp: 3012-3015, ISSN 0022-3166

Dewey, K.G., Nommsen-Rivers, l.A., Heinig, M.J., Cohen, R.J. (2002). Lactogenesis and infant weight change in the first weeks of life. In. *Integrating Population Outcomes,Biological Mechanisms and Research Methods in the Study of Human Milk and Lactation.* Margarett K. Davis, Charles E. Issaacs, lars A. Hasson, Anne L. Wright, (Eds.), pp. (159-165), Kluwer Academic/plenum Publishers, ISBN 0-306-46736-4, New- York, USA.

Dewey, K..G., Nommsen-Rivers, L.A., Heinig, M.j., Cohen, R.J. (2003). Risk factors for suboptimal infant breastfeeding behavior, delayed onset of lactation, and excess neonatal weight loss. *Pediatrics,* Vol.112, No.3, pp. (607-619), ISSN: 1098-4275.

Devroe, S. (2007). Obstetric anaesthesia and analgesia and breastfeeding, *Euroanesthesia 2007, European Society of Anesthesiology (ESA),* ISSN: 1365-2346. Munich, Germany, 9-12 June 2007.

Driscol, JW. (2008). Psychosocial Adaptation to Pregnancy and Postpartum, In: *Perinatal Nursing,* Simpson KR., Creehan PA., (Eds.), pp. 78-87, Lippincott Williams & Wilkins, ISBN 13: 978-0-7817-6759-0, ISBN 10: 0-7817-6759-8, Phidelphia

Ergöçmen, BA.; Tezcan, S. & Çağatay, P. (2009). Üreme Sağlığı, In: *Turkey Demographic and Health Survey 2008 Report*, 18.07.2011, Available from http://www.hips.hacettepe.edu.tr/TNSA2008-Ana Rapor.pdf

Evans, K.C., Evans, R.G., Royal,R., Esterman, A.J., James, S.L.(2003). Effect of caesarean section on breast milk transfer to the normal term newborn over the first week of life. *Arch Dis Child Fetal Neonatal Ed*, Vol.88, No.5, pp.(380-382), ISSN:1468-2052

Filidel Rimon, O.; Shinwell, ES. (2005). Postpartum Concerns; *In: Multiple Pregnancy, Epidemiology, Gestation & Perinatal Outcome*, Blickstein, I.; Keith LG,(Ed.). pp. 1128-1149, Taylor Francis, ISBN-10 1-84214-239-9, ISBN e-book 0-203-01775, Oxon,UK

Flick, L.; White, DK.; Vemulapalli, C.; Stulac, BB.; Kemp, JS. (2001). Sleep position and the use of soft bedding during bed sharing among African American infants at increased risk for sudden infant death seyndrome. *The Journal of Pediatrics*, 138:338-343, ISSN 0022-3476

Francis, M. (2007). *The Everything Health Guide to Postpartum Care,* Adams Media, an F+W Publications Company, ISBN 13: 978-1-59869- 275-4, Avon, USA.

Gagnon, AJ. & Bryanton, J. (2009). Postnatal Parental Education for Optimizing Infant General Health and Parent-Infant Relationships. *Cochrane Database Syst Rev.* Vol.21, No.1, pp.1-64, ISSN: 1469-493X

Galler, JR.; Harrison, RH. & Ramsey, F. (2006). Bed-sharing, breastfeeding and maternal moods in Barbados. *Infant Behavior and Development*, Vol.29, No.4, pp.526-534, ISSN 0163-6383

Glover, V.; Onozawa, K. & Hodgkinson, A. (2002). Benefits of Infant Massage for Mothers with Postnatal Depression. *Seminars in Neonatology,* Vol.7, No.6, pp.495-500, ISSN 1084-2756

Görak, G. (2002). Ethics in Baby Nursing, In: *Basic Neonatology and Principles of Nursing,* Dağoğlu T, Görak G. (Eds.), pp. 31-40, 785-791, Nobel Medical Publishers, ISBN 975-420-195-8, İstanbul

Grassi, A. (2008). Recognition and Treatment Approaches for Polycystic Ovary Syndrome, In: *Women's Health Report*, 15.07.2011, Available from http://www.womenshealthdpg.org/members/news/Summer_2008.pdf

Güngor, I., Gökyıldız, S., & Nahcıvan, N.O (2004). Opinions of a group of women who had caesarean sections about their births and their problems in the early postpartum period. *Journal of Nursing in İstanbul University College Nursing*. Vol.13(53), pp.185-187. ISSN 2141-2499

Günöz, H.; Saka, N.; Darendeliler, F. & Bundak, R. (2003). Growth, Development and Endocrine, In: *Child Health and Diseases*, Cantez T, Ömeroğlu RE, Baysal SU, Oğuz F. (Eds.), Nobel Medical Publishers, pp. 73-76, ISBN 975-420-273-7, İstanbul

Heck, K.E., Schoendorf K.C., & G.F. Chavez et al. (2003). Does postpartum Length of stay affect breastfeeding duration? A population based study. *Birth*. Vol.30 (3), pp: 153-159. ISSN: 1523-536X

Hofer, MA. (2005). The Psychobiology of Early Attachment. *Clinical Neuroscience Research,* Vol.4, No.5-6, pp.291-300, ISSN 1566-2772

Ilgaz, S. (2000). Ten Questions Ten Answer. *Journal of Continuing Medical Education*, Vol.9, No.10, pp.382-385, ISSN 1300-0853

Imdad, A.; Yakoob, M.Y. & Bhutta, Z.A. (2011). Effect of breastfeeding promotion interventions on breastfeeding rates, with special focus on developing countries. *BMC Public Health* . 11(Suppl 3) :S24 doi:10.1186/1471-2458-11-S3-S24

Ince., N. (1998).Assessment of breastfeeding technigues and breastfeeding concultancy at baby-friendly hospitals in the city of İstanbul. Thesis, University of İstanbul.

Ince, Z. (2001). Anne Sütü ile Beslenme: Sorunlar ve Çözüm Yaklaşımları. 23. Pediatri Günleri ve 3. Pediatri Hemşireliği Günleri Özet Kitabı, İstanbul, 10-13 Nisan 2001

Indriyani, SAK.; Retayasa, IW.; Surjono, A. & Suryantoro P. (2009). Percentage Birth Weight Loss and Hyperbilirubinemia During the First Week of Life in Term Newborns. *Paediatrica Indonesiana,* Vol.49, No.3, pp.149-154, ISSN 0030-9311

Işler, A. (2007). Prematüre Bebeklerde Anne Bebek İlişkisinin Başlatılmasında Yenidoğan Hemşirelerinin Rolü. *Perinatoloji Dergisi,* Vol.15, No.1, pp.1–6, ISSN 1300-5251

Jaffe, AC. (2011). Failure to Thrive: Current Clinical Concepts. *Pediatrics in Review,* Vol. 32, pp.100-108, ISSN 0191-9601

Janke, JR. (1998) Breastfeeding duration following cesarean and vaginal births. *J Nurse Midwifery.* Vol.33, pp: 159-164.ISSN:0091-2182

Janke, J. (2008). Newborn Nutrition, In: *Perinatal Nursing,* Simpson KR., Creehan PA., (Eds.), pp. 582-607, Lippincott Williams & Wilkins, ISBN 13: 978-0-7817-6759-0, ISBN 10: 0-7817-6759-8, Phidelphia

Jansen, J.; Weerth, C. & Walraven, JMR. (2008). Breastfeeding and the mother-infant relationship- a review. *Developmental Review,* Vol.28, No.4, pp.503-521, ISSN: 0273-2297

Jolley, CD. (2003). Failure to Thrive. *Current Problems in Pediatric and Adolescent Health Care,* Vol. 33, No.6, pp.183-206, ISSN 0045-9380

Jonkers, D. (2005). Breastfeeding after a caesarean birth. 18.07.2011, Available from http://www.our-birthmatters.net/pdfs/Breastfeeding_After_a_Caesarean.pdf

Kaplan, M. & Merlob, P. (2008). Israel guidelines for the management of neonatal hyperbilirubinemia and prevention of kernicterus. *Journal of Perinatology,* Vol. 28, No.6, pp.389-397, ISSN 0743-8346

Karlström, A., Engström-Olofsson,R., Norberg,KG, Sjöling, M.,Hildingsson, I. (2007). Postoperative pain after cesarean birth affects breastfeeding and ınfant care. *JOGNN,* Vol.36, No.5; pp. (430-440),ISSN: 1552-6909

Kelley, CG. (October 2003). PCOS and Breastfeeding, In: *Breastfeeding Update,* Vol.3, No.3, 15.07.2011, Available from http://www.breastfeeding.org/uploaded_files/newsletters/newsletter11.pdf

Kirk, AT.; Alder, SC. & King, JD. (2007). Cue-Based Oral Feeding Clinical Pathway Results in Earlier Attainment of Full Oral Feeding in Premature Infants, *Journal of Perinatology,* Vol. 27, No. 9, pp.572-578, ISSN 0743-8346

Kliegman, RM. (2002). Diseases of the Fetus and Newborn, In: *Nelson Essential of Pediatrics,* Behrman RE, Kliegman RM, (Eds.), pp.179-186, 226-229, W.B. Saunders Company, ISBN 0-7216-9406-3, Philadelphia, Pensilvania

Korter, D. (July/August 1998). Birth After Cesarean: A Primer for Success. 04.08.2011, Available from http://birthingalternatives.com/Resources/Cesarean/Birth%20After%20Cesarean.pdf

Krugman, SD. & Dubowitz, H. (2003). Failure to Thrive. *American Family Physician,* Vol.68, No.5, pp.879-884, ISSN 0002-838X

Kroeger, M., &Smith, L.J. (2004). *Impact of birthing practices on breastfeeding:Protecting the mother and baby continuum.* Sudbury, MA: Jones and Bartlett Publishers.ISBN: 978-0-7637-6374-9

Kurul, SZ. (2011). Nörolojik Gelişme Geriliği Riski Olan Süt çocuklarının Erken Belirlenmesinin Önemi ve Klinisyenin Rolü, 14.07.2011, Available from http://www.deu.edu.tr/UploadedFiles/Birimler/17991/195-205.pdf

Lauwers, J.; Swisher A. (2010).A *Counseling the Nursing Mother: A Lactation Consultant's Guide*, pp: 344-349, Jones & Barlett Learning, ISBN 978-0-7637-8052-4, Canada

Lauwers, J. Swisher, A. (2011). *Counseling the Nursing Mother. A Lactation Consultant's Guide,* (Fifth edition), Jones and Barlett Publishers, ISBN 978-0-7637-8652-4, Sudbury, USA.

Leung, G, M., Lam, TH, Ho, LM.(2002). Breast-feeding and its relation to smoking and mode of delivery. *Obstet & Gynecology*, Vol.99, No.5, pp. (785–94), ISSN:0029-7844

Littleton, Ly.; Engebretso, J. (2002).Lactation and Nursing Support; In: *Maternal, Neonatal and Women's Health Nursing, Volume 1*, pp.955-1009, Delmar, a Division of Thomson Learning Inc., ISBN 0-7668-0121-7, Albany, NY/USA

Lowdermilk, DL. & Perry, SE. (2007). *Maternity & Women's Health Care*. 9 Edition, pp.612-632, Mosby Elsevier, ISBN-10: 0323043674, ISBN-13: 978-0323043670, St. Louis

Maisels, JM. (2006). Neonatal Jaundice. *Pediatrics in Review*, Vol.27, No.12, pp.443-454, ISSN 0191-9601

Maisels, MJ. & Watchko, JF. (2003). Treatment of Jaundice in Low Birthweight Infants. *Archives of Disease in Childhood - Fetal and Neonatal Edition*, Vol.88, No.6, pp.459-463, ISSN 1359-2998, 1468-2052

Maisels, MJ.; Kring, EA. & DeRidder, J. (2007). Randomized Controlled Trial of Light-Emitting Diode Phototherapy. *Journal of Perinatology,* Vol.27, No.9, pp.565-567 ISSN 0743-8346

Maisels, MJ. & McDonagh, AF. (2008). Phototherapy for Neonatal Jaundice. *The New England Journal of Medicine*, Vol.358, No.9, pp.920-928, ISSN 0028-4793

Mannel, R (2011). Defining lactation acuity to improve patient safety and outcomes. *Journal of Human Lactation*. Vol.27(2), pp: 163-70.ISSN:0890-3344

Margarett K. Davis, Charles E. Issaacs, lars A. Hasson, Anne L. Wright, (Eds.), pp. (159-165), Kluwer Academic/plenum Publishers, ISBN 0-306-46736-4, New-York, USA.

Martins, C. & Gaffan, EA. (2000). Effects of Early Maternal Depression on Patterns of Infant-Mother Attachment: A Meta-Analytic Investigation. *Journal of Child Psychology & Psychiatry*, Vol.41, No.6, pp.737-46, ISSN 0021-9630

Matthiesen, AS.; Ransjö-Arvidson, AB.; Nissen, E. & Uvnäs-Moberg, K. (2001). Postpartum maternal oxytocin release by newborns: effects of infant hand massage and sucking. *Birth*, Vol.28, No.1, pp.13-19, ISSN 0730-7659, 1523-536X (online)

Mayberry, L. (2006). Cesarean delivery on maternal request. *Nursing Implications of the 2006 NIH. State of the Science Conference Statement,* MCN *(Special Report for MCN)*, Vol.32, No.5, pp. (286-89),. ISSN: 1539-0683

McFarlin, BL. (2004). Elective Cesarean Birth: Issues and Ethics of an Informed Decision. *Journal of Midwifery & Women's Health*, Vol.49, No.5, pp.421-429, ISSN 1526-9523

Moehler, E.; Brunner, R.; Wiebel, A.; Reck, C. & Resch, F. (2006). Maternal depressive symptoms in the postnatal period are associated with long-term impairment of mother–child bonding. Archives of Women's Mental Health, Vol.9, No.5, pp.273-278, ISSN 1435-1102

Mohrbacher, N., &Stock, J., (2003). *The breastfeeding Answer book*. Schamburg, IL:La Leche League International.ISBN: 0-76-37-4585-5

Murray, SS. & Mckinney, ES. (2006). *Foundations of Maternal–Newborn Nursing*, Fourth Edition, pp. 439-443, 761-780, Saunders Elsevier, ISBN-13: 978-1-4160-0141-6, ISBN - 10: 1-4160-0141-7, St. Louis, Missouri

Neifert, M.(2009).Great Expectations: *The Essential Guide to Breastfeeding*, pp.39-75, Sterling Publishing, ISBN 978-1-4027-5817-1, New York,USA

Negishi, H., Kishida, T., Yamada, H., Hirayama, E., Mikuni,M ., Fujimoto,S.(1999). Changes in uterine size after vaginal delivery and cesarean section determined by vaginal sonography in the puerperium. *Arch Gyenecol Obstet*, Vol.263, No.1-2, pp.(13-16), ISSN:1432-0711, DOI: 10.1007/s004040050253

Newman, B.M., Newman, P.R.(2009). *Development Through Life: A Psychosocial Approch*,(Tenth edition), Wadsworth Cengage Learning, ISBN-13 :978-0-495-5534-0, Belmont, USA.

Neyzi, O. & Ertugrul, T. (2002). *Pediatrics*, 3th ed., Vol. 1, Tayf Offset, ISBN 975-420-120-X, İstanbul

Nolan, A.,Lawrence, C.(2009). A pilot study of a nursing ıntervention protocol to minimize maternal-ınfant separation after cesarean birth. *JOGNN*, Vol.38, No.4, pp.(430-442), ISSN:1552-6909

Olds, SB.; London, ML.; Wieland Ladewig, PA. & Davidson, MR. (2004). *Maternal-Newborn Nursing & Women's Health Care*, Seventh Edition, Prentice Hall, ISBN-10: 0130990094, ISBN-13: 978-0130990099, Pearson, New Jersey

Ozbek, A., Miral, S. (2003). Prematurity in terms of Children Mental Health. *Turkish Pediatric Journal*, Vol.46, No.4, pp.317-327, ISSN 0010-0161

Page-Goertz, S. (2010). Hypoglycemia in the Breastfeeding Newborn. *International Lactation Consultant Association (ILCA)*, 05.07.2011, Available from www.ilca.org/files/education_and.../ Mod%20Hypoglycemia.pdf

Pasupathy, D., Smith, C.S. (2008). Neonatal outcomes with caesarean delivery at term. *Arch Dis Child Fetal Neonatal Ed*, Vol.93, No.3, PP.(174-75), ISSN:1468-2052

Perez-Escamilla, R., Maulen-Radovan, I., Dewey, K.G. (1996). The association between cesarean delivery and breast-feeding outcomes among Mexican women. *Am. J. Public Health*, Vol.86, No.6, pp.(832-836), ISSN: 1541-0048.

Rempel, L.A., &Rempel, J.K. (2011). The breastfeeding team: The role of ınvolved fathers in the breastfeeding family. *Journal of Human Lactation*. Vol.27(2), pp: 115-121. ISSN: 0890-3344

Renfrew, MJ.; Dyson, L.; McCormick, F.; Misso, K.; Stenhouse, E.; King, SE. & Williams, AF. (2010). Breastfeeding Promotion for Infants in Neonatal Units: A Systematic Review. *Child: Care Health and Development*, Vol.36, No.2, pp.165-178, ISSN 0305-1862

Righard, L. (1998). Are breastfeeding problems related to incorrect bresatfeeding technique and the use of pacifiers and bottles. *Birth*. 25(1), pp: 40-46. ISSN: 1523-536X

Ricci, S.S.; Kyle, T. (2008). Nursing Management of the Newborn , *In: Maternity and Pediatric Nursing*, pp. 497-547,Lippincott Williams & Wilkins, ISBN 13:978-0-7817-8055-1, China

Riordan, J., & Koehn, M. (1998). Reliability and validity testing of three breastfeeding asssesment tools. *Journal of Obstetric Gynecology Neonatal Nursing*. Vol.27(3), pp: 236. ISSN: 1552-6909

Riordan, J., Gross,A., Angeron, J., Krumwiede, B., Melin, J. (2000). The effect of labor pain relief medication on neonatal suckling and breastfeeding duration. *J Hum Lact*, Vol.16, No.1, pp.(7-12), ISSN: 1552-1732

Rosenthal, M.S. (2000). *The Breastfeeding Source Book*, (Third edition), The McGraw-Hill Companies. DOI: 10. 1036/0071392254, (Print), ISBN: 0-7373-0509- 6, USA.

Rowe-Murray, H.J., Fisher, J.V.R. (2002). Baby friendly hospital practices: cesarean section is a persistent barrier to early initiation of breastfeeding. *Birth*, Vol.29, No.2, pp.(124-131), ISSN: 1523-536X

Sabuncuoğlu, O. & Berkem, M. (2006). Relationship Between Attachment Style and Depressive Symptoms in Postpartum Women: Findings from Turkey. *Turkish Journal of Psychiatry*, Vol.17, No.4, pp.252-258, ISSN 1300-2163

Sahin, F. (2002). Child Abuse: Medical Diagnosis and Treatment Tips. *journal of Clinical Pediatrics*, Vol.1, No.3, pp.103-106, ISSN 1303-5312

Satar, M. (2001). Ethical Issues in Neonatal Practicals, *Booklet of the 11th National Neonatology Congress*, ISBN 975-482-651-X, Samsun, June 25-28, 2001

Savaşer, S. (2002). Nutrition of the Newborn, In: *Basic Neonatology and Principles of Nursing*, Dağoğlu T, Görak G. (Eds.), pp. 211-242, Nobel Medical Publishers, ISBN 975-420-195-8, İstanbul

Savaşer, S. (2001). Breast Feeding and the Baby-Friendly Hospitals, Booklet of the 11th National Neonatology Congress, ISBN 975-482-651-X, Samsun, June 25-28, 2001

Sayıner, FD., Özerdoğan, N., Giray, S., Özdemir, E. & Savcı A. (2009). Factors Affecting the Preferences in the Shape of Birth of Women. *Journal of Perinatology*, Vol.17, No.3, pp.104-112, ISSN 1300-5251

Sgro, M. & Campbell, D. (2006). Incidence and Causes of Severe Neonatal Hyperbilirubinemia in Canada. *Canadian Medical Association Journal*, Vol.175, No. 6, pp. 587-590, ISSN 1488-2329

Smith, L.J. (2010). *Impact of Birth Practices on Breastfeeding*, (Second edition), Jones and Barlett Publishers, ISBN 978-0-7637-6374-9, Sudbury, USA.

Simpson, K.R. (2008). labor and birth, In: *Perinatal Nursing*, (Third edition), Kathleen Rice Simpson and patricia A. Creehan, (Eds.), pp.(300- 375), Lippincott Williams & Wilkings, ISBN-13: 978-0-7817-6759-0. Phidelphia, USA.

Sivaslı, E. (2009). Prolonged Jaundice in Newborns Babies. *Gaziantep Medical Journal*, Vol.15, No.2, pp.49-55, ISSN 1300-0888

Soysal, A.S., Ergenekon, E., Aksoy, E.& Erdoğan, E. (2000). Study of Birth Type Variable on Attachment Pattern. *Journal of Clinical Psychiatry*, Vol.3, No.2, pp.75-85, ISSN 1302-0099

Soysal, Ş.; Bodur, Ş.; İşeri, E. & Şenol, Ş. (2005). Attachment Process in Infancy: A Review. *Journal of Clinical Psychiatry*, Vol.8, No.2, pp.88-99, ISSN 1302-0099

Steele, M.; Steele, H. & Johansson, M. (2002). Maternal Predictors of Children's Social Cognition: An Attachment Perspective. *Journal of Child Psychology & Psychiatry*, Vol.43, No.7, pp.861-872, ISSN: 0021-9630

Statewide Maternity and Neonatal Clinical Guidelines Program. (2009). Neonatal jaundice: prevention, assessment and management. In: *Maternity & Neonatal*, 05.07.2011, Available from
http://www.health.qld.gov.au/cpic/documents/mguideg_jaundV4.0.pdf

Sözmen, M. (1992). Effects of early suckling of cesarean-born babies on lactation. *Biol Neonate*. Vol.62, pp: 67-68. ISSN: 0006-3126

Tammentie, T.; Tarkka, MT.; Astedt-Kurki, P. & Paavilainen, E. (2002). Sociodemographic Factors of Families related to Postnatal Depressive Symptoms of Mothers. *International Journal of Nursing Practice*, Vol.8, No.5, pp.240-246, ISSN 1322-7114

Tengir, T. & Çetinkaya, Ş. (2008). Methods Used in Nutrition of Newborn and Nursing Care. *Fırat University Health Sciences Journal*, Vol.3, No.9, pp.120-140, ISSN 1306-6366

Tezel, A. (2006). Nurses'/Midwiferys' Responsibilities In The Assessment Of Postpartum Depression. *New Symposium*, Vol.44, No.1, pp.49-52, ISSN: 1300-8773

Tilokskulchai, F., Phatthanasiriwethin, S., Vichitsukon, K. & Serisathien, Y. (2002). Attachment Behaviors in Mother of Premature Infants: A Descriptive Study in Thai Mothers. *Journal of Perinatal & Neonatal Nursing*, Vol.16, No.3, pp.69-83, ISSN 0893-2190, 1550-5073 (online)

The Childbirth Centre Queensway Carleton Hospital. (December 2005). Cesarean Birth, In: *Information for the New Mother & Her Family*, 06.07.2011, Available from http://www.qch.on.ca/Content/File/Childbrith%20Centre/Information%20for%20the%20New%20Mother%20-%20Cesarean.pdf

Thompson, J.F., Heal, L.J., Roberts, C.L., Ellwood, D.A. (2010). Women's breastfeeding experiences following a significant primary postpartum haemorrhage: A multicentre cohort study. *International Breastfeeding Journal*, Vol.5, No.5, pp. (1-12), ISSN: 1746-4358

Trent, ME; Rich, M.; Austin, SB. & Gordon, CM. (2002). Quality of Life in Adolescent Girls With Polycystic Ovary Syndrome. *Archives of Pediatrics and Adolescent Medicine*, Vol.156, pp.556-560, ISSN 1072-4710

Törüner, Ek; Büyükgönenç, L. (2011). *Child Health*, Gökçe Offset, ISBN 978-605-5901-05-9, Ankara

Tüzün, O. & Sayar, K. (2006). Attachment Theory and Psychopathology. *Journal of Psychiatric and Neurological Sciences*, Vol.19, No.1, pp.24-39, ISSN 1309-5749

Towle, M.A. (2009). *Maternal Newborn Nursing Care*. (First edition), Pearson Prentice Hall, ISBN-13: 978-0-13-113730-1, New Jarsey, USA.

Usha Kiran T, Jayawickrama N (2002). Who is Responsible for the Rising Section Rate?. *Journal of Obstetrics & Gynaecology*, Vol.22, No.4, pp.363-365, ISSN 0144-3615

Walker, M. (2011). *Breastfeeding Management for the Clinician*, (Second edition), Jones and Barlett Publishers, ISBN-13: 978-0-7637-6651-1, Sudbury, USA.

Weiss, RE. (2010). *The Better Way to Breastfeeding*, Fair Winds Press, pp. 68-90, ISBN-10 1-59233-422-9; ISBN 13 978-1-59233-422-3

Welan, A., &Lupton, P. (1998). Promoting Succesful breastfeeding among women with a low income. *Midwifery*. Vol.14, pp: 94-100. ISSN:0091-2182

Willis, C.E., Livingstone, V. (1995). İnfant insufficient milk syndrome associated with maternal postpartum hemorrhage. *J. Human Lact*, Vol. 11. Pp. (123-126), ISSN: 1552-1732

Wong, RJ.; Desandre, GH.; Sibley, E. & Stevenson, DK. (2006). Neonatal Jaundice and Liver Disease, In: *Neonatal – Perinatal Medicine: Disease of the Fetus and Infant*, Martin RJ, Fanaroff AA, Walsh MC. (Eds.), pp.1419-1465, Mosby Elsevier, ISBN-10: 0323009298, ISBN-13: 978-0323009294, Missouri, USA

Xie, RH.; He, G.; Koszycki, D.; Walker, M. & Wen, SW. (2009). Prenatal Social Support, Postnatal Social Support, and Postpartum Depression. *Annals of Epidemiology*, Vol.19, No.9, pp.637-643, ISSN: 1047-2797

Vanky, E.; Isaksen, H.; Moen, MH.; Carlsen, SM. (2008). Breastfeeding in Polycystic Ovary Syndrome. *Acta Obstetricia Et Gynecologica Scandinavica*, Vol.87, No.5, pp.531-535, ISSN 0001-6349, 1600-0412 (online)

Vatansever, Ü. & Çelik, H. (2005). Neonatal Presentations to the Pediatric Emergency Department. *Turkish Journal of Emergency Medicine,* Vol.5, No.3, pp.113-117, ISSN 1304-7361

Vieira, T.O., Vieira, G.O., Giugliani, E.R.J., Mendes, C.MC. Martins, C.C., Silva, L.R. (2010).Determinants of breastfeeding initiation within the first hour of life in a Brazilian population: Cross-sectional study. *BMC Public Health,* Vol.10, No.760, pp.(1- 6), ISSN 1471-2458

Vireday, P. (2002). *Breastfeeding after a cesarean.* Retrieved from< http://www.plus-size-pregnancy.org>.

Vincenzo, Z., Giorgia, S., Francesco, C., &Arturo, G et al. (2010). Elective Cesarean Delivery: Does It Have a Negative Effect on Breastfeeding? *Birth.* Vol.37, No. 4, pp: 275-279. ISSN:1523-536X

Yıldız, S. (2001). The responsibility of the nurse in breastfeeding. *Booklet of the 11th National Neonatology Congress* . pp: 247-252, Samsun, Turkey. ISBN-13: 9780826122070

Yiğit, EK.; Tezcan, S. & Tunçkanat, H. (2009). Nutritional Status of Children and Mothers, In: Turkey Demographic and Health Survey 2008 Report, 18.07.2011, Available from http://www.hips.hacettepe.edu.tr/TNSA2008-AnaRapor.pdf

Yılmaz, M.; İsaoğlu, Ü. & Kadanalı S. (2009). Investigation of the Cesarean Section Cases in Our Clinic Between 2002 and 2007. *Marmara Medical Journal,* Vol.22, No.2, pp.104-110, ISSN 1019-1941

Zanardo ,V.,Svegliado, G., Cavallin, F., Giustardi, A., Cosmi, E., Litta, P., Trevisanuto, D. (2010). Elective cesarean delivery: Does it have a negative effect on breastfeeding? *Birth,* Vol.37, No.4, pp. (275–279), ISSN: 1523-536X

(2011). World Health Statistics, 18.07.2011, Available from http://www.who.int/whosis/whostat/EN_WHS2011_Full.pdf s

9

Determining Factors of Cesarean Delivery Trends in Developing Countries: Lessons from Point G National Hospital (Bamako – Mali)

I. Teguete, Y. Traore, A. Sissoko, M. Y. Djire, A. Thera, T. Dolo, N. Mounkoro, M. Traore and A. Dolo

Department of Obstetrics and Gynecology
Faculty of Medicine, Pharmacy and Dentistry
University of Bamako
Mali

1. Introduction

Pregnancy and delivery have been and continue to be a high risk endeavour for women [Rivière, 1959]. This assertion explains the continuous efforts of healthcare workers to maintain pregnancy and delivery in a normal course.

One of the obstetric interventions introduced to address this issue is the cesarean - delivery. Cesarean delivery is defined as the birth of a fetus through incisions in the abdominal wall (laparotomy) and the uterine wall (hysterotomy) [Cunningham, 2001]. Historically, cesarean delivery was associated with a high complication rate, sometimes causing maternal death. In the era of modern medicine, however, cesarean section has become safe and is widely endorsed throughout the world as a strategy to improve pregnancy outcomes [Weil & Fernandez, 1999].

In the past decades, cesarean rates in high income countries have increased considerably, leading some experts to question the benefit of these elective procedures on maternal and neonatal outcome [Howell et al, 2009; Malvasi et al, 2009; Ba'aqeel, 2009; Jain, 2009; Karlström et al, 2010; Klemeti et al, 2010; Bogg, 2010]. Critics of the trend toward unindicated cesarean delivery have coined these procedures "unneCesareans" [Althabe et al, 2004; Cohain, 2009]. Policies targeted to reverse this trend have been generally unsuccessful [Choudhury et al, 2009].

This epidemic increase is even encountered in some developing countries [Belizán et al 1999; Khawaja et al., 2009; Naidoo & Moodley, 2009; Betran et al, 2007; Villar et al., 2006; Onsrud & Onsrud, 1996; Barros et al, 1991; Faundes & Cecatti, 1991]. Reasons behind the high cesarean delivery rates in some developing countries are generally unclear [Wylie & Mirza, 2008]. Doing more to gain more mainly in private practice [Naido & Moodley, 2009; Wylie & Mirza, 2008]; presumption that CD protects against urinary incontinence, pelvic prolapse, and sexual dissatisfaction ; auspicious date of birth; beliefs that babies delivered surgically are smarter…. [Wylie & Mirza, 2008] are some of the unjustified reasons reported.

Most developing countries, however, report cesarean delivery rates well below the acceptable minimum standard of 5% outlined by the WHO. Poor healthcare access, underdeveloped healthcare infrastructure, geographical inaccessibility, cultural mistrust, poverty, and paucity of human health resources are barriers to providing cesarean deliveries to all women who need them [Dumont et al., 2001; De Brouwere et al, 2002; Ronsmans et al, 2002; Kwawukume, 2001]. Large ecological studies in West Africa emphasized this gap by demonstrating increased maternal mortality in settings with a lower percentage of births supervised by a skilled attendant, fewer deliveries performed in-hospital, or a smaller proportion of deliveries performed by cesarean section. Increased access to these services correlated with lower maternal mortality rate [Ronsmans et al, 2003].

Mali is the 3rd poorest nation in the world, with an estimated maternal mortality ratio between 464 and 830 deaths per 100,000 live births [Chou et al, 2010; Samaké et al, 2007]. In 1990, the Mali Ministry of Health developed a healthcare initiative focusing on the maternal and child health. Among the key elements of the Malian healthcare system, is the clear distinction between the three levels of care provision: primary (community health centres), secondary (district referral health centres) and tertiary care (hospitals). Pregnant women are initially supposed to

book at the community health centres (which is the entry point of the healthcare system) with a primary care midwife or obstetric nurse for care provision during pregnancy, birth and the puerperium. These community health centres have the pivotal role of patients selection based on risk assessment. One important innovation of this new policy was the establishment of a referral system for perinatal complications in 1994. To ensure that referral takes place in an optimal fashion, guidelines for consultation and collaboration between community health centres, district referral health centres and hospital have been formulated in the Perinatality Module and in the Standard, Options and Procedures for Reproductive Health Services Manual. In these documents, all professional groups involved in maternity care agreed on the indications for consultation and referral according to the level of care. This program augmented the healthcare system's capacity to manage obstetric emergencies by upgrading referral centres' technical trays including staff training, surgical theatre rehabilitation, creation community health centres in previously inaccessible areas, organisation of transport between the community centres and referral centres, and communities' mobilisation to own the system. The main obstetric emergency encountered was cephalopelvic disproportion and its complications. Cesarean delivery was the main obstetric procedure used to deal with these complications. Lowering of financial barriers to increase access to this major obstetric intervention was one of the strategies of the organisation of the referral system in Mali.

To date, there have not been any in-depth evaluations of cesarean delivery in Mali since the inception of this program. Poor data capture of most population health indicators have called into question the reliability of cesarean delivery reports for other developing countries [Stanton et al, 2005; Holtz and Stanton, 2007]. In this context, large hospital databases of good quality provide a bird's eye view of the national health system and trends in healthcare delivery over time.

This paper aims to assess the trends of cesarean delivery at the Point G national hospital in Bamako, Mali over a period of 2 decades. We explore the impact of sociodemographic, obstetric, and systemic determinants on cesarean delivery rates. Results are discussed in relation to current medical literature available for developing countries and lessons for improvement of current health systems are highlighted.

2. Study settings and design

2.1 Organisation of delivery care at Point G teaching hospital

Point G National Hospital is a tertiary care referral center in Bamako, Mali affiliated with the Faculty of Medicine, Pharmacy, and Odonto-stomatology at the University of Bamako. This hospital provides emergency obstetric services for women referred from other health centers, as well as prenatal care and delivery services for women from urban and rural areas surrounding Bamako. The catchments population in Bamako grew rapidly from 658,275 in 1987 to 1,016,296 in 1998.

The cesarean delivery rate was 6.5% in Bamako versus 1.6% for the national level [Samaké et al, 2007]. Many patients referred to Point G hospital reside in rural areas surrounding Bamako. Thus, rates of early access to care and facility-based delivery among patients at Point G hospital may be lower than those found among residents of Bamako.

The services available at Point G hospital have changed over time, dividing the hospital's history into distinct periods. Among the major events that influenced obstetric admission at Point G hospital, is the National Perinatality Program implemented in 1994, which included organization of a referral system between primary health structures and district referral centers. Access to cesarean delivery was the cornerstone of this organization which improved transport and designed schemes to lower its cost for women in needs. This referral system has been shown to increase access to emergency obstetric care and decrease maternal mortality in rural Mali [Fournier et al, 2009], though its impact on maternal deaths at an urban tertiary care center is unknown. Between 1998 and 2000, an audit of near-miss events was undertaken to improve delivery services. In 2002 the Government of Mali reorganized the healthcare system, integrating the staff of Point G National Hospital with those at Bamako's Gabriel Touré Teaching Hospital.

The obstetrics and gynecology service of Point G teaching hospital was equipped with 1 labor ward containing 3 delivery tables, 30 beds, and a single operating room for scheduled surgeries as well as emergent surgeries from 1985 to 1994. The hospital has an adult intensive care unit (ICU), but no neonatal ICU, and administers a limited blood transfusion service. At Point G National Hospital the general surgery and urology services also provided care during delivery mainly to those women requiring cesarean delivery.

2.2 Obstetric database

A complete database of all obstetric admissions focusing on characteristics of delivered women, mode of delivery, cesarean indications, and maternal, fetal and immediate neonatal outcome was built to include all deliveries recorded at Point G National Hospital between January 1, 1985 and December 31, 2003 (17 721 patients) [Teguete et al, 2010a]. All data were double-entered in Epi6.fr to insure accuracy. Data were collected from these complete obstetric files, as well as hospital birth registries, registries of on-call midwives, surgical reports, admissions records for the intensive care service, records from the internal medicine and urology services, and hospital death records.

2.3 Analysis

We report trends in cesarean delivery rates at Point G National Hospital in Bamako, Mali from 1985 to 2003. Annual cesarean deliveries rates were calculated and grouped by historic time intervals to elucidate changes in cesarean utilization over time. These intervals represent 5 distinct periods in the hospital's history: 1985 to 1990 before the department of obstetrics and gynecology was established by the first Malian professor in this field ; 1991 to 1995 encompassing the introduction of the National Perinatality ProgramProgram; 1996 to 1997 when the service of obstetrics and gynecology functioned at partial capacity due to hospital renovation; 1998 to 2001 immediately after renovation; and 2002 to 2003 when the major obstetric team moved from Point G to Gabriel Touré Teaching Hospital, another teaching hospital in Bamako.

We first computed cesarean delivery rates during the five time periods according to different categories to observe general trends. Cesarean delivery rates were calculated as the percentage of pregnant women delivered after surgical opening of the abdomen. Crude and adjusted odds ratios (OR) were obtained by logistic regression and subsequently transformed into relative risks (because rates of cesarean delivery were more than 10%) by the equation:

$$RR = \frac{OR}{(1-p_0)+p_0 * OR} \quad \text{[Zhang \& Yu, 1998].} \qquad (1)$$

Characteristics considered to be of relevance for cesarean delivery were: maternal age, marital status, ethnic group, parity, hypertension or diabetes in pregnancy, gestational age, number of fetus (single vs. multiple gestations), cesarean delivery indications and referral status.

We then described the contribution of different indications to overall cesarean delivery rates following the rules of the Baltimore group on cesarean indications reporting for developing countries [Stanton et al, 2008]. Interactions of these indications with maternal characteristics have been reported. The next step looked for our practice concerning specific obstetric group. This step focused on the study of cesarean delivery in ten obstetric groups. The definition of these groups appears in table 3. Based on the review of the relevant literature about this topic [Stavrou et al., 2011; Costa et al, 2010; Brennan et al, 2009; McCarthy et al, 2007; Robson, 2001], we focused on the correlation between trends of overall cesarean delivery rates and that of the cesarean delivery rates in term single cephalic nulliparas (TSCN). The term single cephalic nulliparas gathered groups 1 and 2 during the 19 year period. Pearson's correlation coefficient was used to estimate the relationship between overall CS rates and TSCN cesarean delivery rates. Independent Student *t* test was used to compare mean overall CS rates. The coefficient of variation (CV) was calculated as the standard deviation (SD)/mean x 100. The relevant cesarean indications characterising this specific composite group were identified. Finally, we identified individual factors influencing the cesarean delivery rates in our hospital by multilogistic regression using sequential adjustments.

The final section of the analysis dealt with cesarean morbidity and mortality. We considered maternal as well as fetal and neonatal complications. For maternal complications, we estimated rates of intraoperative complications as well as of post-cesarean complications. We defined intraoperative complications as laceration of the uterus (uterine rupture included), cervix, bladder, vagina or bowel, intraoperative blood loss of ≥1000 ml, blood transfusion, and hysterectomy. Post-cesarean complications included post-cesarean infection, hemorrhage, deep venous thrombosis and puerperal psychosis. Regarding post-cesarean infection, we specifically determined surgical infection rate as well as serious infectious morbidity rate. For surgical site infection we adopted the CDC definition as stated by Horan et al. [Horan et al, 1999]. Serious infectious morbidity was defined as bacteremia, septic shock, septic thrombophlebitis, necrotizing fasciitis; peritonitis, or death attributed to infection. Risk factors for intra-operative complications and post-cesarean infection have been studied. We first computed crude odds ratios followed by adjusted odds ratios. We adjusted each factor for potential confounders in a multivariate logistic regression model. The final step in this analysis of maternal complications studied the trends of cesarean related maternal death risk and relationship between cesarean delivery and maternal mortality in a multivariate analysis of primary predictors including antenatal screening, referral status, maternal age, parity and route of delivery. In this analysis adjusted odds ratio have been produced for cesarean delivery. Regarding fetal and neonatal prognosis, we estimated trends of stillbirth rates and neonatal death rates. These indicators were studied by comparing cesarean to vaginal delivery. Stillbirth was defined as Apgar score = 0 immediately after delivery in a live-born-infant. Neonatal deaths are those occurring during the first 28 days following delivery. However, neonatal death rates presented are underestimated since our observation period was limited to the duration of hospitalization at birth; the maximum length of follow up of the neonates was 13 days. Neonates discharged healthy were assumed to have survived to 28 days. Nonetheless, the rates presented give an idea of the size of this important issue.

All calculations were performed using SPSS version 11.0 (SPSS Inc, Chicago, IL). $P<0.05$ was considered statistically significant. The database used for this analysis was reviewed and approved by the ethics committee of the Faculty of Medicine, Pharmacy, and Dentistry at the University of Bamako, Mali.

3. Findings

3.1 Characteristics of deliveries in our teaching hospital

During a nineteen year period from 1985-2003, 17,721 women delivered at Point G Teaching Hospital, 20.2% of whom traveled from other regions in southern Mali. The proportion of women residing outside of Bamako increased significantly from 13.3% of deliveries between 1985 and 1990 to 23.6% during the period 1998 - 2003 ($p <0.001$).Among the women delivering at Point G, 29.9% were referred from outside health institutions. Patients referred for an obstetric emergency represented 18.1% of women delivering while non-emergency referrals constituted 11.8%. Emergency admission rates varied from a minimum of 7.6% of deliveries in 1986 to a maximum of 25.1%of deliveries in 2000. Patients with non-emergent referrals accounted for a minimum of 7.1% of deliveries in 1990 and a maximum of 21% of deliveries in 1998.

Years	Total deliveries	Number of cesarean delivery	Cesarean delivery rates	Odds ratio	Relative risk	P value	% cesarean in TSCN	Contribution Of TSCN to Total deliveries
1985	1056	132	12.5%	Reference			10.3%	19.3%
1986	948	132	13.9%	1.13	1.1	>0,05	14.7%	20.8%
1987	977	173	17.7%	1.51	1.4	<0,001	19.2%	19.8%
1988	1028	172	16.7%	1.41	1.3	<0,05	13.8%	18.3%
1989	1079	220	20.4%	1.79	1.6	<0,001	19.1%	21.7%
1990	982	204	20.8%	1.84	1.7	<0,001	26.3%	20.9%
1991	1066	279	26.2%	2.48	2.1	<0,001	27.5%	23.9%
1992	1114	317	28.5%	2.78	2.3	<0,001	25.9%	19.3%
1993	1169	340	29.1%	2.87	2.3	<0,001	28.6%	21.8%
1994	1041	298	28.6%	2.81	2.3	<0,001	33.7%	19.2%
1995	1098	343	31.2%	3.18	2.5	<0,001	30.4%	21.8%
1996	747	209	28.0%	2.72	2.2	<0,001	28.3%	24.6%
1997	298	110	36.9%	4.10	3.0	<0,001	26.7%	20.0%
1998	944	305	32.3%	3.34	2.6	<0,001	33.0%	24.4%
1999	847	297	35.1%	3.78	2.8	<0,001	40.7%	22.2%
2000	894	262	29.3%	2.90	2.3	<0,001	32.6%	20.6%
2001	1070	352	32.9%	3.43	2.6	<0,001	30.2%	22.7%
2002	660	197	29.8%	2.98	2.4	<0,001	27.5%	21.9%
2003	703	175	24.9%	2.32	2.0	<0,001	22.8%	20.6%
Total	17721	4517	25.5%				Mean= 25.8%	Mean= 21.2%

TSCN : Term Single cephalic nullipara

Table 1. Trends of number of deliveries, rates and risks of cesarean delivery during the study period.

3.2 Cesarean delivery rates

Observed rates of cesarean delivery and relative risk are presented in table 1 above. The coefficient of variation for overall cesarean delivery rates was 27.9, and the ratio of the highest (36.9%) to the lowest (12.5%) was 2.95, indicating significant variability in overall cesarean delivery rates during the 19 years. Using year 1985 as the reference, we noted a striking increase in the cesarean delivery rate through out the study period. Since 1991, the cesarean delivery rate has been sustained at least 100% above that in 1985. Trends in cesarean delivery rates accounting for sociodemographic characteristics and obstetric history are presented in table 2. Globally, cesarean delivery rates increased ($p<0.05$). Observed cesarean rates were relatively higher in the 35 - 50 years old age group, Bambara ethnic group, grandmultiparas, women residing outside of Bamako, and those referred from other health centers. Cesarean delivery rates for unbooked pregnancies varied between 24.5% and 45.0%. Rates for women who followed antenatal screening varied between 15.6% and 31.0%.

3.3 Indications of cesarean delivery

In practice, the decision to perform a cesarean relies on an array of parameters. There is no general consensus universally accepted way of reporting cesarean delivery indications. Absolute numbers and specific cesarean delivery rates per indication / risk factors for cesarean delivery appeared in table 3. We report here 3 systems of reporting these indications:

3.3.1 Classification of cesareans by mutually exclusive clinical indications

Two independent obstetricians were asked to review our database and to point out what was the major factor leading to the decision of cesarean. They reviewed together cases where they found different factors. The results are presented in table 2 below. Of note, pelvic contraction and suspected fetal distress were the most represented and showed an increasing pattern over time.

Indications	1985 – 1990 N=1033	1991 – 1995 N=1577	1996 – 1997 N=319	1998 – 2001 N=1216	2002 – 2003 N=372
Contracted /deformed pelvis	22.2%	22.1%	19.8%	24.2%	26.6%
Uterine rupture	13.7%	17.8%	9.6%	7.4%	4.4%
Major antepartum hemorrhage	5.8%	5.8%	8.3%	4.2%	4.1%
Transverse lie	11.7%	8.2%	7.7%	6.2%	4.7%
Brow presentation	1.9%	0.9%	1.2%	1.1%	0.8%
Prolonged labor	9.7%	4.8%	7.4%	6.5%	7.4%
Previous cesarean	4.1%	3.5%	4.6%	5.5%	10.4%
Previous obstetric fistula	1.3%	0.6%	1.2%	0.5%	1.9%
Suspected fetal distress	22.8%	28.0%	25.9%	29.9%	26.6%
Maternal diseases	3.6%	5.9%	10.8%	12.2%	8.2%
Breech presentation	3.1%	2.4%	3.4%	3.2%	5.5%

Table 2. Trends in the contribution of eleven mutually exclusive clinical indications.

3.3.2 Classification of Baltimore group on cesarean indications

This classification system separates cesarean indications into absolute, maternal, and non-absolute indications. Absolute maternal indications include obstructed labor (including severe deformed pelvis and failed trial of labor), major antepartum hemorrhage and grade 3 or 4 placenta previa, malpresentation (including transverse, oblique, and brow), and uterine rupture. Non-absolute indications include failure to progress in labor (including prolonged labor); failed induction; previous cesarean delivery; genitourinary fistula or third-degree tear repair; antepartum hemorrhage, (excluding those for absolute indications and including abruptio placentae); maternal medical diseases; severe preeclampsia or eclampsia; psychosocial indications including maternal request, "precious" pregnancy; fetal compromise (including fetal distress, cord prolapse, and severe intrauterine growth retardation); and breech presentation.

Globally 66.3% of cesarean deliveries during the 19 years were performed for absolute maternal indications (2993/4517) vs 33.7% for non-absolute indications (1524/4517). The percentage of absolute maternal indications evolved as follow: 66.8% for 1985 - 1990, 74.6% for 1991 - 1995, 63.6% for 1996 - 1997, 59.5% for 1998 - 2001 and 53.8% for 2002 - 2003 ($p<.001$).

Uterine rupture, an absolute indication for cesarean delivery occurred in 2.6% of all the 17721 deliveries and was the indication of 10.1% of the 4517 cesarean deliveries. The time trends of uterine rupture were as follow: 1.8% of all deliveries recorded in 1985 - 1990, 3.9% for 1991 - 1995, 2.7% for 1996 - 1997, 1.5% for 1998 - 2008 and 0.7% for 2002 - 2003. Of all women with uterine rupture, 94.7% of cases were diagnosed at admission examination in referred patients (92.5% with patients referred emergently).

Uterine rupture occurred in 87.4% (415/475) of cases in an unscarred uterus vs 12.6% (60/475) in a scarred uterus. Observed risk factors for primary uterine rupture included: contracted pelvis, 12.0% (57/475); fetal macrosomia 9.7% (46/475); contracted pelvis associated with macrosomia 3.4% (16/475). Malpresentation was recorded in 12.4% (59/475). Dystocia associated with oxytocin and / or traditional medicines labor augmentation has been observed in 12.6% of cases (60/475). Grandmultiparity (≥7 deliveries in obstetric history) accounted for 12.4% (59/475) of all uterine ruptures while short interpregnancy interval has been observed in 12.0% of all uterine ruptures (57/475). Central placenta previa and twin pregnancy accounted for 1.9% (9/475) each while abruptio placentae has been observed in 1.1% (6/4475). Finally, the cause of 8% of uterine ruptures was unknown (38/475). For cases of uterine rupture secondary to a uterine scar, previous cesarean delivery was the most represented, 11.4% (54/475) followed by previous uterine rupture, 1.3% (6/475). No case of uterine rupture secondary to previous myomectomy was reported.

Six conditions representing 86.2% of cesareans for non-absolute indications included: suspected fetal distress (33.7%), previous cesarean delivery (25.6%), breech presentation (10.1%), eclampsia (5.9%) genitourinary fistula (5.9%) and twin pregnancy (5.1%). Percentages of cesarean deliveries for genitourinary fistula, twin pregnancy, and fetal distress did not show a clear trend. The contributions of breech presentation, eclampsia and previous cesarean delivery, however, increased over time. In 1985 - 1990, 2.90% of cesarean deliveries were performed primarily because of breech presentation; this rate reached 5.64% during 2002 - 2003. These rates were 1.06% and 4.30% respectively for eclampsia and 7.84% and 16.66% for previous cesarean delivery.

Three major indications, when present, gave a 70%-90% likelihood that the woman would receive cesarean. These included cephalopelvic disproportion (CPD), malpresentation, and previous cesarean delivery. 64-85% of women with antepartum hemorrhage were delivered by cesarean section. These four indications accounted for 66.5% of all cesarean deliveries.

Characteristics	1985 - 1990 N=6070	1991 – 1995 N = 5488	1996 – 1997 N = 1045	1998 – 2001 N=3755	2002 – 2003 N=1363
Age groups					
13 - 19 yrs	15.9% (1088)	25.2% (1113)	27.2% (180)	31.6% (707)	24.5% (257)
20 - 34 yrs	16.5% (4087)	28.3% (3558)	28.9% (718)	31.6% (2473)	26.8% (890)
35 - 50 yrs	19.2% (895)	33.5% (817)	40.8% (147)	36.4% (575)	31.8% (216)
Ethnic groups					
Bambara	18.2% (2649)	32.5% (2462)	31.3% (460)	35.4% (1572)	32.2% (605)
Peuhl	18.1% (895)	27.4% (828)	30.1% (163)	31.2% (574)	27.8% (194)
Malinke	15.4% (930)	28.3% (736)	32.6% (129)	33.2% (446)	22.9% (123)
Soninke	17.4% (471)	27.4% (402)	28.8% (80)	28.3% (364)	16.7% (131)
Dogon	14.4% (180)	19.6% (214)	20.0% (50)	23.3% (219)	24.4% (90)
Sonrhaï	12.5% (256)	25.1% (183)	43.2% (37)	32.0% (122)	20.0% (41)
Senoufo	15.0% (100)	18.6% (97)	26.9% (26)	27.2% (81)	21.4% (30)
Bobo	13.0% (130)	15.4% (123)	25.0% (24)	29.3% (41)	22.2% (14)
Bozo	24.4% (45)	25.3% (79)	45.5% (11)	23.7% (38)	14.3% (18)
Maure	15.4% (13)	17.3% (52)	40.0% (5)	31.4% (51)	9.5% (21)
Minianka	23.3% (30)	19.3% (57)	0% (6)	43.5% (23)	21.3% (21)
Others	17.0% (371)	25.9% (255)	27.8% (54)	31.3% (224)	27.3% (75)
Region					
Bamako	11.7% (5265)	18.1% (4194)	23.4% (798)	25.3% (2794)	20.5% (1088)
Kayes	54.2% (24)	56.3% (48)	87.5% (8)	50.0% (24)	80.0% (5)
Koulikoro	51.5% (701)	63.3% (1108)	53.1% (213)	53.8% (865)	55.2% (262)
Sikasso	64.8% (54)	74.1% (81)	46.2% (13)	48.3% (29)	00.0% (5)
Segou	35.3% (17)	59.0% (39)	50.0% (10)	45.8% (24)	33.3% (3)
Mopti	40.0% (5)	33.3% (9)	00.0% (1)	37.5% (8)	00.0% (0)
Others	00.0% (4)	55.6% (9)	50.0% (2)	36.4% (11)	-----
Parity					
0	18.3% (1481)	28.9% (1376)	29.2% (295)	33.5% (1089)	25.2% (359)
1 - 6	16.4% (3906)	27.2% (3559)	30.3% (669)	31.5% (2417)	28.3% (918)
≥ 7	16.3% (683)	35.4% (553)	33.8% (81)	35.4% (249)	22.9% (86)
Antenatal booking					
Yes	15.6% (5218)	17.0% (4334)	28.1% (881)	31.0% (3222)	26.3% (1188)
No	25.9% (852)	24.5% (1154)	45.0% (164)	40.5% (533)	33.7% (175)

Characteristics	1985 - 1990 N=6070	1991 – 1995 N = 5488	1996 – 1997 N = 1045	1998 – 2001 N=3755	2002 – 2003 N=1363
Referral status					
Emergency Ref	59.7% (827)	73.6% (1149)	59.8% (241)	60.1% (826)	62.9% (214)
Non emergency ref.	55.4% (496)	45.2% (662)	65.3% (95)	47.8% (695)	69.8% (149)
Self referral	5.6% (4747)	11.9% (3677)	15.9% (709)	17.4% (2234)	13.4% (1000)
Indications					
CPD	87.1% (470)	91.1% (731)	88.4% (129)	90.2% (553)	88.4% (172)
Antepartum hemorrhage	64.7% (150)	75.4% (203)	84.3% (46)	64.8% (128)	75.9% (29)
Malpresentation	72.2% (212)	85.0% (234)	87.8% (234)	86.7% (135)	81.6% (38)
Breech presentation	32.9% (155)	44.2% (206)	48.1% (52)	51.1% (180)	41.0% (78)
Hypertension	23.3% (227)	42.7% (330)	53.5% (86)	42.0% (441)	30.3% (145)
Eclampsia	29.7% (37)	63.9% (36)	59.1% (22)	53.1% (64)	69.2% (26)
Diabetes in pregnancy	25.0% (8)	38.1% (21)	50.0% (2)	55.6% (18)	62.5% (8)
Previous uterine rupture					
Previous cesarean	100% (7)	88.9% (9)	100% (1)	80% (5)	----
Obstetric fistula treated	73.7% (278)	74.9% (458)	82.5% (97)	77.8% (451)	81.6% (179)
Uterine prolapse treated	85.4% (48)	81.0% (42)	90.0% (10)	96.2% (26)	100% (16)
Cord prolapse	78.6% (14)	86.7% (15)	100% (2)	81.8% (11)	0.0% (2)
Cardiac disease	54.8% (42)	67.3% (52)	80.0% (5)	75.0% (32)	25.0% (4)
Post-term (induction)	7.7% (13)	60.0% (15)	50.0% (2)	37.0% (27)	0.0% (8)
Suspected Fetal	39.4% (33)	57.8% (45)	57.1% (7)	64.2% (34)	52.6% (19)
distress	36.4% (772)	48.1% (1142)	48.4% (213)	51.2% (732)	51.2% (205)
Twin pregnancy	24.8% (149)	32.9% (152)	33.3% (33)	41.5% (106)	37.5% (40)
PROM	32.7% (110)	55.3% (170)	64.3% (28)	50.0% (164)	31.4% (86)
Preterm labor	17.0% (570)	24.5% (486)	32.2% (115)	28.9% (419)	23.4% (124)

CPD: cephalopelvic disproportion Antepartum hemorrhage: placenta praevia and placental abruption.
PROM: Premature rupture of membranes
Percentages represents the cesarean delivery rate for each category. Numbers between parentheses correspond to the total number of delivery in each category.

Table 3. Trends in cesarean delivery rates (total number of deliveries in each category) for sociodemographic, pregnancy and delivery characteristics by time period.

3.3.3 Robson's ten group classification

To further examine trends in cesarean delivery according to patient demographics, we classified our population following Robson's rules (table 4). Collectively, groups 1, 3 and 5 constituted 78.2% of deliveries. Their cesarean delivery rates are 22.6%, 13.2% and 76.4% while their contributions to total cesarean deliveries were respectively 18.14%, 26.54% and 20.86%. Although group 2 and 4 had high levels of cesarean delivery rates (91.9% and 46.3% respectively), they contributed only 8.95% of total cesarean deliveries.

Trends in cesarean delivery rates for each of the ten groups appear in figure 2. There were no significant changes in abdominal delivery for Robson's group 2 (Nulliparous, single gestation, cephalic presentation, ≥ 37 weeks gestational age, induced or cesarean delivery before labor) and group 5 (Previous cesarean delivery, single gestation, cephalic presentation, ≥ 37 weeks gestational age). We observed an increasing cesarean delivery rates for groups 4, 8 and 9. Group 9 presented a two pattern aspect with rates shifting from around 75% before 1990 to around 85% thereafter.

To further understand variations in obstetric practice in our hospital, groups 1 (spontaneously laboring term nulliparas) and 2 were combined as a composite variable, the term TSCN (table 1). The annual TSCN cesarean delivery rate and contribution of TSCN to hospital deliveries are documented in Table 1. The mean cesarean delivery rate in TSCN was 25.8% (range, 10.3% -40.7%). The CV for TSCN cesarean delivery rates was 29.5%, again indicating significant variation between different years. The 19 year trends of cesarean delivery rate in TSCN follows a pattern similar to that of overall cesarean delivery rate (Table 1). Figure 1 demonstrates positive correlation between the overall and TSCN cesarean delivery rates over time (Slope = 0.876). Linear regression model suggested that 77% of the variation of the overall cesarean delivery rates can be explained by the variation observed in TSCN cesarean delivery rates ($p<0.001$). Our analyses suggest that the increase in overall cesarean delivery rate was not related to changes in obstetric groups since the proportion of all deliveries that were TSCN did not vary substantially. The average proportion of TSCN in this study was 21.2% (range, 18.3 -24.4%) with a coefficient of variation of only 8.4% (Table 1).

Of note, 57.9% of cesareans in the TSCN group were indicated because of CPD (this represented 31.4% of all cesareans for CPD). One third of all cesarean deliveries indicated for eclampsia occurred in TSCN but this contributes only 3.2% to TSCN cesarean deliveries.

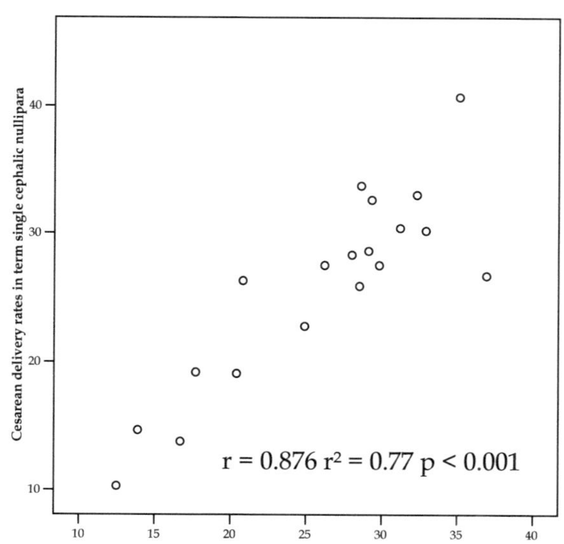

Fig. 1. Correlation between overall cesarean delivery rates and cesarean delivery rates in TSCN.

Robson's classification	Prevalence[1] of Robson groups	% Cesarean delivery[2]	Contribution of each group to total cesarean delivery[3].
Group 1. Nulliparous, single cephalic, ≥ 37 weeks, in spontaneous labor	20.3%	22.6%	18.14%
Group 2. Nulliparous, single cephalic, ≥ 37 weeks, induced or CS before labor	1%	91.9%	3.82%
Group 3. Multiparous (excluding prev. CS), single cephalic, ≥ 37 weeks, in spontaneous labor	51%	13.2%	26.54%
Group 4. Multiparous (excluding prev. CS), single cephalic, ≥ 37 weeks, induced or CS before labor	2.8%	46.3%	5.13%
Group 5. Previous CS, single cephalic, ≥ 37 weeks	6.9%	76.4%	20.86%
Group 6. All nulliparous breeches	0.8%	39.6%	1.27%
Group 7. All multiparous breeches (including prev. CS)	2.3%	45.1%	4.08%
Group 8. All multiple pregnancies (including prev. CS)	2.5%	29.7%	2.94%
Group 9. All abnormal lies (including prev. CS)	2.9%	80%	9.11%
Group 10. All single cephalic, ≤ 36 weeks (including previous CS)	9.5%	21.6%	8.06%
Total	N= 17721	-	N= 4517

[1]Calculated by total women in each group by the total number of deliveries
[2]Calculated by dividing the total number of cesarean in each group by the total number of women in each group
[3].Calculated by dividing numbers of cesarean per group by the total number of cesarean delivery (N=4517)

Table 4. Prevalence of Robson ten groups ; cesarean delivery rate by group and contribution of each group to cesarean delivery.

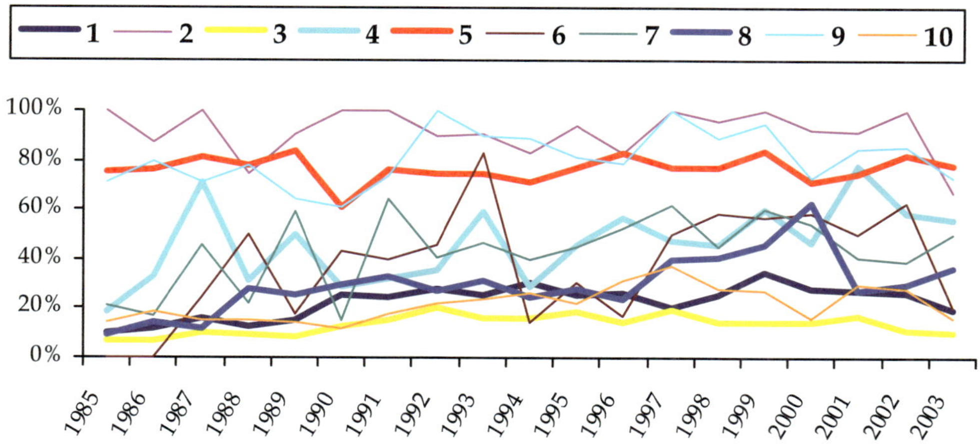

Fig. 2. Nineteen year trends of cesarean delivery rates per Robson's group.

3.4 Multivariate analysis

Finally, we performed multilogistic regression with sequential adjustment to identify explanatory factors for increased cesarean delivery rates. Unadjusted analysis revealed a 100% increase in the rates of cesarean delivery (2003 vs 1985, RR = 2). The best model identified referral status, cephalopelvic disproportion and history of previous cesarean delivery as 3 factors to account for the observed increases in overall cesarean delivery rates. However, this model explained less than half of the observed increase (Figure 4). Of note, controlling for maternal age, parity and marital status didn't affect the observed increase. Controlling for cephalopelvic disproportion alone explained 32% of the increase since we found an adjusted relative risk of 1.68. Adjusting simultaneously for cephalopelvic disproportion, referral status and previous cesarean delivery further decrease the adjusted relative risk to 1.58. We couldn't build another model better than this last one.

As expected, higher levels of abdominal delivery were observed in referred patients (table 2). Since 1986, 60 to 70% of emergency admissions during labor have resulted in cesarean delivery. The cesarean delivery rates for referred patient without emergency fluctuated from 40%-60%. Cesarean delivery rates for direct admissions were ≤ 10% before 1994 and 10-20% thereafter (figure 3).

Cephalopelvic disproportion was a common indication for cesarean delivery, with a mean rate of 39.6% of women delivering abdominally having some degree of CPD. The percentage of CPD in cesarean deliveries ranged from 30.3% in 1985 to 48.8% in 1999. Contracted pelvis constituted 87% of all CPD. Of note, 63.5% of all contracted pelvis were recorded in the referred patients, who generally came from poor rural environments. The high incidence of uterine rupture among this group may correlate with severity of pelvis contraction.

There were 1465 deliveries in which the mother had a history of previous cesarean delivery. An elective cesarean delivery was decided for 858. Common indications for elective cesarean delivery were cephalopelvic disproportion (n=655), abnormal fetal presenting part (112), history of vesico-vaginal fistula (n=36), history of uterine prolapse (n=4), "precious" pregnancy (n=4), post-term pregnancy (n=7), and premature rupture of membranes (n=40). Among the 607 suitable for a trial of scar, 120 were emergency referrals with conditions such as a bleeding placenta praevia, a sudden rise in the blood pressure/eclampsia, or a suspected fetal distress leading to an emergency cesarean delivery. Finally, only 487 trials of scar have been undertaken (one third of all scarred uteri). We recorded 244 vaginal deliveries (50.1%) while 243 were emergency cesarean delivery (49.9%). Two (2) cases of uterine dehiscence occurred (0.4% of the 487 trials of scar) and 1 case of maternal death (0.2%, denominator = 487 trials of scar). There were 25 perinatal deaths (5.1%).

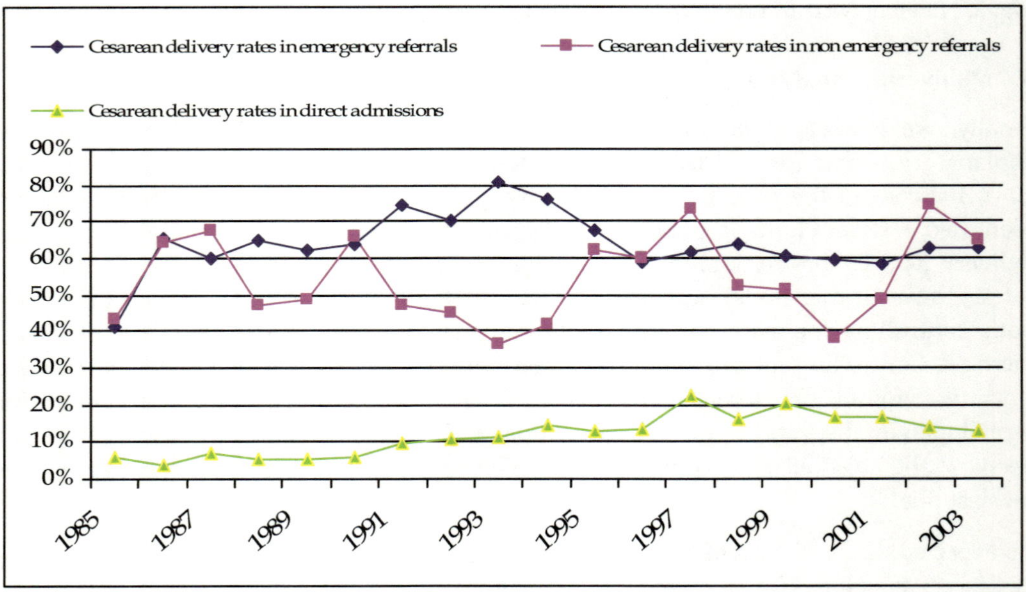

Fig. 3. Trends in cesarean delivery rates by referral status.

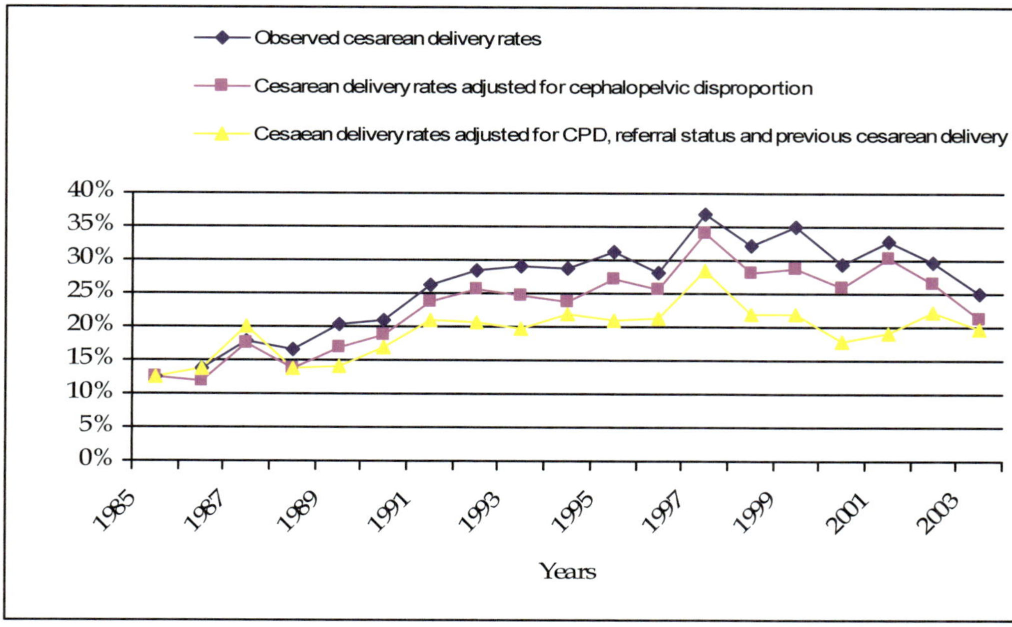

Fig. 4. Observed rates of cesarean delivery and sequentially adjusted rates for changes in cephalopelvic disproportion, mode of admission and history of cesarean delivery.

3.5 Complications of cesarean delivery

3.5.1 Maternal complications

3.5.1.1 Intraoperative surgical complications

We defined intraoperative complications as laceration of the uterus (uterine rupture included), cervix, bladder, vagina or bowel, intraoperative blood loss of ≥1000 ml, blood transfusion, and hysterectomy. Overall, 13.2% (596/4517) of the women undergoing a cesarean delivery had at least one of the above complications. The most common events were uterine rupture (9.2%, 417/4517), hemorrhage (2.4%, 111/4517), hysterectomy (2.1%, 96/4517); urinary tract injury (0.4%, 18/4517), and anesthesia-related complications (0.3%, 15/4517).

Table 5 presents an analysis of factors influencing the occurrence of intraoperative complications. Univariate analyses found four risk factors for intraoperative complications: admission during the active phase of labor (cervical dilatation ≥4cm), transverse lie, total length of labor more than 24 hours, and emergent referrals. However, in multivariate analyses, only emergent referral remained a significant risk factor with a 3.4 folds increase in the odds of intra-operative adverse events. Removing referral status from the multivariate analysis allowed two factors to be linked to intraoperative complications: ruptured membranes at admission (OR=2.1 [1.2 - 3.7], p<0.01) and total length of labor (OR=1.9 [1.1 - 3.5], p<0.05).

Factors	Crude OR	95% CI OR	P	AOR	95% CIAOR	p
Cervical dilatation at time of intervention						
0 – 3 cm	Reference	---	---	Ref	---	---
4 – 10 cm	2.5	1.9 – 3.1	<0.001	1.6	0.8 – 2.9	>0.05
Fetal presentation						
Cephalic	Reference	---	---	Ref	---	---
Breech	0.8	0.6 – 1.2	>0.05	0.8	0.2 – 2.7	>0.05
Transverse	1.5	1.1 – 1.9	<0.05	0.9	0.4 – 2.1	>0.05
Total length of labor						
<12 hours	Reference	---	---	Ref	---	---
12 – 24 hours	1.4	0.9 – 2.1	>0.05	0.9	0.5 – 1.6	>0.05
>24 hours	3.5	2.3 – 5.3	<0.05	1.5	0.8 – 2.8	>0.05
Membranes status						
Not ruptured	Reference	---	---	Ref	---	--
Ruptured	3.0	2.4 – 3.8	<0.001	1.5	0.8 – 2.8	>0.05
Preterm delivery						
No	Reference	---	---	Ref	---	---
Yes	0.6	0.4-0.9	<0.001	0.3	0.1 – 0.4	>0.05
Referral status						
Self-referred	Reference	---		Ref	---	
Referred with emergency	5.1	3.9 – 6.5	<0.001	3.4	1.7 – 6.8	<0.001
Referred without emerg.	0.7	0.4 – 0.9	<0.01	0.8	0.2 – 2.9	>0.05
Body mass index						
<35.0 kg/m^2	Reference	---	Ref	---	---	--
≥ 35 Kg/m^2	1.3	0.5 – 2.9	>0.05	2.1	0.4 – 10.2	>0.05
Intraoperative adhesions						
No	Reference	---	Ref	---	---	---
Yes	0.8	0.6-1.2	>0.05	1.7	0.8 – 3.9	>0.05

CI: confidence interval OR: odds ratio AOR: adjusted odds ratio CIAOR: confidence interval of the adjusted odds ratio

Table 5. Risk factors for intraoperative surgical complications.

3.5.1.2 Post-cesarean complications

Post-cesarean infection

The incidence of post-partum infection among cesarean deliveries was 20.1% (910/4517) compared to 3.9% (509/13204) for vaginal deliveries (OR= 6.3 [5.6 - 7.1], p<0.001). Of the 4517 cesarean deliveries, 17.5% (790/4517) met the criteria for surgical site infection as defined by CDC. Endometritis, peritonitis, post-partum urinary tract infection and serious infectious morbidity were more linked to abdominal route of delivery (table 6).

Risk factors for post-cesarean infection identified in a univariate analysis were: emergent referral, younger maternal age (13 - 19 years old), nulliparity, ruptured membranes at admission, abnormal amniotic fluid coloration, and prolonged labor (total length ≥ 12 hours). In multivariate analyses, only 3 factors remained significantly associated with postpartum infection: abnormal amniotic fluid coloration, ruptured membranes before admission and duration of labor >24 hours (table 7).

	Cases per Cesarean Delivery (%), n=4517	Cases per Vaginal Delivery (%), n=13204	OR (95% CI)
Endometritis	11.1 (n=500)	3.3 (n=436)	3.6 [3.2 - 4.2]
Wound infection	6.8 (n=305)	---	---
Peritonitis	4.0 (n=18)	0.02 (n=2)	26.4 [6.1 - 113.9]
Urinary tract infection	0.7 (n=35)	0.2 (n=24)	4.3 [2.5 - 7.2]
Serious infectious morbidity¥	2.7 (n=123)	0.1 (n=8)	46.2 [22.6 - 94.5]

¥Defined as bacteremia, septic shock, septic thrombophlebitis, necrotizing fasciitis; peritonitis, or death attributed to infection

Table 6. Post-Partum Infectious Complications by Delivery Route.

Postpartum hemorrhage: Recorded rates were comparable between cesarean delivery and vaginal delivery, 1.7% vs 1.4% (P>0.05).

Deep venous thrombosis. Only 11 cases have been recorded during the study period; 9 in cesarean deliveries vs 2 in vaginal deliveries (OR = 13.2 [2.8 - 61.0]).

Puerperal psychosis. In 19 years, 6 cases occurred, 5 after cesarean delivery and 1 post-vaginal delivery (OR = 14.6 [1.7 - 125.3].

Risk factors	Unadjusted Odds ratio	95% CI	P	AOR	95%CI	P
Referral status						
Self admission	1.0	1.3 – 1.9	<0.01	1.0	0.6 – 1.3	>0.05
Referred emergently	1.6	0.4 – 0.7	<0.01	0.9	0.5 – 1.5	>0.05
Referred without	0.5			0.9		
Maternal age						
20 – 34 years	1.0	1.1 – 1.6	>0.01	1.0	0.5 – 1.6	>0.05
13 – 19 years	1.4	0.7 – 1.1	>0.05	0.9	0.9 – 1.8	>0.05
35 – 50 years	0.9			1.1		
Parity						
1 – 6	1.0	1.1 – 1.4	< 0.05	1.0	0.4 – 1.8	>0.05
Nulliparous	1.2	0.8 – 1.3	>0.05	0.8	0.7 – 1.5	>0.05
≥ 7	1.0			1.02		
Body Mass Index (BMI)						
<35 Kg/m^2	1.0	0.2 – 0.9	<0.05	1.0	0.2 – 2.1	>0.05
≥35 Kg/m^2	0.4			0.6		
Membranes status at						
admission	1.0	2.8 – 3.9	<0.001	1.0	1.3 – 3.7	<0.01
Non ruptured	3.3			1.9		
Ruptured						
Amniotic fluid color at						
admission	1.0	2.7 – 3.9	<0.001	1.0	1.5 – 3.2	<0.001
Normal	3.3			2.2		
Abnormal						
Cervical dilatation at						
admission	1.0	1.2 – 1.7	<0.001	1.0	1.01 – 2.1	<0.05
0 – 3 cm	1.8			1.4		
4 – 10 cm						
Duration of labor						
< 12 hours	1.0	1.1 – 1.9	<0.05	1.0	0.9 – 1.9	>0.05
12 – 23 hours	1.4	1.9 – 3.6	<0.05	1.3	1.4 – 3.4	<0.001
≥ 24 hours	2.7			2.2		
Induction of labor						
No	1.0	0.6 – 1.8	>0.05	1.0	0.3 – 3.6	>0.05
Yes	1.04			1.1		
Antepartum hemorrhage						
No	1.0	0.1 – 0.3	<0.001	1.0	0.01 – 0.4	<0.01
Yes	0.2			0.05		
Per/postpartum						
hemorrhage	1.0	0.9 – 2.5	>0.05	1.0	0.3 – 4.1	>0.05
No	1.5			1.1		
Yes						

CI = Confidence Interval AOR: Adjusted odds ratio

Table 7. Risk factors for post-partum infection.

3.5.1.3 Maternal mortality and cesarean delivery

During the 19 year period, 417 maternal deaths were recorded. Among these maternal deaths, 348 occurred per or postpartum (83.4%). The majority of these delivery period deaths, 70.1% (244/348), were associated with cesarean delivery. Thus, 5.4% (244/4517) of cesarean deliveries resulted in a maternal death. The corresponding rate for vaginal delivery was 0.9% (104/13204).

Twelve of the 244 maternal deaths associated with cesarean delivery occurred before the intervention was performed (4.9%). A similar proportion occurred during cesarean. The vast majority of maternal deaths were recorded in the post-cesarean period (90.1%).

The absolute number and risk of cesarean-related maternal deaths shows a sharp decrease beginning in 1994 (Figure 5).

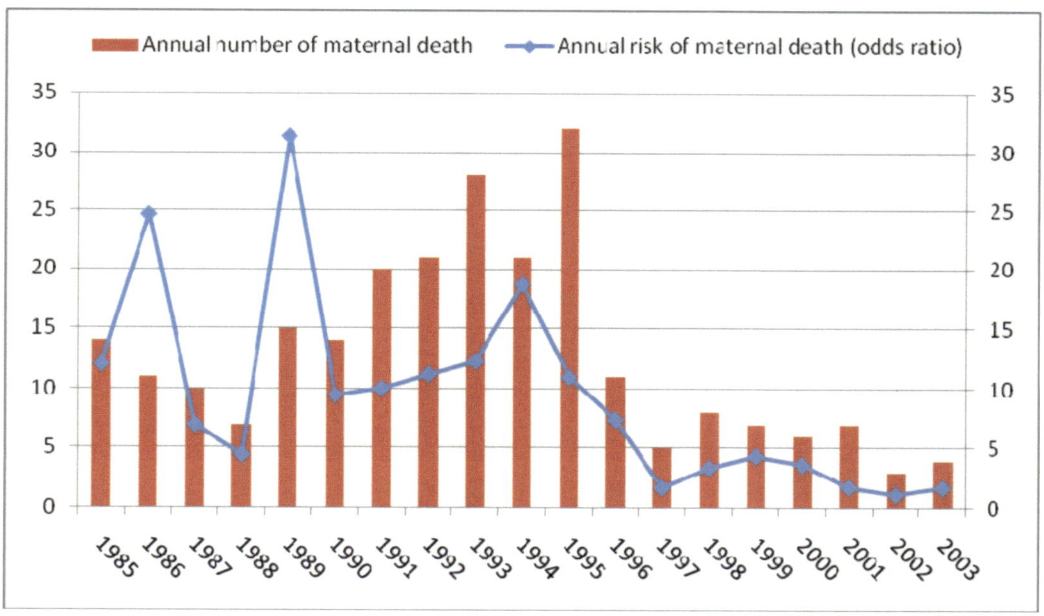

Fig. 5. Trends of annual number and risk of cesarean related maternal deaths.

Table 8 presents case fatality rates for direct and indirect maternal complications by route of delivery. The vast majority of maternal complications (91.8% for cesarean delivery, 83.9% for vaginal delivery) and maternal deaths (95.5% for cesarean delivery, 87.5% for vaginal delivery) were the consequences of direct maternal complications. The overall case fatality rate was 6.9% (244/3548) for cesarean delivery compared to 2.9% (104/3597) for vaginal delivery. In the cesarean delivery group among direct maternal complications, uterine rupture had the highest fatality rate (23.2%). There was a consistent decrease in the incidence and case fatality rates of uterine rupture in women delivered abdominally (figure 6). The incidence decreased from 10.5% for the period 1985 - 1990 to 4.5% for the period 2002 - 2003. The case fatality rates decreased from 29.9% to 6.9% in the same time periods.

Causes	CESAREAN DELIVERY			VAGINAL DELIVERY		
	Total number	Death	Case rate fatality	Total number	Death	Case rate fatality
Direct maternal complications						
hemorrhage	377	45	11.9%	491	40	8.1%
Hypertension and complications	374	17	4.5%	1196	24	2.0%
Dystocia	1096	5	0.5%	475	2	0.4%
Uterine rupture	455	101	23.3%	20	0	0.0%
Postpartum infection	910	57	6.2%	480	25	5.2%
Other direct causes	45	8	17.8%	356	0	0.0%
Indirect maternal complications						
HIV	6	0	0.0%	7	0	0.0%
Malaria	135	0	0.0%	170	2	1.2%
Hemoglobinopathy	24	1	4.2%	49	0	0.0%
Anemia	43	1	2.3%	215	0	0.0%
Cardiac disease	25	7	28.0%	59	5	8.5%
Diabetes	17	0	0.0%	23	0	0.0%
Hepatitis	1	0	0.0%	5	0	0.0%
Other indirect causes	40	2	5.0%	51	6	11.8%
Total	3548	244	6.9%	3597	104	2.9%

Table 8. Absolute numbers of cases, number of deaths and case fatality rates of direct and indirect maternal complications for cesarean delivery and vaginal delivery.

We examined the relationship between cesarean delivery and maternal death in the context of other known primary predictors (table 9). Cesarean delivery remained strongly associated with maternal death even after controlling for antenatal screening, referral status, maternal age, parity, abruption, placenta previa, hypertensive disorders, and malpresentation.

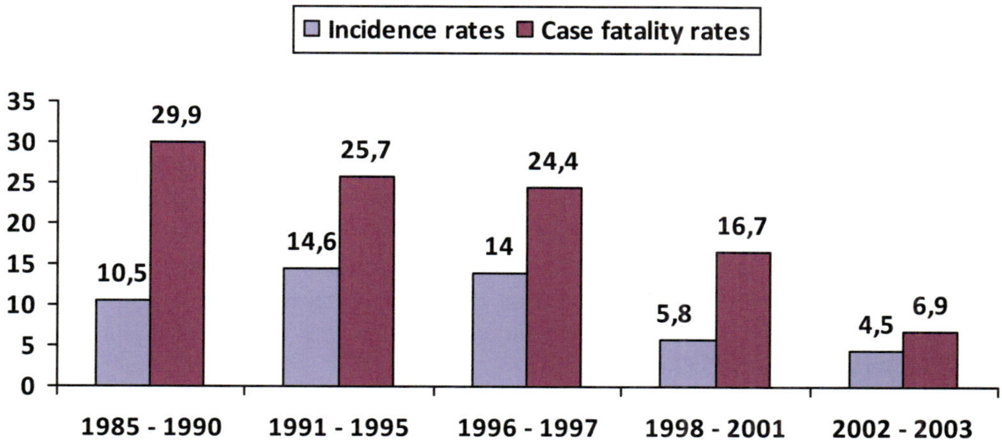

Fig. 6. Time trends of uterine rupture incidence rate and case fatality rates among 4517 cesarean deliveries at Point national hospital, Bamako, Mali, 1985 - 2003.

Variables	Crude OR	95% CI	Adjusted OR	95% CI
Antenatal screening				
No	7.0	5.7 - 8.7		
Yes	1.0			
Referral status				
Referred emergently	25.7	18.7 - 35.4		
Referred without emergency	3.2	1.9 - 5.2		
Self admission	1.0			
Maternal age				
35 - 50 years	0.8	0.6 - 1.2		
13 - 19 years	1.6	1.2 - 2.0		
20 - 34 years	1.0			
Parity				
Nullipara	0.9	0.7 - 1.2		
Grandmultipara	1.2	0.9 - 1.8		
Multipara	1.0			
Route of delivery				
Cesarean delivery	7.2	5.7 - 9.1	2.8*	- 3.8
Vaginal delivery	1.0			

* Controlling for antenatal screening, referral status, maternal age, parity, CPD, placental abnormalities (abruption and previa), hypertensive disorders, and malpresentations.

Table 9. Odds ratios with 95% confidence interval for maternal death for primary predictors.

3.5.2 Perinatal complications

3.5.2.1 Stillbirth rates

Overall, the stillbirth rate for cesarean delivery was 19.3% vs. 7.3% for vaginal delivery (p<0.001). Since 2000, the gap between the two curves narrowed significantly (figure 7). Gestational age-specific stillbirth rates are shown in table 10. Preterm stillbirth rates were comparable for the two routes of delivery or higher in the vaginal route. However, there was a statistically significant difference for term stillbirth rates with higher rates observed in the cesarean delivery group. The risk of stillbirth associated with cesarean delivery was high in univariate analysis (2.9 [2.7 - 3.2]). However, after adjusting for maternal age, parity, referral status, CPD, antepartum hemorrhage, hypertension in pregnancy, malpresentation and uterine rupture, the risk disappeared and cesarean delivery ws shown to be protective against stillbirth (aOR = 0.36 [0.30 – 0.42]).

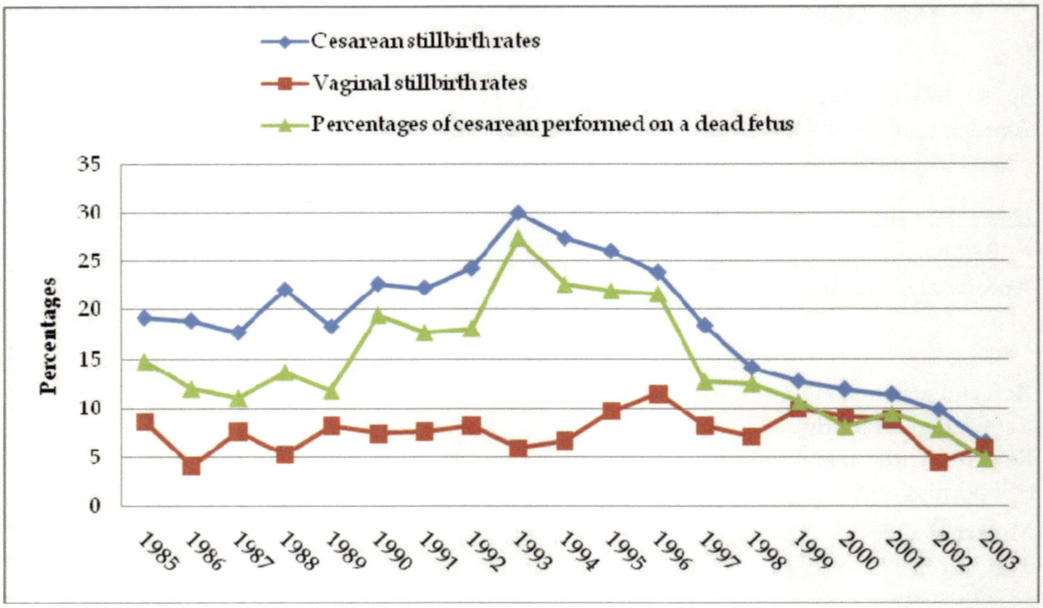

Fig. 7. Time trends of stillbirth rates for cesarean and vaginal delivery, Point G teaching hospital, 1985 - 2003.

3.5.2.2 Neonatal mortality

Neonatal mortality rates over time are shown in Figure 8. Rates were generally higher for cesarean delivery compared to vaginal delivery. Neonatal death rates didn't vary significantly over time for either route of delivery. As expected, the younger the gestational age, the higher the neonatal death rate (Table 10). Univariate analysis revealed an increased risk of neonatal death when the delivery route was abdominal as compared to vaginal route (Table 11). However, after adjusting for maternal (age, parity, referral status), pregnancy (gestational age at delivery, booking status) and fetal / neonatal (suspected fetal distress during labor characterized by an abnormal heart beat rate and / or an abnormal amnionic fluid color, birth weight) characteristics, there was no association between cesarean delivery and neonatal death (table 11). Risk factors for neonatal death in the multivariate analysis included suspicion of fetal distress, very low birth weight and emergently referred women in labor.

	Cesarean delivery					Vaginal delivery					
Weeks of pregnancy	Total birth	Live births	Still-births	%* Still-births	N.* Deaths	% N.* Deaths	Total birth	Live births	Still-births	% Still births*	N. * Deaths	% N.* deaths
22 weeks	1	0	1	100	-	-	28	6	22	78.6	5	83.3
23 weeks	2	0	2	100	-	-	5	0	5	100	0	-
24 weeks	2	0	2	100	0	-	42	11	31	73.8	6	54.5
25 weeks	4	3	1	25.0	1	33.3	24	9	15	62.5	2	22.2
26 weeks	4	3	1	25.0	0	0.0	35	19	16	45.7	3	15.8
27 weeks	1	1	0	0.0	0	0.0	29	18	11	37.9	3	16.7
28 weeks	37	17	20	54.1	6	35.3	146	50	96	65.8	8	16.0
29 weeks	16	6	10	62.5	1	16.7	46	28	18	39.1	2	7.1
30 weeks	23	15	8	34.8	2	13.3	76	56	20	26.3	9	16.1
31 weeks	8	7	1	12.5	1	14.3	36	23	13	36.1	2	8.7
32 weeks	34	23	11	32.4	2	8.7	44	30	14	31.8	11	36.7
33 weeks	25	17	8	32.0	1	5.9	87	61	26	29.9	2	3.3
34 weeks	68	53	15	22.1	1	1.9	192	145	47	24.5	7	4.8
35 weeks	67	59	8	11.9	3	5.1	171	138	33	19.3	4	2.9
36 weeks	184	154	30	16.3	10	6.5	470	421	49	10.4	7	1.0
37 weeks	385	332	53	13.8	8	2.4	913	849	64	7.0	10	1.2
38 weeks	1390	1178	212	15.3	36	3.1	4182	3994	188	4.5	32	0.8
39 weeks	1080	866	214	19.8	19	2.2	3581	3433	148	4.1	25	0.7
40 weeks	779	609	170	21.8	24	3.9	2326	2230	96	4.1	21	0.9
41 weeks	177	133	44	24.9	5	3.8	394	380	14	3.6	3	0.8
42 weeks	103	61	42	40.2	4	6.6	122	107	15	12.3	1	0.9
>42 weeks	75	66	9	12.8	1	1.5	63	60	3	4.8	1	1.7

N. death= neonatal death. % N. death = percentage of neonatal death compute by dividing number of neonatal deaths by number of live birth. % stillbirth = percentage of stillbirth computed by dividing numbers of stillbirth by total number of birth

Table 10. Total numbers of births, stillbirth, and stillbirth rates and neonatal death for cesarean and vaginal delivery, Point G teaching hospital, 1985 -2003.

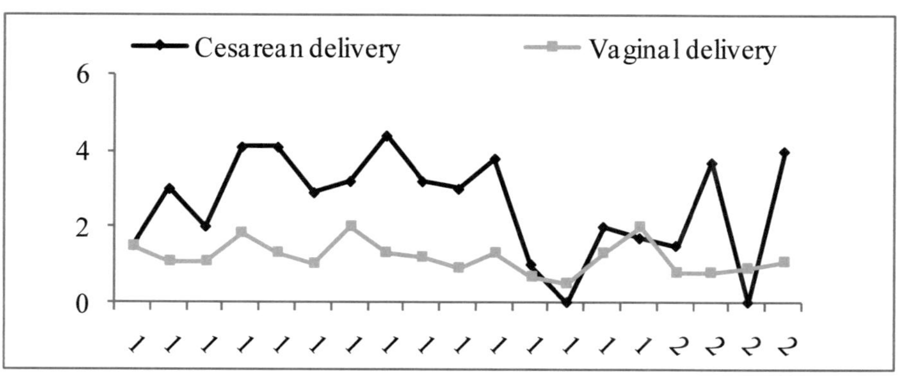

Fig. 8. Neonatal death rates for cesarean and vaginal delivery.

	Unadjusted odds ratio			Adjusted odds ratio		
Factors	OR	95% CIor	P value	AOR	95% CIaor	P value
Route of delivery						
Vaginal delivery	1.0			1.0		
Cesarean delivery	2.6	2.1 - 3.3	<0.001	0.9	0.6 - 1.2	>0.05
Antenatal booking						
Yes	1.0			1.0		
No	3.1	2.3 - 4.1	<0.001	1.5	1.1 - 2.1	<0.01
Maternal age						
20 - 34 years old	1.0			1.0		
13 - 19 years old	2.1	1.6 - 2.7	<0.001	1.3	0.9 - 1.9	>0.05
≥ 35 years old	1.3	0.9 - 1.9	>0.05	1.4	0.9 - 2.2	>0.05
Maternal parity						
1 - 6	1.0			1.0		
0	1.7	1.3 - 2.2	<0.001	1.2	0.9 - 1.7	>0.05
≥ 7	1.2	0.7 - 1.8	>0.05	0.7	0.4 - 1.3	>0.05
Referral status						
Self admission	1.0			1.0		
Referred emergently	7.6	5.9 - 9.9	<0.001	2.6	1.9 - 3.7	<0.001
Referred without emergency	2.5	1.7 - 3.6	<0.001	1.5	0.9 - 2.2	>0.05
Birth weight						
≥ 2500 grs	1.0			1.0		
500 - 999 grs	47.9	28.5 - 80.6	<0.001	8.8	3.2 - 24.3	<0.001
1000 - 1499 grs	16.1	10.6 - 24.6	<0.001	4.3	1.9 - 9.4	<0.001
1500 - 1999 grs	5.3	3.5 - 8.1	<0.001	1.6	0.8 - 3.1	>0.05
2000 - 2499 grs	1.6	1.1 - 2.4	<0.05	0.9	0.5 - 1.5	>0.05
Gestational at delivery						
≥ 37 weeks	1.0			1.0		
22 - 27 weeks	29.9	17.4 - 51.1	<0.001	2.1	0.8 - 5.8	>0.05
28 - 32 weeks	11.6	8.2 - 16.5	<0.001	2.2	1.1 - 4.6	<0.05
33 - 36 weeks	2.6	1.8 - 3.7	<0.001	1.6	0.9 - 2.9	>0.05
Antepartum hemorrhage						
Yes	4.9	3.2 - 7.7	<0.001	1.4	0.8 - 2.3	>0.05
No	1.0			1.0		
Suspect fetal distress						
Yes	20.8	14.3 - 30.3	<0.001	20.6	14.2 - 30.1	<0.001
No	1.0			1.0		

OR : odds ratio CI : confidence interval AOR : adjusted odds ratio

Table 11. Predictors of neonatal mortality, Point G national hospital, Bamako, Mali, 1985 - 2003.

4. Discussion

4.1 Strengths and limitations

We report here an analysis of deliveries during a nineteen year period in a teaching hospital in Mali (West Africa). Our main findings are: (1) a striking increase in cesarean delivery rates throughout the study period; (2) women in labor referred with an emergency condition not only constituted the largest proportion of cesarean deliveries but also this mode of admission seriously jeopardized the maternal as well as the perinatal prognosis; (3) the two most common indications for cesarean delivery were cephalopelvic disproportion and previous cesarean delivery; (4) there were very low rates of planned cesarean delivery as expressed by the small contribution of Robson groups 2 and 4.

While the majority of women delivering at Point G National Hospital originate from Bamako, the substantial proportion of women referred from other regions and the sociodemographic characteristics of the pregnant women in this setting provide a perspective on hospital-based obstetric care in the whole country up to 2003. Since 2003, Mali has instituted important changes in the delivery of obstetric care. In 2004, a nationwide emergency obstetric and neonatal care program was put in place to reinforce the perinatality program. In 2006, the Malian government began to provide medically indicated Cesarean deliveries free of charge in public hospitals and referral district health centers, increasing access and leading to subsequently higher Cesarean delivery rates (Teguete et al, 2010b). Additionally, since 2002, major staffs of the department of obstetrics and gynecology have been appointed to Gabriel Toure teaching hospital, a nearby hospital of the Malian capital city with easier accessibility. These aspects are not covered by the database used here.

Trends in Cesarean delivery rates after 2003 can be examined through an improved and adapted obstetric database installed at Gabriel Touré teaching hospital after the transfer of staff. This database contains more than 400 variables related to patients' demographic, medical and obstetric factors as well as pregnancy outcomes [Teguete et al, 2008; Teguete et al, 2009]. Rates of Cesarean delivery at the Gabriel Touré teaching hospital increased from 21% in 2003 to 32% in 2009 (Teguete I. et al, 2010b). After sequential adjustment for maternal demographic, obstetric, and referral characteristics as described above, 19% of the observed increase remained unexplained (figure 9), compared to 58.5% for the Point G database. CPD, referral status and previous cesarean delivery were the major determinants of cesarean delivery, as at Point G teaching hospital. These findings will be the core of the following comments.

4.2 Cesarean delivery rates in developing countries

The current situation of cesarean delivery rates in developing countries is very complex with large differences between countries, within countries, and between health centers [Fesseha et al, 2011; Cissé et al, 1998]. A large ecological cross-sectional study reported that, in low income countries where cesarean deliveries rates are less than 10%, as section rates increase, neonatal and maternal mortality decrease [Althabe et al, 2006]. Our database revealed a sharp increase in the rates of hospital cesarean delivery, similar to those observed in many teaching hospital maternity wards in Africa [Muganyizi & Kidanto, 2009; Geidam et al, 2009; Kwawukume, 2001]. However, countrywide cesarean delivery rates remain under the minimum level of 5% advised by the WHO for optimal obstetric care (table 12).

Rural populations remain underserved in many developing countries [Leone et al, 2008, Kizonde et al, 2006]. A recent regional meeting for the final evaluation of the "Initiative 2010" aimed at reducing maternal mortality ratios and neonatal mortality rates by 50% by 2010 reported that among 17 West and Central African countries evaluated; only five had national cesarean delivery rates of 5% or more [Ba, 2011]. Thus, in sub-Saharan Africa where coverage in healthcare service is low, initiatives to increase cesarean rates are ongoing in order to meet the millennium development goals [El-Khoury et al, 2011]. At the same time, there are calls for caution [Mbaye et al, 2011; Fesseha et al 2011] to prevent high unnecessary cesarean rates like those observed in many developed countries as well as some developing countries [Khawaja et al, 2004].

Countries	Teaching hospital	District hospital /Rural area	Country level
Tanzania	Muganyizi & Kidanto, 2009 1999: 15.1% 2005: 25.6%	Stein, 2008 1986 – 1994: 9.4% 1995 – 1999: 20.3%	Wenjuan et al, 2011 1992 – 1993: 2.9% 2004 – 2005: 4.0%
Nigeria	Ijaiya & Aboyeji 2001 1990: 3.8% 1999: 20.7% Geidam et al, 2009 2000: 7.2% 2003: 13.3% 2005: 13.9%	Ikeako, 2009 2005 – 2009 : 10.4%	Wenjuan et al, 2011 1990: 2.5% 2003: 1.9% 2008: 2.1%
Ghana	Kwawukume, 2001 1988: 25.2% 1995: 17.7% 1999: 23.8%	Buekens et al, 1998 1998 = 2.8%	Wenjuan et al, 2011 1993: 4.8% 2003: 4.4% 2008: 7.2%
Mali	Our study, 2011 1985: 12.5% 1988: 16.7% 1990: 20.8% 1999: 35.1% 2003: 24.9%	Maïga et al, 1999 1993 – 1995: 1%	El-Khoury et al, 2011 2005: 0.9% 2006: 1.6% 2007: 2.1% 2008: 2.2% 2009: 2.3%
Burkina Faso	Bambara et al, 2007 2000 : 11.3%	Buekens et al, 2003 1999 = 1.0%	Wenjuan et al, 2001 1993: 1.6% 2003: 0.7
Senegal	Cissé et al 2004 1992 : 12% 1996: 17.5% Ngom et al, 2001 2001: 25.1%	Cissé, 1998 1996 : 0.1% - 0.7%	Wenjuan et al, 2011 1992 – 1993: 2.5% 2005: 3.9%
Madagascar	Andriamady et al, 2001 1998 : 6.8%	Robitail et al, 2004 1997 : 0.7% 1999: 0.58% 2000: 0.67% 2001: 0.71%	1997: 0.6% Wenjuan et al, 2011 1993: 1.1% 2008 – 2009: 1.7%
Kenya	Wanyonyi et al, 2007 1996: 20.4% 2001: 25.9% 2004: 38.1%	Buekens et al, 2003 1993: 4.1% 1998: 5.7%	Wenjuan et al, 2011 1993: 6.0% 2003: 4.9% 2008: 7.2%
Namibia		van Dillen J, 2007 2001 – 2002 : 7.9%	Wenjuan et al, 2011 1992: 7.2% 2006 – 2007: 13.6%

Table 12. Cesarean delivery rates in different settings of selected sub-saharan african countries.

4.3 Referral system and cesarean delivery

Like in many developing countries, access to healthcare for the poor and underserved remains insufficient in Mali.

After the publication of the now famous article "Where is the M in MCH?" [Rosenfield & Maine, 1985], and the introduction of the Safe Motherhood Initiative in Nairobi in 1987, maternal mortality reduction in sub-Saharan Africa garnered increased attention and commitment [UN. Report, 1994]. In this context, maternal and child protection have become major targets in the implementation of the healthcare system by the Malian government.

Many developing countries paid special attention to the organisation of the referral system to improve maternal and child healh [Rudge et al, 2011]. Likewise, the National Perinatality Program of Mali was conceived in 1994 and organised the referral system to improve the environment of perinatal care. Reported interventions at the community level focused on (1) educational activities to raise awareness of danger signs and encourage the use of obstetric services; (2) reducing geographical and financial barriers through emergency loan schemes / subvention and (3) improving transport and communication [Kandeh et al, 1997; Nwakoby et al 1997]. This policy led to an increase in cesarean delivery rates in rural district hospitals [De Brouwere, 1997], but it was very difficult to implement in large cities like Bamako. The high incidence at Point G of uterine rupture, a preventable end stage obstetric morbidity, demonstrates the unmet needs of cesarean delivery.

Thus, like in many developing countries [Sørbye et al, 2011], access to emergency obstetric care is unsatisfactory in Mali and unequal. Despite a national obstetric referral system, many birthing women (often without complications or known risk factors) bypass referring facilities to get access directly to the higher level of obstetric care. On the other hand, many women without access to care have to travel long distances to access care during labor and delivery. Difficulties related to referral health systems are frequently reported in sub-Saharan Africa [Cissé et al; 1998] and were common features in our hospital before 1994. Large population based studies emphasize the need to ensure that the women least likely to seek care are not marginalized [Jacqueline et al., 2003], requiring a functional referral system.

In Mali, access to cesarean delivery was a priority of referral system organisation from its inception. This system may be partially responsible for the decreased risk of caesarean-related maternal death after 1994 as well as the downward trend in post-cesarean stillbirth rates. However, the risk of maternal death when caesarean delivery is needed is still high despite adjustment for other factors. The unsatisfactory initial impact of cesarean delivery on maternal and fetal / neonatal health led the Malian government to make it free of charge. Many other countries engaged in such political commitment to eliminate financial barriers. However some authors reported that, although removing user fees has the potential to improve access to health services especially for the poor, it is not appropriate in all contexts [James et al, 2006]. Similarly, simulations have found that decreasing the price of Cesarean delivery has minor effects, suggesting that greater increases in access to care would come from investment in the improvement of healthcare structures and care processes [Mariko, 2003]. Developing countries face serious issues in this respect, due to the lack of and inequitable distribution of human resources. For example, in 2002 in Mali, 265 midwives were posted in Bamako or in regional hospitals, while only 164 were working at the peripheral level. As a result, only 24% of deliveries were attended by a skilled professional. Similar figures have been reported from Tanzania [Olsen et al., 2005]. Many basic health facilities do not even have a midwife, so, many patients have to come directly to the tertiary hospital or go nowhere at all [Gerein N et al, 2006]. Many strategies have been or are being tested to solve this problem. Unfortunately, there is no one single-bullet solution [Dayrit et al, 2010]. These gaps contribute to the poor performance of the health system [Lawn J E., 2009]. Thus, a holistic approach has to be considered for better strengthening of the health system in order to meet the performance goals of the WHO schematic framework [WHO, 2007]

4.4 Cephalopelvic disproportion

The expression cephalopelvic disproportion (CPD) came into use prior to the 20th century to describe obstructed labor due to disparity between the dimensions of the fetal head and maternal pelvis that preclude vaginal delivery. This term, however, originated at a time when the main indication for cesarean delivery was overt pelvic contracture due to rickets (Olah & Neilson, 1994). CPD can be due to a contracted pelvis or a disproportionately large fetal head and is thus not limited to primary cesarean delivery only [Carbone B., 2000].

In a systematic review of cesarean delivery for maternal indication, Dumont A. et al [Dumont al, 2001] found that cephalopelvic disproportion was the commonest indication, and 1.4% to 8.5% of all deliveries resulted in cesarean birth for this indication. Similarly, a large population based study in West Africa reported that 1% of all deliveries were complicated by CPD [Ould El Jouda D et al, 2001]. The proportion of all cesarean deliveries due to contracted pelvis (a sub-entity of CPD) has been reported to be between 20% in Senegal [Bouillin et al, 1994] and 37.3% in Bobo Dioulasso, Burkina Faso [Bambara et al, 2007]. Comparable trends have been reported in Senegal with mean rates of 31.3% for CPD ranging from 26% to 34.9% between 1992 and 2001 [Cissé et al, 2004; N'Gom PM et al, 2004], as well as Ethiopia (34% [Fesseha et al, 2011]). Similar high incidence rates of CPD have been reported in non sub-Saharan developing countries [Festin et al, 2009]. Our data pointed out the importance of contracted pelvis in CPD. Cephalopelvic disproportion was a major indication of cesarean delivery in our hospital from 1985 to 2003. A mean rate of 39.6% of women who delivered abdominally had some degree of CPD, ranging from 30.3% to 43.4% between 1985 and 2003. In addition, in our study contracted pelvis constituted the vast majority of all CPD (87%). 63.5% of all contracted pelvis cases were found in patients referred most commonly from poor rural settings. The high incidence rates of uterine rupture (an end stage of obstructed labor) recorded in this group may correlate with severity of pelvis contraction and confirmed the close link between referred patients during labor / delivery and need of cesarean reported elsewhere [Amelink - Verburg et al, 2009].

The cause of high rates of contracted pelvis in rural areas may be due to several factors such as genetics, increasing recognition, or the impact of resource scarcity on the female bony pelvis [Cissé et al, 2004; Kurki, 2011]. Special attention must be devoted to malnutrition in sub-Saharan Africa. Malnutrition prevalence remains unfortunately high; the proportion of the population with low daily caloric intake exceed 30% in many countries, and this trend is mirrored by the prevalence of low weight in children under five years old [USAID / West Africa professional paper series, 2008]. Consequently, prevention of obstructed labor can be achieved only through a multidisciplinary approach aimed in the short term at identifying high-risk cases and in the long term at improving nutrition. Early motherhood should be discouraged, and efforts are needed to improve nutrition during infancy, childhood, early adulthood, and pregnancy. Improving the access to and promoting the use of reproductive and contraceptive services will also help reduce the prevalence of this complication [Konje & Ladipo, 2000].

4.5 Previous cesarean delivery

One third of our patients with a history of previous cesarean delivery were allowed a trial of labor (TOL), and the probability of successful vaginal delivery in this group was 50.1%. In our guidelines for trial of labor after cesarean birth (TOLAC), neither labor induction nor labor augmentation were permitted. No TOLAC was attempted when the number of previous cesarean delivery was >1 or in the case of a previous history of uterine rupture. These strict criteria explained our relative low rate of TOLAC.

In a meta-analysis of 963 papers, the range for TOLAC and VBAC rates was large (28-82 percent and 49-87 percent, respectively). Predictors of women having a TOL were having a prior vaginal delivery and settings of higher-level care, namely tertiary care centers [Guise et al, 2010]. Similar findings have been reported in sub-Saharan [Boulvain et al, 1997]; the percentage of TOL ranged from 37% to 97% across reports, with probability of successful vaginal delivery of 69% (95% CI 63-75%). Maternal mortality among all women with a previous cesarean section was 1.9/1000 (95% CI 0-4.3). Uterine rupture and scar dehiscence occurred in 2.1% (95% CI 1.0-3.2). With our restrictions on VBAC, we recorded fewer vaginal deliveries, but also less uterine rupture / dehiscence, as was found in rural Zimbabwe [Spaans et al, 1997]. In settings where such cautions were not applied, higher morbidity levels were observed [Olagbuji et al., 2010, Adanu & McCarthy, 2007; Olusanya & Solanke, 2009; Sepou et al, 2003; Nwokoro et al 2003; Oboro et al, 2010; Wanyonyi & Karuga, 2010]. A large multicenter propective study in a western country with a uniform and well organised delivery care system emphasized the greater perinatal risk associated with a trial of labor [Landon et al, 2004]. Although these findings can be a subject of debate [Greene, 2004]; they must be considered and women deserve to be well informed of the risks and benefits of TOL and VBAC [Kraemer et al, 2004]. A recent systematic review suggests that VBAC is a reasonable choice for the majority of women and found that adverse outcomes were rare for both elective repeat cesarean delivery and trial of labor [Guise JM et al., 2010a, 2010b]. The need for studies identifying patients at greatest risk is of primary importance in sub-Saharan Africa where high levels of morbidity are often reported.

Overall, in sub-Saharan Africa a selective policy of trial of labor after a previous cesarean delivery has a success rate comparable to that observed in developed countries. Vaginal birth after cesarean appears to be relatively safe and applicable in this context and contributes significantly to the global cesarean delivery rate.

4.6 Low rates of elective delivery

There are many reports emphasising on the high levels of emergency delivery in sub-Saharan hospitals and health centres [Fesseha et al, 2011; Shah et al, 2009; Wylie & Mirza, 2008; Dumont et al, 2001]. In contrast to wealthier countries, planned delivery remains an underused option in Sub-Saharan Africa [Stavrou E. P. et al, 2011]. For example, during the two decades at Point G teaching hospital, only 212 pregnant women underwent labor induction. In many sub-Saharan African countries, labor induction is not common as necessary medications are not readily available. Before the year 2000, oxytocine was the only medication available in Mali for labor induction and was only used for very favorable cases with a Bishop cervical score ≥ 7. Despite the lower rates of labor induction, we observe a mean rate of post-induction cesarean delivery of approximately 90% (Robson group 2). High levels of cesarean delivery following labor induction in nulliparas have been qualified as universal [Brennan et al, 2009 ; Main et al., 2006; McCarthy et al, 2007; Robson, 2001; Costa et al 2010; Yeast et al, 1999]

Unpublished data from the WHO Global Survey on Maternal and Perinatal Health, which included 373 health-care facilities in 24 countries and nearly 300 000 deliveries, showed that 9.6% of the deliveries involved labor induction. Overall, the survey found that facilities in African countries tended to have lower rates of induction of labor (lowest: Niger, 1.4%) compared with Asian and Latin American countries (highest: Sri Lanka, 35.5%) [WHO, 2010].

One point is that many indications of labor induction are associated with preterm delivery. The lack of neonatal resuscitation facilities [Hofmeyr et al, 2009] and the poor outcomes of preterm neonates lead many sub-saharan obstetric teams to avoid preterm labor induction or preterm elective cesarean delivery. Even in hospitals, staffs are frequently not trained in resuscitation and equipment is not available. A national service provision assessments in 6 African countries demonstrated that only 2%-12% of personnel conducting births had been trained in neonatal resuscitation and only 8%-22% of facilities had equipment for newborn respiratory support [Wall et al, 2009]. This important gap certainly impacts clinical decision making in Sub-Saharan obstetric units.

Therefore, it is a challenge for healthcare workers and policymakers dealing with pregnancy management in developing countries to examine critically ways to increase percentage of planned delivery. This challenge can be met firstly with preventive measures at a public health level (e.g. counselling and education), at the pregnant women's level (e.g. improved utilisation of the antenatal care services), and at the caregiver's level (e.g. better selection of cases in order improve the percentage of pregnant referred without emergency, an overt contracted pelvis mustn't begin labor at the level of primary care where obstetric surgery is not available).

5. Conclusion

From 1985 to 2003, cesarean delivery rates at Point G National Hospital increased substantially. Most of the increase in cesarean delivery rates is explained by higher proportions of outside referrals, cephalopelvic disproportion, and history of previous cesarean delivery. The increased cesarean delivery rate cannot, however, be fully explained by these factors or other characteristics collected by this study, and is likely the multifactorial impact of psychosocial determinants of healthcare utilization and systemic problems of healthcare delivery. These variables are beyond the scope of this study. Future ecological studies addressing clinical, financial, and geographical considerations as well as cultural acceptability of cesarean delivery are needed. Since emergency referrals for caesarean during delivery significantly worsen the maternal and fetal prognosis, more widespread access to facilities capable of performing caesarean sections as well as earlier referrals of high risk pregnancies from primary health centers before the onset of complications would likely lead to substantial improvements in maternal and neonatal outcomes. A holistic need assessment will govern improved healthcare delivery strategies and aid progress towards meeting the millennium development goals in developing countries.

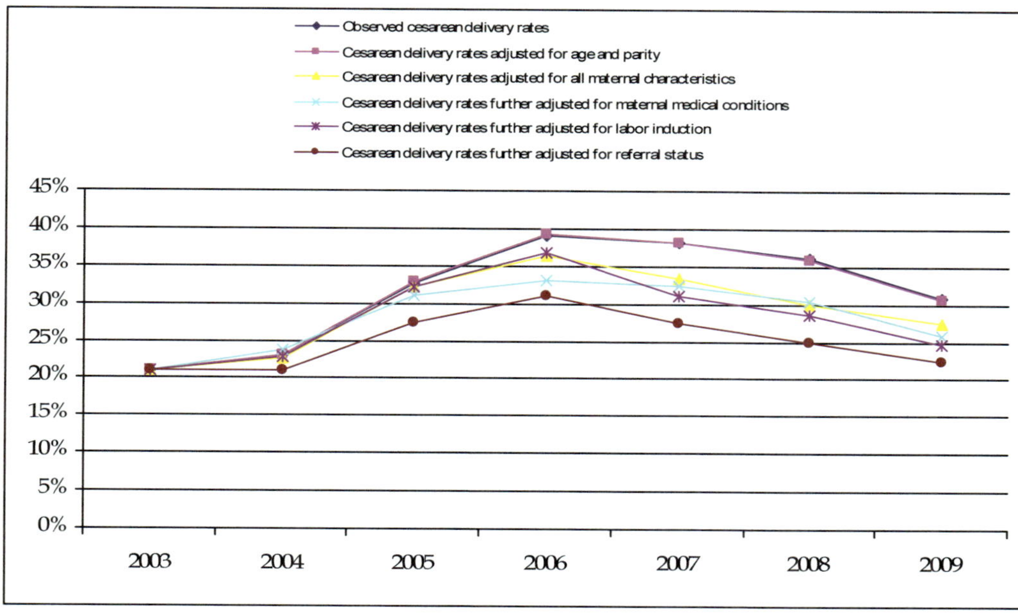

Fig. 9. Observed rates of cesarean delivery and adjusted rates after sequentially adjusting for age, parity, maternal conditions, obstetric practice and referral status (Teguete I. et al, 2010b).

6. Acknowledgments

To Evan and Lauren Oreinstein, for their valuable contribution to this work.

To all the medical students who participated in the Point G obstetric database completion: Seydou Traore, Sekou Coulibaly, Marie Lea Dakouo, Aïssata Nene Bah, Seydou Fané, Amadou Fomba, Adama Diarra, Nouhoum Camara, Yakouni dite Hawa Dougnon, Sandrine Eyoko.

7. References

Adanu R.M.K. & McCarthy M.Y. (2007); Vaginal birth after cesarean delivery in the West African setting. *International Journal of Gynecology and Obstetrics* Vol .98, No 3, (September 2007), pp. (227-231). PMID: 17603060.

Althabe F, Belizán J, Villar J, Alexander S, Bergel E, Ramos S, Romero M, Donner A, Lindmark G, Langer A, Farnot U, Cecatti JG, Carroli G. & Kestler E. (2004). Latin American Cesarean Section Study Group: Mandatory second opinion to reduce rates of unnecessary cesarean sections in Latin America: a cluster randomised controlled trial. *Lancet,* Vol 363, No 9425, (June 2004), pp. (1934-1940). PMID: 15194252.

Althabe F, Sosa C, Belizán JM, Gibbons L. & Jacquerioz F. (2006). Cesarean section rates and maternal and neonatal mortality in low-, medium-, and high-income countries: an ecological study. *Birth,* Vol. 33, No 4, (December 2006), pp. (270-277). PMID: 17150064.

Amelink-Verburg MP, Rijnders ME, Buitendijk SE. A trend analysis in referrals during pregnancy and labor in Dutch midwifery care 1988-2004. *BJOG,* Vol 116, No 7, (June 2009), pp. (923-32). PMID: 19522796

Andriamady Rasoarimahandry CL, Andrianarivony MO & Ranjalahy RJ. (2001). Indications and prognosis of cesarean section at Befelatanana maternity unit--Central University Hospital of Antananarivo (apropos of 529 cases, during the year 1998). *Gynecol Obstet Fertil.* Vol. 29, No 12, (December 2001), pp. (900-4). PMID : 11802553.

Ba K. S. (2011). Evaluation Finale de l'Initiative Vision 2010. Réunion d'Evaluation Finale de la VISION 2010 BAMAKO 1 - 6 Octobre 2011

Ba'aqeel H.S. (2009). Cesarean delivery rates in Saudi Arabia: A tenyear review. *Annals of Saudi Medicine* Vol. 29, No 3, (May - June 2009), pp. (179-183). PMID : 19448379.

Bambara M, Fongan E, Dao B, Ouattara H, Lankoande J. & Kone B. (2007). La césarienne en milieu africain: à propos de 440 cas à la maternité du CHUSS de Bobo-Dioulasso (Burkina Faso). *Méd Afrique Noire,* Vol. 54 No 6, (2007), pp. (343-348).

Barros FC, Vaughan JP, Victora CG & Huttly SRA. (1991). Epidemic of Cesarean sections in Brazil. *Lancet,* Vol 338, No 8760, (July 1991), pp. (167-169). PMID: 1677075.

Béla G., Péter N. & János T. (2009). Trends in prevalence of cesarean section in Uzsoki Hospital between 1st January, 1999 and 30th june, 2009. Analysis of some suspected factors. *Magyar Noorvosok Lapja* Vol. 72 No 6, (2009), pp. (269-272).

Belizán J. M., Althabe F., Barros F. C. & Alexander S. (1999). Rates and implications of cesarean sections in Latin America: ecological study. *BMJ* 1999; Vol. 319, No 7222, (November 1999) pp. (1397–402). PMID: 10574855.

Bell J, Curtis SL & Alayón S. (2003). Trends in delivery care in six countries. *DHS analytical studies* Calverton, MD: ORC Macro, No. 7, (2003), p. 62.

Betran AP, Merialdi M, Lauer JA, Bing-Shun W, Thomas J, Van Look P & Wagner M. (2007) Rates of cesarean section: analysis of global, regional and national estimates. *Paediat Perinatal Epidemiol* Vol. 21 No 2, (March 2007), pp. (98-113), PMID: 17302638.

Bogg L., Huang K., Long Q., Shen Y. & Hemminki E. (2010). Dramatic increase of Cesarean deliveries in the midst of health reforms in rural China. *Social Science & Medicine,* Vol. 70, No 10, (May 2010) pp. (1544–1549), PMID: 20219278.

Bouillin D, Fournier G, Gueye A, Diadhiou F & Cissé CT. (1994) Epidemiological surveillance and obstetrical dystocias surgery in Senegal. *Sante,* Vol. 4, No 6, (November - December 1994), pp. (399-406), PMID : 7850191.

Boulvain M, Fraser WD, Brisson-Carroll G, Faron G & Wollast E. (1997). Trial of labor after cesarean section in sub-Saharan Africa: a meta-analysis. *Br J Obstet Gynaecol.* Vol 104, No 12 (December 1997), pp. (1385-1390), PMID: 9422017.

Brennan DJ, Robson MS, Murphy M, et al. (2009). Comparative analysis of international cesarean delivery rates using 10-group classification identifies significant variation in spontaneous labor. *Am J Obstet Gynecol* Vol. 201, No 3, (September 2009), pp. (308.e1-8), PMID:19733283.

Buekens P., Curtis S. & Alayón S. (2003) Demographic and Health Surveys: cesarean section rates in sub-Saharan Africa. *BMJ* Vol 326, No 7381, (January 2003), p. 136, PMID: 12531845.

Carbone B. (2000). Recommandations pour la pratique clinique. Indications de césarienne en cas de dystocie.*J Gynecol Obstet Biol Reprod;* Vol 29, No Suppl. n° 2, (2000), pp. (68 - 73).

Chaillet N, Dumont A. (2007). Evidence-Based Strategies for Reducing Cesarean Rates: A Meta Analysis. *Birth* Vol 34, No 1, (March 2007), pp. (53-64), PMID: 17324180.

Chou D. et al. (2010). Trends in Maternal Mortality: 1990 to 2008. World Health Organization: Geneva 2010.

Choudhury A.P., Dawson A.J. (2009). Trends in indications for cesarean sections over 7 years in a Welsh district general hospital. *Journal of Obstetrics and Gynaecology,* Vol 29, No 8, (November 2009), pp. (714-717), PMID: 19821664.

Cissé C.T., Faye E.O., de Bernis L., Dujardin B., Diadhiou F. (1998). Césariennes au Sénégal : couverture des besoins et qualité des services. *Cahiers Santé* Vol. 8, No 5, (September - October 1998), pp. (369-377) PMID : 98504015.

Cissé CT, Ngom PM, Guissé A, Faye EO, Moreau JC. (2004). Thinking about the evolution of cesarean section rate at University Teaching Hospital of Dakar between 1992 and 2001. *Gynecol Obstet Fertil.* Vol 32, No 3, (March 2004) pp. (210-217), 15123118.

Cohain J.S. (2009). Documented causes of unneCesareans. *Midwifery today with international midwife,* Vol. 63, No 92, (Winter 2009), pp. (18-19), PMID: 20092138.

Commission de l'Union Africaine. Réunion du Comité des experts de la troisième réunion conjointe en 2010 de la Conférence des ministres de l'économie et des finances de l'Union africaine et de la Conférence des ministres africains des finances, de la planification et du développement économique de la Commission économique pour l'Afrique. Rapport 2010 sur l'évaluation des progrès accomplis par l'Afrique vers la réalisation des Objectifs du Millénaire pour le développement. Lilongwe (Malawi) 25 -28 mars 2010.

Costa M. L., Cecatti J. G., Souza J. P., Milanez H. M. & Gülmezoglu A. M. (2010) Using a Cesarean Section Classification System based on characteristics of the population as a way of monitoring obstetric practice. *Reproductive Health* Vol 7, No 13, (June 2010), doi:10.1186/1742-4755-7-13 PMID: 20579388.

Cunningham FG, Gant NF, Leveno KJ, Gilstrap III LC, Hauth JC & Wenstrom KD. (2001). Williams Obstetrics. (21st Edition). McGraw-Hill, New York, 1668 p.

Dayrit MM, Dolea C. & Braichet JM. (2010). One piece of the puzzle to solve the human resources for health crisis. *Bull World Health Organ.* Vol. 88, No 5, (May 2010), p: 322 PMID : 20461216.

De Brouwere V. (1997). Appui à la mise en ouvre et à l'évaluation du système de référence avec la périnatalité comme porte d'entrée dans le Cercle. *UNICEF Mali,* 1997.

De Brouwere V, Dubourg D, Richard F. & Van Lerberghe W. (2002). Need for cesarean sections in west Africa. *The Lancet* Vol 359, No 9310 (March 2002) pp : 974 - 975, PMID : 11918936.

Dumont A., de Bernis L., Bouvier-Colle M-H & Bréart G, for the MOMA study group (2001). Cesarean section rate for maternal indication in sub-Saharan Africa: a systematic review. *The Lancet*, Vol. 358, No 9290, (October 2001), pp. (1328–334), PMID: 11684214.

El-Khoury M, Gandaho T, Arur A, Keita B, & Nichols L. (2011). Improving Access to Life-saving Maternal

Health Services: The Effects of Removing User Fees for Cesareans in Mali. Bethesda, MD: *Health Systems 20/20*, April 2011, Abt Associates Inc.

Faundes A, Cecatti JG. (1993). Which policy for Cesarean section in Brazil? An analysis of trends and consequences. *Health Policy Plann* Vol. 8 No 1, (March 1993), pp. (33-42).

Fesseha N., Getachew A., Hiluf M., Gebrehiwot Y., Bailey P. (2011). A national review of cesarean delivery in Ethiopia. *International Journal of Gynecology and Obstetrics* Vol. 115, No 1, (October 2011) pp. (106–111), PMID: 21872239.

Festin MR, Laopaiboon M, Pattanittum P, Ewens MR, Henderson-Smart DJ, Crowther CA; SEA-ORCHID Study Group. (2009) Cesarean section in four South East Asian countries: reasons for, rates, associated care practices and health outcomes. *BMC Pregnancy Childbirth.* Vol. 9, No 9, (May 2009) p:17, PMID: 19426513.

Fournier P, Dumont A, Tourigny C, Dunkley G & Dramé̀c S. (2009). Improved access to comprehensive emergency obstetric care and its effect on institutional maternal mortality in rural Mali. *Bull World Health Organ* Vol. 87, No 1, (January 2009), pp. (30–8), PMID: 19197402.

Geidam A.D., Audu B.M., Kawuwa B.M. & Obed J.Y.(2009) Rising trend and indications of cesarean section at the university of Maiduguri teaching hospital, Nigeria. *Annals of African Medicine*, Vol. 8, No 2, (April – June 2009) pp. (127-132). PMID: 19805945.

Gerein N, Green A, Pearson S. (2006). The implications of shortages of health professionals for maternal health in sub-Saharan Africa. *Reprod Health Matters* Vol. 14, No 27, (May 2006) pp. (40-50). PMID: 16713878.

Graham W. (1998). The scandal of the century. *Br J Obstet Gynaecol* Vol. 105, No 4, (April 1998), pp. (375-376). PMID: 9609258.

Greene M. (2004). Vaginal Birth After Cesarean Delivery Revisited. *New England Journal of Medicine* Vol. 351, No 25, (December 2004), pp. (2647-2649). PMID: 15598961.

Guihard P, Blondel B (2001).Trends in risk factors for cesarean sections in France between 1981 and 1995: lessons for reducing the rates in the future. *BJOG*. Vol. 108, No 1, (January 2001), pp. (48-55). PMID: 11213004.

Guise JM, Eden K, Emeis C, Denman MA, Marshall N, Fu RR, Janik R, Nygren P, Walker M, McDonagh M. (2010a). Vaginal birth after cesarean: new insights. *Evid Rep Technol Assess (Full Rep)*. No. 191, (March 2010), pp. (1-397). PMID : 20629481.

Guise JM, Denman MA, Emeis C, Marshall N, Walker M, Fu R, Janik R, Nygren P, Eden KB, McDonagh M. (2010b). Vaginal birth after cesarean: new insights on maternal and neonatal outcomes. *Obstet Gynecol.* Vol. 115, No 6, (June 2010), pp. (1267-78). PMID: 20502300.

Hofmeyr GJ, Haws RA., Bergström S, Lee ACC, Okong P, Darmstadt GL., Mullany LC., Shwe Oo EK, & Lawn JE. (2009). Obstetric care in low-resource settings: What, who, and how to overcome challenges to scale up? *International Journal of Gynecology and Obstetrics* Vol. 107, Suppl 1, (October 2009), pp. (S21–S45). PMID: 19815204.

Holtz SA & Stanton CK. (2007). Assessing the quality of cesarean birth data in the Demographic and Health Surveys. *Stud Fam Plann*. Vol 38, No 1, (March 2007); pp. (47-54). PMID: 17385382.

Horan TC, Gaynes RP, Martone WJ, Jarvis WR, Emori TG. (1992) CDC definitions of nosocomial surgical site infections, 1992: a modification of CDC definitions of surgical wound infections. *Infect Control Hosp Epidemiol* Vol. 13, N°10: (October 1992), pp. (606-8). PMID: 1334988

Hosmer DW Jr, Lemeshow S. (1989). *Applied logistic regression*. pp. (131–3), John Wiley & Sons, New York.

Howell S., Johnston T., MacLeod S.-L. (2009) Trends and determinants of cesarean sections births in Queensland, 1997-2006. *Australian and New Zealand Journal of Obstetrics and Gynaecology* Vol. 49, No 6, (December 2009), pp. (606-611). PMID: 20070708.

Ijaiya M.A. and Aboyeji P.A. (2001). Cesarean delivery: the trend over a ten-year period at Ilorin, Nigeria. *The Nigerian Journal of Surgical Research*, Vol. 3, No 1 (March 2001), pp. (11 - 18).

Ikeako LC, Nwajiaku L, Ezegwui HU. (2009). Cesarean section in a secondary health hospital in Awka, Nigeria. *Niger Med J* Vol. 50, No…, (2009), pp. (64-67).

Jain N.J., Kruse L.K., Demissie K., Khandelwal M. (2009). Impact of mode of delivery on neonatal complications: Trends between 1997 and 2005. *Journal of Maternal-Fetal and Neonatal Medicine* Vol. 22, No 6, (June 2009), pp. (491-500). PMID: 19504405.

James C D., Hanson K, McPake B., Balabanova D., Gwatkin D., Hopwood I. Kirunga C., Knippenberg R.,

Meessen B., Morris S.l S., Preker A, Souteyrand Y., Tibouti A., Villeneuve P.l & Xu K. (2006). To Retain or Remove User Fees? Reflections on the Current Debate in Low- and Middle-Income Countries. *Appl Health Econ Health Policy* Vol. 5, No 3, (2006), pp. (137-153). PMID: 17132029.

Kandeh HB, Leigh B, Kanu MS et al. (1997). Community motivators promote use of emergency obstetric services in rural Sierra Leone. The Freetown/Makeni PMM Team. *International Journal of Gynaecology and Obstetrics* Vol. 59, Suppl 2, (November 1997), pp. (S209-18). PMID: 9389633.

Karlström A., Ra°destad I., Eriksson C., Rubertsson C., Nystedt A., and Hildingsson I. (2010). Cesarean Section without Medical Reason, 1997 to 2006: A Swedish Register Study. *Birth* Vol. 37, No 1, (March 2010), pp (11 - 20). PMID: 20402717.

Khawaja, M., Choueiry, N., Jurdi, R. (2009). Hospital-based cesarean section in the Arab region: An overview. *Eastern Mediterranean Health Journal*, Vol. 15, No 2, (March - April 2009), pp. (458-469). PMID : 19554995.

Khawaja M, Kabakian-Khasholian T, Jurdi R. (2004). Determinants of cesarean section in Egypt: evidence from the demographic and health survey. *Health Pol* Vol. 69, No 3, (September 2004), pp. (273-281). PMID: 15276307.

Kizonde K, Kinekinda X, Kimbala J, Kamwenyi K. (2006). La césarienne en milieu africain; exemple de la maternité centrale Sendwe de Lubumbashi, R. D. Congo. *Méd Afrique Noire* Vol. 53, No 5, (2006), pp. (293-298).

Klemetti, R., Che, X., Gao, Y., Raven, J., Wu, Z., Tang, S., Hemminki, E. (2010). Cesarean section delivery among primiparous women in rural China: an emerging epidemic. *American Journal of Obstetrics and Gynecology* Vol. 202, No 1, (January 2010), pp. (65.e1-65.e6). PMID: 19819416.

Konje J C and Ladipo O A. Nutrition and obstructed labor (2000). *Am J Clin Nutr* Vol 72, Suppl 1, (July 2000); pp. (291S–7S). PMID: 19871595.

Kowalewski A., Jahn A., Kimatta S.S. (2000). Why Do At-Risk Mothers Fail To Reach Referral Level? Barriers Beyond Distance and Cost. *Afr J Reprod Health,* Vol. 4, No 1, (2000), pp. (100-109).

Kraemer D. F., Berlin M., and Guise J-M. The relationship of health care delivery system characteristics and legal factors to mode of delivery in women with prior cesarean section: a systematic review. *Women's Health Issues* Vol. 14, No 3, (May - June 2004), pp. (94–103). PMID: 15193637.

Künzel W., Herrero J., Onwuhafua P., Staub T., Hornung C. (1996) Maternal and perinatal health in Mali, Togo and Nigeria. *European Journal of Obstetrics & Gynecology and Reproductive Biology,* Vol. 69, No 1, (1996) pp. (11-17). PMID: 8909951.

Kurki H.K. (2011). Compromised skeletal growth? Small body size and clinical contraction thresholds for the female pelvic canal. *Int. J. Paleopathol.* (2011), doi:10.1016/j.ijpp.2011.10.004

Kwawukume E. Y. (2001). Cesarean section in developing countries. *Best Practice & Research Clinical Obstetrics & Gynaecology,* Vol. 15, No. 1, (February 2001), pp. 165 - 178. PMID: 11359321.

Landon MB, Hauth JC, Leveno KJ, Spong CY, Leindecker S, Varner MW, et al. (2004). Maternal and perinatal outcomes associated with a trial of labor after prior cesarean delivery. *N Engl J Med.* Vol. 351, No 25, (December 2004), pp. (2581-9). PMID: 15598960.

Leone T., Padmadas S S., Matthews Z. (2008). Community factors affecting rising cesarean section rates in developing countries: An analysis of six countries. *Social Science & Medicine,* Vol 67, No 8, (October 2008) pp. (1236–1246). PMID: 18657345.

Mariko M. (2003). Quality of care and the demand for health services in Bamako, Mali: the specific roles of structural, process, and outcome components. *Social Science & Medicine* Vol. 56, No 6, (March 2003), pp. (1183–1196). PMID: 12600357.

Lawn J E., Kinney M, Lee A CC, Chopra M, Donnay F, Paul V. K., Bhutta Z A., Bateman M, Darmstadt G L. (2009). Reducing intrapartum-related deaths and disability: Can the health system deliver? *International Journal of Gynecology and Obstetrics* Vol. 107, Suppl. 1, (October 2009), pp. (S123–S142). PMID: 18815205.

Lawn J. E., Lee A. CC, Kinney M., Sibley L., Carlo W. A., Paul V. K., Pattinson R., Darmstadt G. L. (2009). Two million intrapartum-related stillbirths and neonatal deaths: Where, why, and what can be done? *International Journal of Gynecology and Obstetrics,* Vol. 107, Suppl. 1, (October 2009) ; pp. (S5–S19). PMID : 19815202.

Maiga Z, Traoré Nafo F & El Abassi A (1999) La réforme du secteur santé au Mali (1989-1996). *Studies in Health Services Organisation & Policy* 12. ITGPress, Antwerpen.

Main EK, Moore D, Farrell B, et al. (2006). Is there a useful cesarean birth measure? Assessment of the nulliparous term singleton vertex cesarean birth rate as a tool for obstetric quality improvement. *Am J Obstet Gynecol* Vol 194, No 6, (June 2006), pp. (1644-51), discussion (1651-2). PMID: 16643812.

Malvasi A., Tinelli A., Guido M., Zizza A., Cotrino G., Vergari U. (2009). The increasing trend in cesarean sections in south eastern italy: Medical and biopolitical analysis of causes and possible mechanisms for its reduction. *Current Women's Health Reviews* Vol. 5, No 3, (2009), pp. (176-183)

Mbaye EM, Dumont A, Ridde V, Briand V. (2011). Doing more to earn more: cesarean sections based on three cases of exemption from payment in Senegal. *Sante Publique*. Vol. 23, No 3, (May-June 2011), pp. (207-19). PMID: 21896215.

McCarthy FP, Rigg L, Cady L, Cullinane F. (2007). A new way of looking at Cesarean section births. *Aust N Z J Obstet Gynaecol* Vol 47, No 4, (August 2007), pp. (316-20). PMID: 17627688.

Menacker F, Declercq E, Macdorman MF. (2006). Cesarean delivery: background, trends, and epidemiology. *Semin Perinatol.* Vol. 30, No 5, (October 2006), pp. (235-41). PMID: 17011392.

Muganyizi P. S and Kidanto H. L. (2009). Impact of change in maternal age composition on the incidence of Cesarean section and low birth weight: analysis of delivery records at a tertiary hospital in Tanzania, 1999–2005. *BMC Pregnancy and Childbirth,* Vol. 9, (July 2009), p 30. PMID: 19622146.

Naidoo N., Moodley J. (2009). Rising rates of Cesarean sections: an audit of Cesarean sections in a specialist private practice. *SA Fam Pract* Vol. 51, No 3, (2009), pp. (254-258).

Ngom PM, Cisse CT, Cisse ML, Faye EO, Moreau JC. (2004). Epidemiology and prognosis of cesarean sections in University Hospital of Dakar. *Dakar Med.* Vol. 49, No 2, (2004), pp. (116-20). PMID: 15786620.

Nwakoby B, Akpala C, Nwagbo D et al. (1997). Community contact persons promote utilization of obstetric services, Anambra State, Nigeria. The Enugu PMM Team. *International Journal of Gynaecology and Obstetrics* Vol. 59, Suppl. 2, (November 1997), pp. (S219-24). PMID: 9389634.

Nwokoro C. A., Njokanma O. F., Orebamjo T., and Okeke G. C. E. (2003). Vaginal birth after primary cesarean section: the fetal size factor. *Journal of Obstetrics and Gynaecology,* Vol. 23, No. 4, (July 2003) pp. (392–393). PMID: 12881079.

Oboro V., Adewunmi A., Ande A, Olagbuji B., Ezeanochie M. & Oyeniran A. (2010). Morbidity associated with failed vaginal birth after cesarean section. *Acta Obstetricia et Gynecologica.* Vol. 89, No 9, (September 2010), pp. (1229–1232). PMID: 20804350.

Olagbuji B., Ezeanochie M.& Okonofua F. (2010). Predictors of successful vaginal delivery after previous cesarean section in a Nigerian tertiary hospital. *Journal of Obstetrics and Gynaecology,* Vol 30, No 6, (August 2010), pp. (582–585). PMID: 20701507.

Olah KSJ, Neilson J. (1994). Failure to progress in the management of labor. *Br J Obstet Gynaecol* Vol. 101, No 1, (January 1994), pp. (1 - 3). PMID: 8297861.

Olsen OE, Ndeki S, Norheim OF. (2005). Human resources for emergency obstetric care in northern Tanzania: distribution of quantity or quality? *Hum Resources Health* Vol. 3, No 5, (July 2005): 12 p. [Available from: www.human-resources-health.com/content/3/1/5] PMID: 16053519.

Olusanya B O., Solanke O A. (2009). Adverse neonatal outcomes associated with trial of labor after previous cesarean delivery in an inner-city hospital in Lagos, Nigeria. *International Journal of Gynecology and Obstetrics* Vol. 107, No 2, (November 2009), pp. (135–139). PMID: 19647823.

Onsrud L, Onsrud M. (1996). Increasing use of cesarean section, even in developing countries. *Tidsskr Nor Laegeforen* Vol. 116, No 1, (January 1996), pp. (67-71). PMID: 8553342.

Ould El Jouda D., Bouvier-Colle M.-H., MOMA Group. (2001). Dystocia: a study of its frequency and risk factors in seven cities of west Africa. *International Journal of Gynecology & Obstetrics* Vol 74, No 2 (August 2001), pp. (171 - 178). PMID: 11502297.

Riviere M. (1959). Mortalité maternelle au cours de l'état gravido-puerpéral, avortement exceptés. *Bull soc, gynécol Obstét., Congrés de Paris* No 11, (1959), pp. (141-272).

Robitail S, Gorde S, Barrau K, Tremouille S, Belec M. (2004). How much does a cesarean section cost in Madagascar? Socio-economical aspects and cesarean sections rate in Toamasina, Madagascar 1999-2001. *Bull Soc Pathol Exot.* Vol. 97, No 4, (November 2004), pp. (274-9). PMID: 17304751.

Robson MS. (2001). Classification of Cesarean Sections. *Fetal and Maternal Medicine Review* Vol 12, No 1, (January 2001), pp. (23-39).

Ronsmans C, Damme W V., Filippi V, Pittrof R. (2002). Need for cesarean sections in West Africa. *The Lancet* Vol 359, No 9310, (March 2002), p 974. PMID: 11861198.

Ronsmans C., Etard J. F., Walraven G., Høj L., Dumont A., de Bernis L. and Kodio B. Maternal mortality and access to obstetric services in West Africa. *Tropical Medicine and International Health.* Vol. 8, No 10, (October 2003), pp. (940–948). PMID: 14516306.

Rosenfield A, Maine D. (1985). Maternal mortality – a neglected tragedy. Where is the M in MCH? *Lancet* Vol. 2, No 8446, (July 1985), pp. (83-85). PMID: 2861534.

Rudge MV, Maesta I, Moura PM, Rudge CV, Morceli G, Costa RA, Abbade J, Peracoli JC, Witkin SS, Calderon IM,

Group C. (2011). The safe motherhood referral system to reduce cesarean sections and perinatal mortality - a cross-sectional study [1995-2006]. *Reprod Health.* Vol. 23, No 1, (November 2011), pp. (34). PMID: 22108042.

Samaké S, Traoré SM, Ba S, Dembélé É, Diop M, Mariko S, et al. (2007). Demography and Health SurveyMali 2006. Bamako: *Cellule de Planification et de Statistique, Ministère de la Santé* (2007).

Sepou A, Nguembi E, Yanza M-C, Penguélé A, Ngbalé R., Kouabosso A., Domandé-Modanga Z., Gaunefet C, Nali M. N. (2003) Utérus cicatriciel : suivi de 73 parturientes à la Maternité centrale de Bangui (République centrafricaine). *Cahiers d'études et de recherches francophones / Santé 2003.* Vol. 13, N. 4, (2003), pp. (231-3).

Shah A., Fawole B., M'Imunya J. M., Amokrane F., Nafiou I., Wolomby J-J., Mugerwa K., Neves I., Nguti R., Kublickas M., Mathai M. Cesarean delivery outcomes from the WHO global survey on maternal and perinatal health in Africa. *International Journal of Gynecology & Obstetrics*, Vol. 107, No 3, (December 2009), pp. (191-197). PMID: 19782977.

Sørbye I K, Vangen S, Oneko O, Sundby J and Bergsjø P. (2011). Cesarean section among referred and selfreferred birthing women: a cohort study from a tertiary hospital, northeastern Tanzania. *BMC Pregnancy and Childbirth* Vol. 11, No 55, (July 2011), PMID: 21798016. http://www.biomedcentral.com/1471-2393/11/55

Spaans W. A., van der Velde F. H., & van Roosmalen J. (1997). Trial of labor after previous cesarean section in rural Zimbabwe. *European Journal of Obstetrics & Gynecology and Reproductive Biology* Vol. 72, No 1, (March 1997), pp. (9 – 14). PMID: 9076415.

Stanton C.K., Dubourg D., De Brouwere, V., Pujades, M. & Ronsmans C. (2005). Reliability of data on cesarean sections in developing countries. *Bulletin of the World Health Organization* Vol 83, Vol 6, (June 2005), pp. (449-455). PMID: 15976896.

Stanton C., Ronsmans C., and the Baltimore Group on Cesarean. (2008). Recommendations for Routine Reporting on Indications for Cesarean Delivery in Developing Countries. *Birth* Vol. 35, No 3, (September 2008), pp. (204 - 2011). PMID: 18844646.

Stavrou E. P., Ford J. B., Shand A. W., Morris J. M., Roberts C. L. (2011). Epidemiology and trends for Cesarean section births in New South Wales, Australia: A population-based study. *BMC Pregnancy and Childbirth* Vol. 11, No 8, (January 2011). PMID: 21251270.

Stein W., Katundo I., Byengonzi B. (2008). Cesarean Rate and Uterine Rupture: A 15-year Hospital-Based Observational Retrospective Study in Rural Tanzania. *Z Geburtshilfe Neonatol* Vol. 212, No 6, (2008), pp. (222-225). PMID: 19085739.

Teguete I., Mounkoro N., Traore Y., Dolo T., Kayenta K., Diallo A., Sissoko A., Djire M., Traore M., Dolo A. Malaria and pregnancy at Gabriel Toure Teaching Hospital in Bamako between 2003 and 2007. *Journal de la SAGO*, Vol. 9, No 1, (2008), pp. (12-16).

Teguete I., Mounkoro N., Traore Y., Dolo T., Kayentao K., Sissoko A., Traore M., Dolo A. (2009). O928 Malaria and pregnancy at the Gabriel Toure teaching hospital in Bamako (Mali) between 2003 and 2007. *International Journal of Gynecology & Obstetrics*, Vol. 107, Suppl. 2, (October 2009), Page S357.

Teguete I., Traore Y., Dennis N., Mounkoro N., Traore M. and Dolo A. (2010). A 19-year retrospective investigation of maternal mortality at Point G National Hospital, Bamako, Mali. International Journal of Gynaecology and Obstetrics, Vol: 108, No 3, (March 2010), pp. (194 - 198). PMID: 19944419.

Teguete I, Mounkoro N, Traoré Y, Dolo T, Sissoko A, Djire MY Traoré M, Dolo A. Influencing factors of delivery rates at Gabriel Toure Teaching hospital, Bamako, Mali. Proceedings of the XIth African Society of Gynecology and Obstetrics (SAGO). Libreville (Gabon), November 22nd - 26th, 2010b. Abstract book, page 20.

UN. (1995). Report of the International Conference on Population and Development, (ICPD), Cairo, 5-13 September 1994, Programme of Action of the International Conference on Population and Development. *UN*, New York, 1995.

van Dillen J, Meguid T, Petrova V & van Roosmalen J.(2007) Cesarean section in a semi-rural hospital in northern Namibia. *BMC Pregnancy Childbirth* Vol 72, No 2, (March 2007), 6 p. [Available from: www.biomedcentral.com/1471-2393/7/2] PMID: 17346332.

Villar J, Valladares E, Wojdyla D, Zavaleta N, Carroli G, Velazco A, Shah A, Campodonico L, Bataglia V, Faundes A, Langer A, Narvaez A, Donner A, Romero M, Reynoso S, de Padua KS, Giordano D, Kublickas M, Acosta A, for the WHO 2005 global survey on maternal and perinatal health research group. (2006). Cesarean delivery rates and pregnancy outcomes: the 2005 WHO global survey on maternal and perinatal health in Latin America. *Lancet* Vol 367, No 9535, (2006), pp. (1819-29). PMID: 16753484.

Wall S. N., Lee A. CC., Niermeyer S., English M., Keenan W. J., Carlo W., Bhutta Z. A., Bang A., Narayanan I., Ariawan I. & Lawn J. E. (2009). Neonatal resuscitation in low-resource settings: What, who, and how to overcome challenges to scale up? *International Journal of Gynecology and Obstetrics* Vol. 107, Suppl. 1, (October 2009), pp. (S47–S64). PMID: 19815203.

Wanyonyi S. Z. & Karuga R. N. (2010). The utility of clinical care pathways in determining perinatal outcomes for women with one previous cesarean section; a retrospective service evaluation. *BMC Pregnancy and Childbirth,* Vol. 10, No 62, (October 2010), PMID: 20946628.

Wanyonyi S, Sequeira E, & Obura T. (2006). Caesarian section rates and perinatal outcome at the Aga Khan University Hospital, Nairobi. *East Afr Med J* Vol. 83, No 12, (December 2006), pp. (651-658). PMID: 17685209.

Weil O & Fernandez H. (1999). Is safe motherhood an orphan initiative? *Lancet,* Vol. 354, No 9182, (September 1999), pp. (940–43). PMID: 10489970.

Wenjuan W, Alva S., Wang S., & Fort A. (2011). Levels and Trends in the Use of Maternal Health Services in Developing Countries. *DHS Comparative Reports* 2011; No. 26. Calverton, Maryland, USA: ICF Macro.

West African regional food for peace office. (2008). Understanding Child Malnutrition in the Sahel: A Case Study from Goundam Cercle, Timbuktu Region, Mali. *USAID / West Africa professional paper series* N°6 (June 2008).

WHO (2010). Global Survey on Maternal and Perinatal Health. Induction of labor data. Geneva, World health Organization, 2010 (available at: http://www.who.int/reproductivehealth/topics/best_practices/global_survey)

World Health Organization. (2007). Everybody's business: Strengthening health systems to improve health outcomes. WHO's framework for action. *Geneva: WHO*; 2007

Wylie B. J. & Mirza F. G. (2008). Cesarean Delivery in the Developing World. *Clinics in Perinatology,* Vol. 35, No 3, (September 2008), pp. (571-582). PMID: 18952023.

Yeast J. D., Jones A., & Poskin M. (1999). Induction of labor and the relationship to cesarean delivery: A review of 7001 consecutive inductions. *Am J Obstet Gynecol,* Vol 180, No 3 Pt 1, (March 1999), pp. (628-33). PMID: 10076139.

Zhang J. & Yu KF. (1998). What's the relative risk? A method for correcting the odds ratio in cohort studies of common outcomes. *JAMA* Vol. 280, No 19, (November 1998), pp. (1690–1). PMID: 9832001.